Applications of AI for Interdisciplinary Research

Applying artificial intelligence (AI) to new fields has made AI and data science indispensable to researchers in a wide range of fields. The proliferation and successful deployment of AI algorithms are fuelling these changes, which can be seen in fields as disparate as healthcare and emerging Internet of Things (IoT) applications. Machine learning techniques, and AI more broadly, are expected to play an ever-increasing role in the modelling, simulation, and analysis of data from a wide range of fields by the interdisciplinary research community. Ideas and techniques from multidisciplinary research are being utilised to enhance AI; hence, the connection between the two fields is a two-way street at a crossroads. Algorithms for inference, sampling, and optimisation, as well as investigations into the efficacy of deep learning, frequently make use of methods and concepts from other fields of study. Cloud computing platforms may be used to develop and deploy several AI models with high computational power. The intersection between multiple fields, including math, science, and healthcare, is where the most significant theoretical and methodological problems of AI may be found. To gather, integrate, and synthesise the many results and viewpoints in the connected domains, refer to it as interdisciplinary research. In light of this, the theory, techniques, and applications of machine learning and AI, as well as how they are utilised across disciplinary boundaries, are the main areas of this research topic.

- This book apprises the readers about the important and cutting-edge aspects of AI applications for interdisciplinary research and guides them to apply their acquaintance in the best possible manner.
- This book is formulated with the intent of uncovering the stakes and possibilities involved in using AI through efficient interdisciplinary applications.
- The main objective of this book is to provide scientific and engineering research on technologies in the fields of AI and data science and how they can be related through interdisciplinary applications and similar technologies.
- This book covers various important domains, such as healthcare, the stock market, natural language processing (NLP), real estate, data security, cloud computing, edge computing, data visualisation using cloud platforms, event management systems, IoT, the telecom sector, federated learning, and network performance optimisation. Each chapter focuses on the corresponding subject outline to offer readers a thorough grasp of the concepts and technologies connected to AI and data analytics, and their emerging applications.

Applications of AI for Interdisciplinary Research

Edited by
Sukhpal Singh Gill

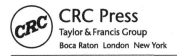

CRC Press

Taylor & Francis Group

Boca Raton London New York

CRC Press is an imprint of the
Taylor & Francis Group, an **informa** business

Designed cover image: Getty Images

First edition published 2025
by CRC Press
2385 NW Executive Center Drive, Suite 320, Boca Raton FL 33431

and by CRC Press
4 Park Square, Milton Park, Abingdon, Oxon, OX14 4RN

CRC Press is an imprint of Taylor & Francis Group, LLC

ISBN: 9781032733302 (hbk)
ISBN: 9781032740102 (pbk)
ISBN: 9781003467199 (ebk)

DOI 10.1201/9781003467199

Typeset in Minion
by KnowledgeWorks Global Ltd.

Contents

Preface

THIS BOOK PROVIDES A COMPREHENSIVE TEXT AND REFERENCE COVERING THE scientific and engineering research on technologies in the fields of artificial intelligence (AI) and data science and how they can be related through interdisciplinary applications and similar technologies. It provides up-to-date knowledge of various advancements in AI and discusses solutions for various important domains (such as cloud computing, edge computing, security, healthcare, federated learning, finance and economics, natural language processing (NLP), and emotional intelligence). The objective of this book is to provide a one-volume source of technical insight into applications of AI for interdisciplinary research, including current state-of-the-art requirements, performance, evaluation, and challenges. This book is based on the research work conducted at the Network Research Group, Queen Mary University of London, and aims to provide scientific and engineering research on technologies in the fields of AI and data science and how they can be related through interdisciplinary applications and similar technologies, covering various important domains:

- The applications of AI in the healthcare domain, especially cardiovascular risk assessment using biomedical indicators, skin lesions, cancer, and thyroid.

- The utilisation of the latest machine learning modes for NLP involves focusing on opinion mining and the visualisation of news Really Simple Syndication (RSS) feeds for efficient information gain.

- Applications of AI in economics and finance include prediction of real estate prices, stock market prices, and household financial expenditures.

- The prediction of household financial expenditure and healthcare status for heart and cancer patients using federated learning and cloud computing.

- Analyse the performance of machine learning models for data visualisation in small- and medium-sized enterprises (SMEs) using different cloud providers, such as Google or Amazon Web Services.

- Focusing on enhancing data security for cloud computing, exploring fraud detection approaches in federated learning, and improving edge node protection in edge computing using AI.

- Conducting predictive analytics for optical interconnection network performance optimisation in the telecom sector using machine learning.

- Designing a machine learning-based model for emotional intelligence to study emotional state inference using mobile sensing.

- Developing machine-learning-based mobile and Internet of Things (IoT) applications such as social event tracking systems.

This book is essential for graduate and postgraduate students in computer science and engineering, applied computer science, data science, and business analytics. It also links fundamental principles to advanced technical content from experts in the field for enthusiasts and professionals looking to learn more. Furthermore, this book helps researchers publish novel studies on developing AI model applications in multidisciplinary research.

Acknowledgements

This book is based on research that was carried out at the Network Research Group at Queen Mary University of London. The research focused on applications of artificial intelligence (AI) for interdisciplinary research, such as cloud computing, edge computing, security, healthcare, and natural language programming (NLP), from the year 2020 to the present day. I would like to express my appreciation to Prof. Steve Uhlig, who is the Head of the Networks Research Group, for motivating me to initiate the investigation, continue working on it, and ultimately publish it.

I would like to express my gratitude to the Master of Science students from the School of Electronic Engineering and Computer Science at Queen Mary University of London who have made significant contributions to this book as leading authors. A huge debt of appreciation is owed to Dr. Rupinder Kaur of Kings Education London for all of her academic assistance; she was always pushing me to think critically, offering insightful criticism, and proofreading my work.

I am thankful to Muhammed Golec, who has read and commented on several chapters. As an additional expression of gratitude, I would like to thank Dr. Elliott Morsia, Commissioning Editor; Shamayita Dey, Editorial Assistant; and everyone else at CRC Press for having faith in my work and being so accommodating.

Lastly, I want to express my deepest appreciation to my parents and all of my family members for their unwavering support and affection. Without each of them, I would not have been able to finish writing this book.

Sukhpal Singh Gill
School of Electronic Engineering and Computer Science
Queen Mary University of London
London, United Kingdom

Editor

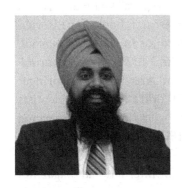

Dr. Sukhpal Singh Gill is an Assistant Professor in Cloud Computing at the School of Electronic Engineering and Computer Science (EECS), Queen Mary University of London (QMUL), UK, and is a member of the Network Research Group. Prior to this, Dr. Gill held positions as a research associate at Evolving Distributed Systems Lab at the School of Computing and Communications, Lancaster University, UK, and as a postdoctoral research fellow at the Cloud Computing and Distributed Systems (CLOUDS) Laboratory, School of Computing and Information Systems, The University of Melbourne, Australia. He was awarded Fellow of the Higher Education Academy (FHEA) in 2022 after passing PGCAP/PGCert with Distinction. He has published his PGCAP/PGCert work in highly ranked education conferences and journals such as *IEEE EDUCON* (the top conference for education papers with an acceptance rate 26%), Wiley *Computer Applications in Engineering Education* (Impact Factor = 2.1), and *ITNOW* published by the British Computer Society (BCS). Before joining CLOUDS Lab, Dr. Gill also worked in the Computer Science and Engineering Department of Thapar University, India, as a lecturer. Dr. Gill received his Bachelor's degree in Computer Science and Engineering from Punjab Technical University with Distinction in 2010. Then he obtained the Degree of Master of Engineering in Software Engineering (Gold Medalist), as well as a Doctoral Degree specialisation in Autonomic Cloud Computing from Thapar University. He was a Department of Science & Technology (DST) Inspire Fellow during his doctorate work and worked as a senior research fellow (Professional) on a DST Project, Government of India. Dr. Gill was a research visitor at Monash University, University of Manitoba, University of Manchester, and Imperial College London. He was a recipient of several awards, including the QMUL Education Excellence Award 2023, Elsevier Internet of Things Editor's Choice Award 2024, Elsevier Best Paper Award 2023, Distinguished Reviewer Award from Software: Practice and Experience (Wiley), 2018; Best Paper Award in Australasian Symposium on Parallel and Distributed Computing (AusPDC 2023) at ACSW 2021; and the EECS Award for the "Widest Academic Staff Contribution", QMUL in 2023. He has also served as the PC member for venues such as *IEEE PerCom, UCC, CCGRID, CLOUDS, ICFEC*, and *AusPDC*. His one review paper has been nominated and selected for the ACM 21st Annual Best of Computing Notable Books and Articles as one of the notable items published in computing 2016. He has co-authored 180+ peer-reviewed papers (with 9000+ citations and an H-index 50 as per Google Scholar) and has published in prominent international journals and conferences such as *IEEE TCC, IEEE TSC, IEEE TSUSC, IEEE TCE, ACM TOIT, IEEE TII, IEEE TNSM, IEEE IoT Journal, Elsevier JSS/FGCS, IEEE/ACM UCC* and *IEEE CCGRID*. Dr. Gill served as a Guest Editor for *SPE (Wiley), JCC Springer Journal, Sustainability Journal (MDPI),* and *Sensors Journal (MDPI)*. He is a regular reviewer for *IEEE TPDS, IEEE TSC, IEEE TNSE, IEEE TSC, ACM CSUR,* and *Wiley SPE*. Dr. Gill has reviewed more than 650 research articles for high-ranked journals and prestigious conferences as per Web of Science. He has edited research books for Elsevier, Springer, and CRC Press. Dr. Gill is serving as an Associate Editor in *IEEE IoT Journal, Elsevier IoT Journal, Wiley SPE Journal, Wiley ETT Journal,* and *IET Networks Journal*. Dr. Gill is serving as an Editor-in-Chief for *IGI Global IJAEC* and Area Editor for Springer *Cluster Computing Journal*. His name appears in the list of the World's Top 2% of Scientists released by Stanford University and Elsevier BV (2022 and 2023). Dr. Gill has been serving as an editorial board member for *IGIGLOBAL JOEUC,* and *MECS IJEME*. One of his articles published by the *IEEE Internet of Things* journal is highlighted in *IEEE Spectrum* (the world's leading engineering magazine). Dr. Gill wrote articles for international magazines such as *Ars Technica, Tech Monitor, Cutter Consortium,* and *ICT Academy*. He has been interviewed by Tallinn University, Estonia, to talk about "The capabilities and limitations of ChatGPT for Education". His research interests include cloud computing, fog computing, software engineering, Internet of Things, and energy efficiency. For further information, please visit www.ssgill.me.

Contributors

Ahmed M. Abdelmoniem
Parinaz Banifatemi
Jisma Choudhury
Muhammed Golec
Sukhpal Singh Gill
Aswin Kumar Govindan
Waleed Ul Hassan
Ho Kuen Lai
Shai Lynch
Shabnam Manjuri
Diogo Mota
Sindhu Muthumanickam
Usman Naeem
Muhammad Usman Nazir
Karan Pardeshi
Jairaj Patil
Sai Siddharth Ponugoti
Neelam Rathore
Tanjina Rhaman
Suganya Senguttuvan
Satyam Sharma
School of Electronic Engineering and Computer Science
Queen Mary University of London
London, United Kingdom

I

Healthcare

CHAPTER 1

Machine Learning-Based Prediction of Thyroid Disease

Tanjina Rhaman and Sukhpal Singh Gill

1.1 INTRODUCTION

In present-day society, the introduction of machine learning (ML) has increased the potential for understanding, managing, and treating different health conditions. Artificial intelligence (AI) and ML technologies continue to prevail in medical fields, and this is creating more room for innovative and evidence-based outcomes and healthcare solutions [1]. In today's medical world, ML has been successfully used to make accurate predictions and identify thyroid disease. Research by Fallahi et al. [2] claimed that through ML, there are different algorithms that improve the learning, prediction, and assessment capacity. These include decision trees, k-nearest neighbour (KNN), support vector machines (SVMs), and artificial neural networks (ANNs) [3]. For thyroid disease, its incidence and prevalence can be accurately assessed using these different ML algorithms. Different researchers and academicians have dedicated time to understanding how ML can contribute to positive outcomes in the prediction and diagnosis of thyroid disease. ML algorithms allow for the opportunity to develop accurate models for the early diagnosis of both hyperthyroidism and hypothyroidism [4]. These algorithms can leverage large datasets and identify patterns that may not be easily identifiable through traditional diagnostic methods, thus leading to an earlier diagnosis [5]. Hyperthyroidism and hypothyroidism are two distinct thyroid disorders that result from an imbalance in thyroid hormone production. Whereas excessive hormone synthesis and release characterize hyperthyroidism, inadequate hormone production causes hypothyroidism. Graves' disease is one of the most common causes of hyperthyroidism, and the leading symptoms include anxiety, heat intolerance, rapid heart rate, and significant weight loss [6]. Hyperthyroidism and hypothyroidism usually affect a significant percentage of individuals. According to Salman and Sonuç [7], men have at least a tenth of the thyroid prevalence compared with women. Due to a deficiency in iodine, goitre or active thyroid modules may be common in some regions, with at least 15% prevalence. Early detection of the diseases, diagnosis, and care are vital in preventing their progression and possible death. According to the National Health Service (NHS), approximately 1 in 20 people in the United Kingdom experience some form of thyroid

DOI: 10.1201/9781003467199-2

disease, with women more likely to develop the condition than men. Statistics show that thyroid-based diseases must be taken seriously.

1.1.1 Motivation and Our Contributions

The desire to enhance early detection and treatment of this prevalent condition is the motivation behind this chapter on ML-based prediction of thyroid disease. Healthcare professionals may be able to spot patterns and risk factors such as depression, fatigue, and weight gain that are not immediately obvious through conventional diagnostic techniques by using ML algorithms to analyse patient data [8]. For patients with thyroid disease, this might result in earlier and more accurate diagnoses as well as better treatment outcomes, therefore avoiding surgery in the long term. The ultimate objective of using technology is to raise the standard of patient care and enhance general health outcomes.

The main contributions to this work are to

- Improve the reliability of diagnosis for thyroid-related illnesses using ML,

- Propose models that improve the accuracy of predicting thyroid disease,

- Identify important features for the feature selection to give a higher accuracy, and

- Explain how using ML by shedding light on the complicated interaction of factors and using a powerful classifier can aid in the medical diagnosis of thyroid disease.

1.2 RELATED WORK

This section discusses the literature review under various subsections.

1.2.1 Thyroid Disease and Machine Learning

This literature review examines the use of ML techniques in the early diagnosis and prediction of thyroid disease, an endocrine disorder affecting millions worldwide. A study by Chaganti et al. [9] was conducted using a comprehensive approach that encompassed selective feature extraction together with ML algorithms. The objective was to develop accurate prediction models that can help medical practitioners distinguish different states of thyroid disease. Following the selected aspects of ML, the models, such as random forest (RF), had 98% accuracy, SVMs had 85% accuracy, and logistic regression had 91.3% accuracy. Despite the accuracy variations, the specificity of the results was an indication of the efficiency of predicting thyroid using ML algorithms. In this study, the findings varied due to feature selection factors including thyroid-stimulating hormone (TSH), age, gender, and triiodothyronine (T3) uptake. To improve the accuracy of the ML models, features such as lifestyle, family history, and other environmental factors could have been considered. The inclusion of risk factors allowed for accurate predictions. Thus, throughout this study, it is evident that medical practitioners can use ML approaches to improve decisions and enhance patient care.

To better understand thyroid diseases, Razia et al. [10] aimed to use ML models to predict disease outcomes. With the help of classification algorithms, they used different types of ML techniques, including supervised, unsupervised, deep learning, reinforcement, and semi-supervised. The algorithms they used for diagnosing diseases include principal component analysis (PCA), linear discriminant analysis (LDA), decision trees, k-means, and KNN. Their research established that ML attempts to find a correlation between the numerical attributes of inputs and outputs based on previous data. This can be used to predict diseases, including those related to the thyroid.

1.2.2 Hyperthyroidism and Machine Learning

Hyperthyroidism is a condition whereby the body produces an excess of thyroid hormones, specifically thyroxine (T4) and T3. Graves' disease is the most common cause of hyperthyroidism, and it is an autoimmune disorder where the body develops antibodies that stimulate the thyroid gland, leading to thyroid hormone overproduction [11]. As the research and technology in ML continue to improve, developments have allowed for a superior understanding of hyperthyroidism. With the help of ML, a study by Fallahi et al. [2] revealed that this offers an opportunity to develop accurate models that can facilitate the early diagnosis of hyperthyroidism. This can be attributed to the algorithms that leverage compound datasets, making it possible to identify patterns not easily identifiable using traditional diagnostic approaches.

According to Salman and Sonuç [7], ML can be effective in understanding hyperthyroidism, and they collected data from 1250 people from different age groups. They compared patients' data with health data, including age, T4 and T3 analysis, and a host of other characteristics. The key findings, with the help of SVM, RFs, decision trees, and logistic regression, revealed that different ML techniques are accurate in the diagnosis of hyperthyroidism. The RF had an accuracy of 98.93, which showed the precision and accuracy of ML algorithms. The research outcomes were similar to those of the study by Chiu et al. [12], which also sought to identify the key markers to detect hyperthyroidism early. In the study, the authors claim that the use of different ML methods can help with early prediction. They also used algorithms, including decision trees and RF, to make accurate predictions. The findings revealed that the RF can be accurately used to predict hyperthyroidism with an accuracy of 97.4%.

1.2.3 Hypothyroidism and Machine Learning

Hypothyroidism, on the other hand, is a condition where the body produces an insufficient number of thyroid hormones. Chronic autoimmune thyroiditis, or Hashimoto's thyroiditis, is the most common cause of primary hypothyroidism, which results from a malfunctioning thyroid gland [13]. Research by Bhattacharya et al. [5] sought to predict hypothyroidism using clinical and demographic features through ML. They used techniques such as decision trees, RFs, and SVM to make accurate predictions of hypothyroidism. The researchers used laboratory-based test results and characteristics of patients to arrive at deductions on how ML improves hypothyroidism prediction. A similar study [14] also used attributes such as TSH, age, sex, free thyroxine, and anti-thyroid peroxidase (anti-TPO) antibodies to predict cases of hypothyroidism accurately with ML. The prediction outcomes from decision trees, RF, SVMs, and k-star classifier predict the risk and occurrence of hypothyroid. From their findings, RF and decision trees had accuracy scores of 99.44 and 98.97% consecutively. This shows that ML techniques can be used to make better predictions of hypothyroidism, resulting in better treatment outcomes.

Another research by Hossain et al. [15] sought to create a predictive analysis of hyper- and hypothyroidism using ML. The authors use different ML algorithms to make predictions of hyper- and hypothyroidism. These algorithms included RF classifier, naïve Bayes classifier, SVM, and KNN. Further, using different characteristics and behaviour of the collected database, features such as T3, total thyroxine (TT4), TSH, and free T4 index (FTI) are the most effective in the diagnosis of thyroid disease. Their research revealed that RF gives a maximum accuracy score of 91.42% and a precision of 92%. Further, Chaganti et al. [9] found that ML is effective in examining and predicting thyroid diseases. By conducting a literature search of articles about thyroid disease detection, the outcomes revealed that ML can be more effective in thyroid cancer detection with an accuracy of 64.3%.

1.2.4 Risk Factors Associated with Hyperthyroidism and Hypothyroidism

Hyperthyroidism and hypothyroidism, according to Hossain et al. [15], are among the common thyroid gland illnesses that have been found in 110 countries worldwide. The condition has put more than 1.6 billion people in danger. Most cases have been found in Latin America, Africa, and Asia. Currently, doctors believe that despite the differences in the symptoms of hyperthyroidism and hypothyroidism, a lack of concentration on hypothyroidism could result in obesity. To diagnose hyperthyroidism, blood tests measure T3, T4, and TSH levels. Other diagnostic methods used include radioactive iodine scans and ultrasounds [6]. Common treatment options include radioactive iodine therapy, taking anti-thyroid medications, and sometimes thyroidectomy, depending on disease severity.

Hypothyroidism, on the other hand, is grouped into primary and secondary hypothyroidism. Chronic autoimmune thyroiditis, or Hashimoto's thyroiditis, is the most common cause of primary hypothyroidism, which results from a malfunctioning thyroid gland [13]. Secondary hypothyroidism may arise from pituitary or hypothalamic dysfunction. Symptoms of hypothyroidism include cold intolerance, constipation, depression, fatigue, and weight gain [13]. Diagnostic methods, such as laboratory tests to measure T4 and TSH levels, are used to confirm hypothyroidism. Levothyroxine replacement therapy, a synthetic thyroid hormone, is the mainstay of treatment for hypothyroidism [16]. Therefore, to lower the incidence and mortality rates caused by thyroid disease, disease detection has been perceived as an important consideration for modern healthcare organizations. With the help of ML models, the computational complexity of these algorithms makes them effective for the prediction of thyroid diseases. Table 1.1 compares the proposed work with existing works based on key parameters.

TABLE 1.1   Comparison of Proposed Work with Existing Works

Work	Algorithms	Accuracy
Aversano et al. [4]	Decision tree, naïve Bayes, k-nearest neighbours, random forest, XGB, AdaBoost, gradient boost.	61%, 53%, 81%, 58%, 72%, 58%, 58%.
Chaganti et al. [9]	Random forest, gradient boost, AdaBoost, logistic regression, supportive vector machine	98%, 97%, 97%, 85%, 85%.
Proposed work	XGBoost, AdaBoost, random forest	99%, 99%, 99%.

1.3 METHODOLOGY

This section discusses the methodology used to conduct this study.

1.3.1 Dataset Description

The datasets used in this investigation have been from the well-known UCI thyroid illness datasets (Datasets - UCI Machine Learning Repository [17]). The primary dataset in this collection, which consists of 9172 distinct observations with 31 unique characteristics for each one, contains a variety of thyroid illness datasets. The fundamental goal of this research is to classify thyroid illnesses based on these characteristics. The relevance of characteristics is an important consideration in establishing the best collection of criteria for accurate thyroid disease categorization [18]. As shown in Table 1.2, the dataset's attributes include Boolean (M, F, f, t), continuous (float, int), and string values. To assess the relevance

TABLE 1.2   Feature Description in the Thyroid Dataset

Feature Name	Feature Value
Age	Continuous
Sex	M, F.
On thyroxine	f, t.
Query on thyroxine	f, t.
On antithyroid medication	f, t.
Sick	f, t.
Pregnant	f, t.
Thyroid surgery	f, t.
I-131 treatment	f, t.
Query hypothyroid	f, t.
Query hyperthyroid	f, t.
Lithium	f, t.
Goitre	f, t.
Tumour	f, t.
Hypopituitary	f, t.
Psych	f, t.
TSH measured	f, t.
TSH	Continuous.
T3 measured	f, t.
T3	Continuous.
TT4 measured	f, t.
TT4	Continuous.
T4U measured	f, t.
T4U	Continuous.
FTI measured	f, t.
FTI	Continuous.
Thyroxine-Binding Globulin (TBG) measured	f, t.
TBG	Continuous.
Referral source	WEST, STMW, SVHC, SVI, SVHD, and others.

(Continued)

TABLE 1.2 (*Continued*)   Feature Description in the Thyroid Dataset

Feature Name	Feature Value
Target	Hyperthyroid conditions (A, B, C, D)
	Hypothyroid conditions (E, F, G, H)
	Binding protein (I, J)
	General health (K)
	Replacement therapy (L, M, N)
	Discordant results (R)
Patient_ID	Continuous

of these qualities, this research employs a feature-based approach. The classification challenge, which focuses on the health disorders and diagnosis classes provided by the dataset, is the essence of this endeavour [19]. When looking at the class counts, it should be noted that a significant number of the samples are classified as "no condition". Individuals who do not have thyroid illness are classified as having this condition. The dataset, on the other hand, allows for a variety of diseases such as primary hypothyroidism, balanced hypothyroidism, increased binding proteins, and associated non-thyroidal sickness, among others. The data preparation approach is used to solve the issue of unbalanced classes. The proposed technique includes feature selection and preprocessing stages that result in a balanced thyroid illness classification dataset. While the "no condition" categorization predominates in the dataset, researchers should not disregard the nuanced situations of concurrent non-thyroidal disease, in which individuals have changed thyroid levels as a result of chronic illness but do not have primary thyroid malfunction. The primary dataset contains 9173 patient records. 6771 of which are for normal people with no signs of thyroid illness. The rest of the data are classified as primary hypothyroidism, compensated hypothyroidism, increased binding proteins, and concomitant non-thyroidal disease. Given the discrepancies associated with thyroid illness distribution, this thorough selection guarantees that the dataset is appropriate for effective model training and validation [20].

1.3.2 Data Processing

The implementation starts with a careful data preprocessing strategy intended to ensure data quality and relevancy. The dataset, which was obtained from the UCI Machine Learning Repository, contains patient information on several thyroid-related disorders. To simplify the study, the first step was to exclude individuals who have been identified as having negative, hyperthyroid, or hypothyroid disorders. This improved dataset has roughly 7500 items, which corresponds to the core topic of this research investigation. To improve the dataset, redundant columns were removed that indicate that blood test values were taken, as these columns provide little value due to the availability of real test measures. Furthermore, for data consistency, outliers were excluded, such as an exceptionally high age value of 6526 years. Individuals beyond the age of 100 are also excluded since their little contribution does not justify potential mistakes. The count and graph of missing values are given in Figures 1.1 and 1.2, respectively.

1.3.3 Feature Analysis

A critical aspect of the work is a thorough examination of hormone level measures, which are critical in understanding thyroid illness. TSH readings that are high indicate primary

	Total	Percent
TBG	7287	0.965677
T3	2209	0.292738
TSH	722	0.095680
T4U	676	0.089584
FTI	669	0.088656
TT4	354	0.046912
sex	250	0.033130
age	4	0.000530
goitre	0	0.000000
psych	0	0.000000

FIGURE 1.1 Percentage of missing values for key features.

hypothyroidism, whereas low levels indicate hyperthyroidism. TSH values between 0.5 and 5.0 mIU/L are considered normal. This investigation extends to T3 assays, with increased total T3 levels indicating hyperthyroidism. In adults, the acceptable range for total T3 levels is 80–220 ng/dL. Similarly, TT4 values were investigated, which are affected by a variety of circumstances, including drugs. Total T4 levels in individuals typically vary from 5.0 to 12.0 g/dL. The research carried out also includes thyroxine utilisation rate (T4U) measures,

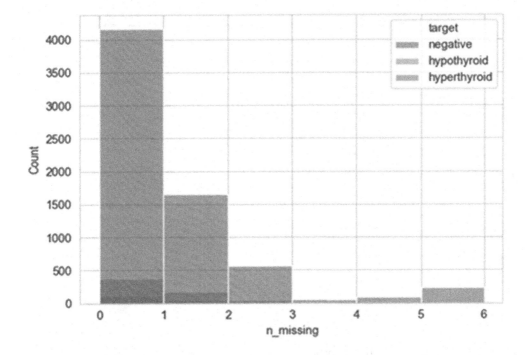

FIGURE 1.2 Class-wise missing values.

which represent the body's efficient use of T4 hormone. Furthermore, the FTI was assessed, which represents unbound T4 and is an indication of thyroid gland function. The typical range for FT4 levels is 0.7–1.9 ng/dL.

1.3.4 Missing Data Handling

Addressing missing data emerged as a critical component of the development process. According to the findings, the bulk of the missing results are related to blood test readings. This disparity might be related to tests not being requested or being documented incorrectly. The technique used includes distinct approaches for certain features. To preserve the data's intrinsic value, important attributes such as T3, TSH, FTI, and TT4 are submitted to imputation. Given the significance of T3 as a predictor, its possible influence on the results necessitates imputation. Furthermore, because of their importance in assessing thyroid function, proposing imputing TSH, FTI, and TT4 was the natural next step. With around 3.31% missing values, the "sex" characteristic requires careful examination. Before deciding if imputation is essential, it is necessary to assess its importance for modelling purposes. In terms of the "age" property, the four missing values are managed by eliminating observations with blatantly inconsistent (extremely big) age values, improving the dataset's coherence and integrity. Figure 1.3 shows the importance of the features discussed in the previous paragraph in numeric form. Further, it is observed that numerical features have a high weight in the classification. Therefore, Figure 1.4 shows the class-wise plot for the numerical attributes.

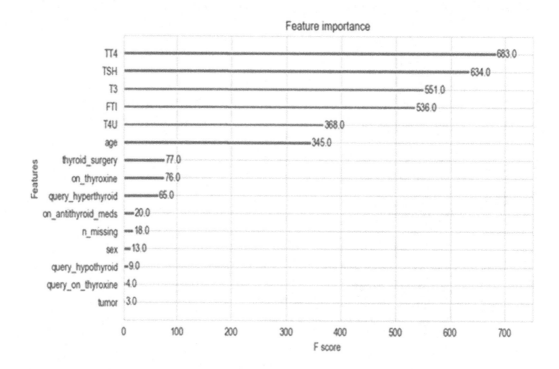

FIGURE 1.3 Measure of feature importance.

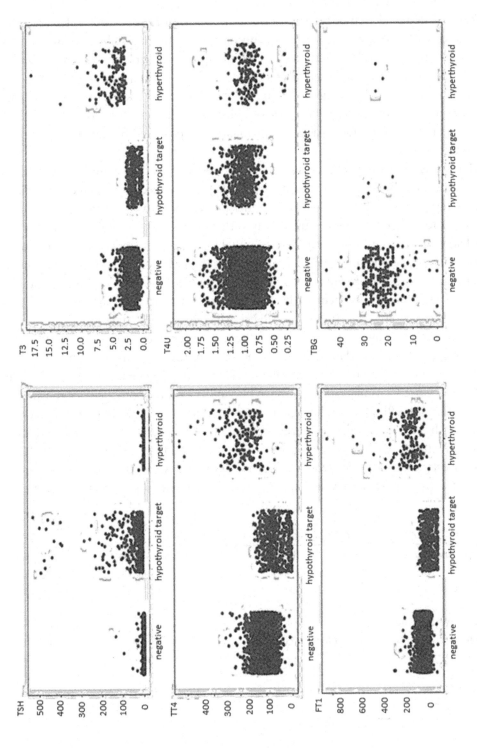

FIGURE 1.4 Scatterplot of numerical features against target classes.

1.3.5 Machine Learning Classifiers

To improve the reliability of diagnosis for thyroid-related illnesses, the initiative was to take the calculated step of revising the feature set used in this study [21]. The intention was to collect a greater range of significant data from the dataset by including a new and comprehensive set of characteristics [22]. This shift from past research allows for enhanced comprehension of the fundamental trends and linkages between the features of the dataset [23]. In addition to improving the feature set, classifiers were chosen based on their success in previous research projects [24]. The established abilities and effectiveness of XGBoost, AdaBoost, and RF in addressing the various issues provided by medical datasets led to their adoption.

Each classifier was examined systematically, testing its performance individually given the overall context of the provided data [21]. The need to recognize each classifier's unique characteristics and determine which model is most effective for the problem drove the decision to investigate them sequentially rather than in an ensemble. XGBoost's ability to deal with missing values and manage unbalanced datasets makes it a good foundation for the investigation. The hyperparameters were then carefully adjusted and evaluated for independence [22]. Following that, the focus was on AdaBoost, a classifier notable for its recursive rectification of incorrectly classified examples. Its novel method of aiding inadequate learning attracted interest in this research for reliable diagnoses [25]. Finally, RF was reviewed, taking advantage of its resilience against overfitting and its ability to cope with high-dimensional data. The last component of this experiment is intended to give a thorough comparison of three different classifiers. The independent classifier implementations acquire legitimacy and relevance by building on best practices established in earlier research [4, 9]. This method guarantees that each model is extensively assessed and helps with the larger objective of precisely diagnosing thyroid-related illnesses. Finally, the research stands out by expanding the feature space and applying a methodical, sequential investigation of three strong classifiers: XGBoost, AdaBoost, and RF. Tables 1.3–1.5 show the hyperparameter values for different implementations of the XGBoost classifier,

TABLE 1.3   Hyperparameter Tuning for XGBoost Classifier

Hyperparameter	Experiment 1	Experiment 2	Experiment 3
objective	'multi:softmax'	'multi:softmax'	'multi:softmax'
num_class	3	3	3
missing	1	1	1
early_stopping_rounds	10	10	
eval_metric	['merror''mlogloss']	['merror''mlogloss']	['merror''mlogloss']
seed	42	42	42
gamma		0	0
learning_rate		0.1	0.1
max_depth		3	5
reg_lambda		1	1
subsample		1	10
colsample_bytree		1	

TABLE 1.4   Hyperparameter Tuning for AdaBoost Classifier

Hyperparameter	Experiment 1	Experiment 2	Experiment 3
base_estimator	DecisionTreeClassifier	DecisionTreeClassifier	DecisionTreeClassifier
max_depth	10	5	10
n_estimators	300	100	500
learning_rate	0.01	0.5	0.5
random_state	42	42	42

TABLE 1.5   Hyperparameter Tuning for Random Forest Classifier

Hyperparameter	Experiment 1	Experiment 2
n_estimators	700	500
random_state	42	42
max_depth	NA	10
min_samples_split	NA	10

AdaBoost classifier, and RF classifier. To obtain the best hyperparameter set, three different experiments were performed for XGBoost and AdaBoost classifiers, whereas for RF, two experiments were performed due to lesser hyperparameters. The last experiment gave a better performance, and the results are considered from this experiment.

In conclusion, a methodically staged implementation path includes data preparation, extensive feature analysis, correcting missing data issues, and deploying the XGBoost classifier. Each stage, when completed thoroughly and precisely, adds to the broader objective of better classifying thyroid-related disorders. This methodology, which was adapted to the dataset's particular properties, not only increases the understanding of thyroid health but also offers a methodical way to solve complicated multiclass classification challenges [26]. This work contributes to the field of medical diagnostics using ML by shedding light on the complicated interaction of factors and using a powerful classifier [27].

1.4 RESULTS

The experimental component of the study was to evaluate the suggested ML approach's effectiveness on the UCI thyroid dataset. Using the proposed technique, the concentration was on attaining a high degree of precision in thyroid illness categorization. With an astounding accuracy of 99%, the acquired findings verify the effectiveness of the technique used. This finding highlights the possible benefits of ML approaches for improving thyroid illness prediction accuracy. An attempt was made to contextualize the result by comparing it with other research, notably research that used ML methods such as RF, SVM, AdaBoost, and decision trees. The prime goal of this study has been the literature study of the already existing models and then the implementation of the best three models from the previous research [25, 27]. Given the statement, the following have been implemented: XGBoost classifier, AdaBoost classifier, and RF classifier. These three have achieved better performance in previous research (see Table 1.6). From the experiments, the XGBoost classifier performs best among other models. Primarily, it is observed that the dataset has imbalanced classes. Given that it is also found that all the models in the study produce

TABLE 1.6   Comparison of Results

Model	Accuracy	Precision	Recall	F1 Score
Decision Tree (Aversano et al.) [4]	0.61	0.63	0.61	0.59
Naïve Bayesian (Aversano et al.) [4]	0.53	0.56	0.53	0.52
KNN (Aversano et al.) [4]	0.81	0.81	0.81	0.80
Random forest (Aversano et al.) [4]	0.58	0.58	0.58	0.57
XGB (Aversano et al.) [4]	0.72	0.73	0.72	0.71
AdaBoost (Aversano et al.) [4]	0.58	0.60	0.58	0.57
Gradient boost (Aversano et al.) [4]	0.58	0.60	0.60	0.59
Random forest (Chaganti et al.) [9]	0.98	0.98	0.98	0.98
Gradient boost (Chaganti et al.) [9]	0.97	0.98	0.98	0.98
AdaBoost (Chaganti et al.) [9]	0.97	0.97	0.97	0.97
Logistic regression (Chaganti et al.) [9]	0.85	0.85	0.85	0.85
SVM (Chaganti et al.) [9]	0.85	0.85	0.85	0.85
CNN (Chaganti et al.) [9]	0.93	0.94	0.92	0.93
Proposed XGB	0.99	0.97	0.99	0.98
Proposed AdaBoost	0.99	0.92	0.94	0.93
Proposed random forest	0.99	0.95	0.91	0.93

99% accuracy on the given feature set, the individual class accuracies have an observable gap due to the imbalanced nature of the data. Therefore, it is seen in the experiments that classes with fewer instances have a low recall rate (Table 1.6). Also, as observed in Figure 1.5, there is a smooth line. In contrast, in Figures 1.6–1.8, it can be concluded that despite the high accuracy given in Figure 1.6 for RF, Figure 1.7 shows a low learning rate for class 2. Similarly, Figure 1.8 shows a spike in the loss curve/error rate curve

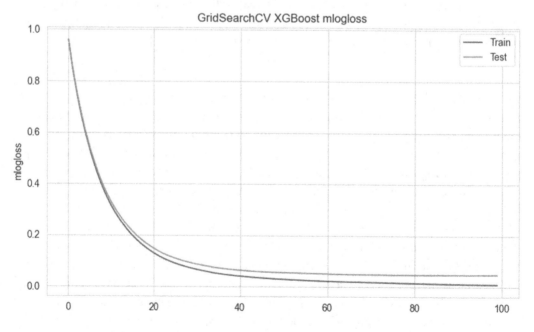

FIGURE 1.5   Learning curve for experiment 3 in terms of loss.

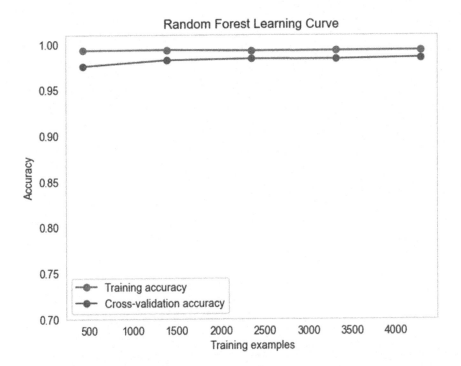

FIGURE 1.6   Learning curve for random forest in terms of accuracy.

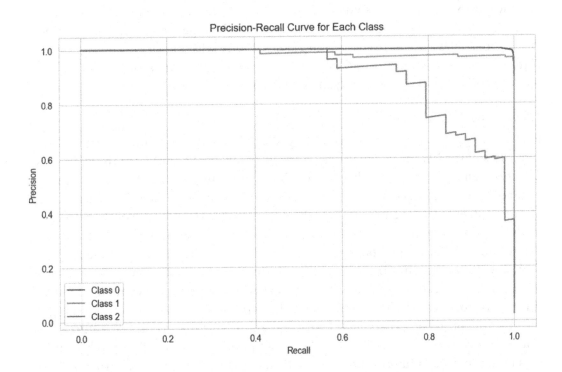

FIGURE 1.7   Precision recall curve for random forest.

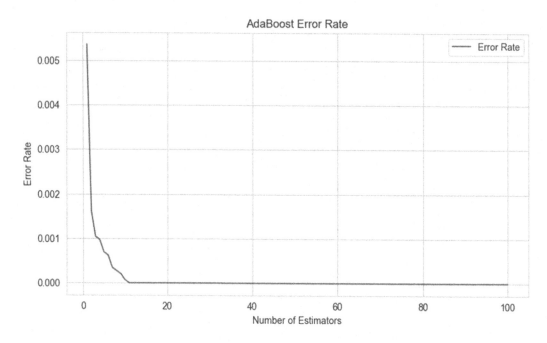

FIGURE 1.8   Learning curve for AdaBoost classifier in terms of loss.

for AdaBoost due to fewer instances of class 2. When compared with previous investigations, this study attained an accuracy of 99%, which greatly beats the stated accuracy in other works. Notably, earlier studies using various ML techniques generated accuracies of roughly 97%, highlighting the significant leap that the suggested methodology brings. This demonstrates the effectiveness of the careful feature selection, preprocessing, and use of the XGBoost classifier. Table 1.6 shows the comparison of the obtained results with the previous research applying ML to the thyroid dataset.

1.5 CONCLUSIONS

Findings imply that combining feature significance selection with the intrinsic characteristics of the XGBoost classifier significantly improves accuracy in thyroid illness detection. This finding highlights the possibilities of using advanced ML techniques to enhance medical diagnosis. The considerable amount that indicates that the accuracy of this work outperforms previous results demonstrates the promise of the technique in the field of thyroid illness categorization. This result not only shows advances in ML techniques but also emphasizes the significance of specialized methodology for dealing with the peculiarities of medical information. In conclusion, a 99% accuracy in thyroid illness categorization on the UCI dataset establishes a new standard in contrast to previous research that used other ML techniques. This achievement highlights the potential of the proposed technique, emphasizing the importance of feature selection, preprocessing, and classifier selection in improving accuracy. This study contributes to the continued improvement in the field of medical diagnostics through ML by beating established standards.

1.6 FUTURE WORK

One angle that can be further investigated is the presence of secondary thyroid diseases in patients with hypothyroidism. Understanding if there is a particular additional thyroid disease that can affect hypothyroidism can provide valuable insights. It is not uncommon for patients to suffer from multiple thyroid diseases simultaneously. This discovery emphasizes the potential of advanced ML techniques for improving medical diagnoses. Further work can also be explored using deep neural networks [27]. They are trained as part of deep learning, a subset of ML, to recognise intricate patterns in data. Traditional ML techniques have been employed in the past to forecast thyroid illness [26]. The model's accuracy can be increased by utilising deep learning techniques like convolutional neural networks (CNNs), recurrent neural networks (RNNs), and autoencoders [28]. These methods help the model become more generalizable to new data by teaching it complex representations of the data [25].

REFERENCES

[1] Gill, S. S., Xu, M., Ottaviani, C. et al. (2022). AI for next generation computing: Emerging trends and future directions. *Internet of Things*, 19, 100514.

[2] Fallahi, P., Ferrari, S. M., Ruffilli, I. et al. (2016). The association of serum TSH with exercise capacity in patients with Hashimoto's thyroiditis. *European Journal of Endocrinology*, 174(3), 325–331.

[3] Tuli, S., Basumatary, N., Gill, S. S. et al. (2020). HealthFog: An ensemble deep learning based smart healthcare system for automatic diagnosis of heart diseases in integrated IoT and fog computing environments. *Future Generation Computer Systems*, 104, 187–200.

[4] Aversano, L., Bernardi, M. L., Cimitile, M. et al. (2021). Thyroid disease treatment prediction with machine learning approaches. *Procedia Computer Science*, 192, 1031–1040. https://doi.org/10.1016/j.procs.2021.08.106

[5] Bhattacharya, S., Verma, A., Sinha, V. et al. (2017). Predictive data mining for medical diagnosis: An overview of heart disease prediction. *International Journal of Computer Applications*, 166(4), 20–23.

[6] Biondi, B., Kahaly, G. J., & Robertson, R. P. (2019). Thyroid dysfunction and diabetes mellitus: Two closely associated disorders. *Endocrine Reviews*, 40(3), 789–824.

[7] Salman, K., & Sonuç, E. (2021). Thyroid disease classification using machine learning algorithms. *Journal of Physics: Conference Series*, 1963(1), 012140. https://doi.org/10.1088/1742-6596/1963/1/012140

[8] Tuli, S., Tuli, S., Wander, G. et al. (2020). Next generation technologies for smart healthcare: Challenges, vision, model, trends and future directions. *Internet Technology Letters*, 3(2), e145.

[9] Chaganti, R., Rustam, F., De La, T. et al. (2022). Thyroid disease prediction using selective features and machine learning techniques. *Cancers*, 14(16), 3914. https://doi.org/10.3390/cancers14163914

[10] Razia, S., Siva Kumar, P., & Rao, A. S. (2020). Machine Learning Techniques for Thyroid Disease Diagnosis: A Systematic Review. *In Studies in Computational Intelligence* (pp. 203–212). Springer International Publishing. https://doi.org/10.1007/978-3-030-38445-6_15

[11] Taylor, P. N., Albrecht, D., Scholz, A. et al. (2013). Global epidemiology of hyperthyroidism and hypothyroidism. *Nature Reviews Endocrinology*, 14(5), 301–316.

[12] Chiu, C. Y., Yen, J. C., Hu et al. (2021). Deep learning for identifying markers for early hyperthyroidism diagnosis. *Healthcare*, 9(1), 48.

[13] Chaker, L., Bianco, A. C., Jonklaas, J. et al. (2016). Hypothyroidism. *The Lancet*, 388(10055), 1155–1166.

[14] Chanprapaph, K., Iamsumang, W., Wattanakrai, P. et al. (2018). Thyroid autoimmunity and autoimmunity in chronic spontaneous urticaria linked to disease severity, therapeutic response, and time to remission in patients with chronic spontaneous urticaria. *BioMed Research International*, 2018, 9856843.

[15] Hossain, M. B., Shama, A., Adhikary et al. (2023). An Explainable Artificial Intelligence Framework for the Predictive Analysis of Hypo and Hyper Thyroidism Using Machine Learning Algorithms. In *Human-Centric Intelligent Systems*. Springer Science and Business Media LLC. https://doi.org/10.1007/s44230-023-00027-1

[16] Jonklaas, J., Bianco, A. C., Bauer et al. (2014). Guidelines for the treatment of hypothyroidism. *Thyroid*, 24(12), 1670–1751.

[17] Datasets - UCI Machine Learning Repository (1987). Available at: https://archive.ics.uci.edu/ datasets (Accessed: 20 August 2023).

[18] Liu, C., Xie, L., Kong, W. et al. (2019). Prediction of suspicious thyroid nodule using artificial neural network based on radiofrequency ultrasound and conventional ultrasound: A preliminary study. *Ultrasonics*, 99. https://doi.org/10.1016/j.ultras.2019.105951

[19] Desai, F., Chowdhury, D., Kaur, R. et al. (2022). HealthCloud: A system for monitoring health status of heart patients using machine learning and cloud computing. *Internet of Things*, 17, 100485.

[20] Wajner, S. M., & Maia, A. L. (2012). New insights toward the acute non-thyroidal illness syndrome. *Frontiers in Endocrinology*, 3(JAN). https://doi.org/10.3389/fendo.2012.00008.

[21] Dhillon, A., Singh, A., Vohra et al. (2022). IoTPulse: Machine learning-based enterprise health information system to predict alcohol addiction in Punjab (India) using IoT and fog computing. *Enterprise Information Systems*, 16(7), 1820583.

[22] Moqurrab, S. A., Tariq, N., Anjum et al. (2022). A deep learning-based privacy-preserving model for smart healthcare in internet of medical things using fog computing. *Wireless Personal Communications*, 126(3), 2379–2401.

[23] Iftikhar, S., Golec, M., Chowdhury, D. et al. (2022). FogDLearner: A deep learning-based cardiac health diagnosis framework using fog computing. *Proceedings of the 2022 Australasian Computer Science Week* (pp. 136–144).

[24] Golec, M., Gill, S. S., Parlikad, A. K., & Uhlig, S. (2023). HealthFaaS: AI based smart healthcare system for heart patients using serverless computing. *IEEE Internet of Things Journal*, 10(21), 18469–18476.

[25] Singh, R., & Gill, S. S. (2023). Edge AI: A survey. *Internet of Things and Cyber-Physical Systems*, 3, 71–92.

[26] Gill, S. S., Arya, R. C., Wander, G. S. & Buyya, R. (2019). Fog-based smart healthcare as a big data and cloud service for heart patients using IoT. *In International Conference on Intelligent Data Communication Technologies and Internet of Things (ICICI) 2018* (pp. 1376–1383). Springer International Publishing.

[27] Gill, S. S., & Kaur, R. (2023). ChatGPT: Vision and challenges. *Internet of Things and Cyber-Physical Systems*, 3, 262–271.

[28] Gill, S. S., Wu, H., Patros, P. et al. (2024). Modern computing: Vision and challenges, *Telematics and Informatics Reports*, 13, 1–46.

CHAPTER 2

HeartGuard

A Deep Learning Approach for Cardiovascular Risk Assessment Using Biomedical Indicators Using Cloud Computing

Parinaz Banifatemi and Sukhpal Singh Gill

2.1 INTRODUCTION

Heart diseases consist of a wide range of cardiovascular conditions, ranging from heart attacks to congenital heart defects and heart failure [1]. Patients who are affected by such diseases usually show specific symptoms, such as chest pain, which, along with other biomedical markers, can be vital in diagnosing the risk of heart disease. Because heart disease is the leading cause of mortality all around the globe, it requires a vast understanding and approach for early detection and prevention [1]. Our modern lifestyle alterations, including dietary habits and a lack of physical activity, have resulted in an increase in risk factors such as obesity, diabetes, and high cholesterol levels [2]. However, the advancement of artificial intelligence (AI) and machine learning (ML) has provided unique capabilities to healthcare, enabling the early detection of diseases with remarkable accuracy [3,4]. Considering the fact that heart disease tends to be a "silent killer", the ability to predict it before it shows symptoms is notable in the current healthcare system [5]. Utilising the latest ML/AI models for predicting the risk of heart disease has been explored before; however, identifying and ranking the most significant biomedical markers is still unexplored. This study applies cutting-edge algorithms and techniques to break down vital factors contributing to heart disease [6]. Through a detailed analysis of features such as depression, age, sex, max heart rate achieved, resting blood pressure, and others, we are trying to build a hierarchy of biomarkers based upon their importance.

Although recent eagerness to battle obesity and raise awareness has restricted heart disease rates, the challenge still remains, especially with the availability of multiple treatments including bariatric surgery, gastric bypass surgery, and liposuction [7,8]. In contrast to the previous works, our study highlights determining the most essential biomedical markers, focusing on improving accuracy by considering important factors and ignoring

DOI: 10.1201/9781003467199-3

less important ones. As a result of implementing powerful ML techniques including decision trees, linear classifiers, neural networks, and others, we were able to reach a remarkable accuracy of 97% in predicting the general risk of having heart disease [4]. Based on that, the biomedical markers were ranked, bringing out the most vital contributors such as depression, age, sex, max heart rate achieved, and blood pressure. This introduction sets the stage for an exploration of a novel, cloud-based approach to heart disease prediction that excels at the accuracy of previous methodologies as well as providing unparalleled insights into the key factors leading to heart disease. By focusing on these essential biomarkers, we pave the way for personalised healthcare strategies, foster timely interventions, and potentially save lives [9].

2.2 INNOVATION AND IMPLEMENTATION: ENHANCING HEART DISEASE PREDICTION WITH A CLOUD-DEPLOYED SYSTEM

Heart disease continues to challenge healthcare systems all around the world and causes significant economic struggle and loss of life [10]. Traditional methods of detection and prediction, while valuable, have often fallen short in offering convenient and precise interventions [11]. This study offers an innovative solution that not only leverages state-of-the-art ML techniques but also points out the impact of specific biomedical markers, guiding us to an approach that can redefine early diagnosis and treatment [12]. The architecture of our study is meticulously crafted to offer a comprehensive insight into heart disease prediction and the identification of influential biomedical markers [13]. As depicted in Figure 2.1, our approach commences with an exploratory data analysis (EDA) on a heart dataset. Through this initial analysis, we draw preliminary conclusions and identify key

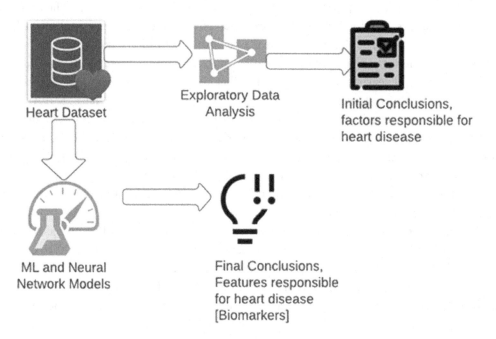

FIGURE 2.1   Proposed architecture.

features that may play a vital role in the occurrence of heart disease. From the same heart dataset, we then apply advanced ML and neural network techniques to extract and rank the biomarkers based on their significance. This twofold approach of conducting EDA to glean initial insights, followed by employing cutting-edge ML and neural networks to further refine the understanding, allows us to offer a robust and innovative solution. The ranked biomarkers provide a targeted and more personalised method of early detection, potentially saving lives and optimising healthcare resources. By coupling traditional analysis with modern computational methods, our study sets a new benchmark in the field of heart disease prediction and treatment.

The contributions of this work are manifold.

2.2.1 Development of a Novel Prediction System

We introduce a new ML and neural network-based intelligent heart disease prediction system, known as HeartGuard. Utilising an amalgamation of decision trees, linear classifiers, and neural networks, the system achieves remarkable accuracy in risk determination.

2.2.2 Feature Importance Analysis

A comprehensive EDA was conducted to identify key biomedical markers responsible for heart disease, such as depression, age, sex, maximum heart rate achieved, and resting blood pressure. The recognition of these factors serves as a pioneering step in risk assessment and personalised medical treatment. In our analysis, several key observations have been derived from a series of figures that elucidate various factors contributing to heart disease susceptibility. These findings reveal a multifaceted relationship between demographic, clinical, and physiological characteristics and the likelihood of heart disease development.

Figure 2.2 provides compelling evidence regarding the gender disparity in heart disease susceptibility, highlighting that males are markedly more prone to this condition. This finding prompts further investigation into the underlying biological, lifestyle, or sociocultural factors that may be responsible for this observed difference between male and female subjects.

Figure 2.3 examines the different levels of chest pain severity and their associations with the likelihood of developing heart disease. Specifically, individuals experiencing level 4 chest pain intensity were found to be more susceptible to heart disease. This relationship not only emphasises the critical importance of pain assessment in clinical settings but also invites further studies to understand the underlying pathophysiology connecting intense chest pain to heart disease.

Figure 2.4 elucidates the correlation between heart disease risk and a particular physiological parameter: the slope of 2.0. This observation raises intriguing questions about the role that this specific slope value plays in heart disease pathogenesis. It may be reflective of certain underlying cardiac conditions that manifest in this particular slope value, warranting further in-depth examination. From Figure 2.4, we can conclude that men are more prone to heart disease.

We have conducted a detailed age-related analysis, revealing that individuals aged between 52 and 63 are more prone to heart disease. This age bracket could be indicative

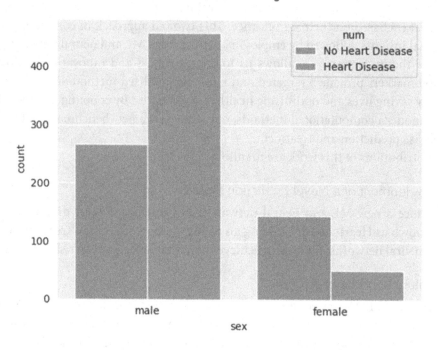

FIGURE 2.2   Count of number of heart patients with respect to the gender.

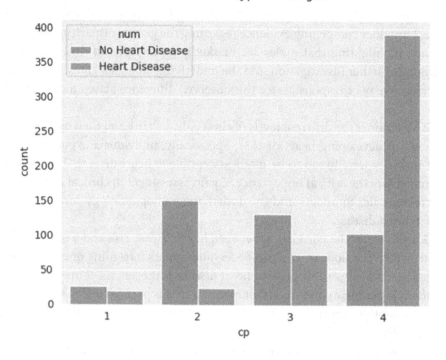

FIGURE 2.3   Count of number of heart patients with respect to the chest pain.

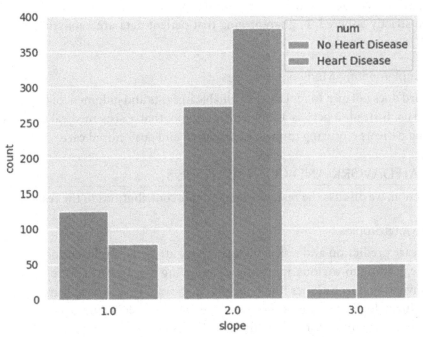

FIGURE 2.4   Count of number of heart patients with respect to the slope.

of a critical period during which genetic, metabolic, lifestyle, and other age-related factors converge to increase vulnerability to heart disease. This observation serves as a vital insight for targeted interventions and preventive measures within this specific age group.

In summary, these figures collectively paint a complex and nuanced picture of heart disease risk. By identifying gender, chest pain intensity, specific physiological parameters, age, and key diagnostic features as critical determinants, this analysis paves the way for a more integrated and multifactorial approach to understanding, diagnosing, and managing heart disease.

2.2.3 Deployment on the Cloud

Uniquely, HeartGuard has been deployed on the Google Cloud Platform (GCP), allowing for real-time predictions [9]. This deployment paves the way for global accessibility and integration into existing healthcare systems, enabling prompt and well-informed medical decisions.

2.2.4 Economic and Social Impact

The implementation of this system can translate into considerable savings for health services [12]. For example, the reduction of avoidable shortcomings in heart failure prediction, which cost the National Health Service (NHS) £21 million in 2019 [14], illustrates the potential fiscal benefits. Additionally, patients stand to gain from early diagnosis, receiving timely and targeted interventions that minimise pain and complications.

2.2.5 Privacy Considerations

Ensuring the protection of patient information is paramount. Legal and ethical guidelines have been strictly adhered to, guaranteeing that patient data are anonymised and confidentiality is maintained.

2.2.6 Complementing Medical Expertise

HeartGuard does not aim to replace the valuable insights and judgment of trained medical professionals. Instead, it acts as a supplementary tool that assists medical practitioners in identifying patients requiring immediate attention and customised care.

2.3 RELATED WORK AND CONTRIBUTIONS

In this section, we discuss the related work and our contributions to the research.

2.3.1 Previous Studies

Heart disease prediction and risk assessment have attracted the attention of researchers worldwide, leading to various approaches employing ML and AI. These range from the use of conventional techniques like *k*-means clustering, DNA-based learning, ensemble learning, fuzzy logic, and more. For instance, ensemble learning using decision trees has shown high accuracy for risk prediction [15], and neural networks have also yielded promising results [7]. Several existing studies have explored hybrid systems combining genetic algorithms, fuzzy logic, and principal component analysis (PCA) with open-source tools like WEKA and KEEL [16]. Another innovative research work [17] looked at the potential of using video imagery to calculate heart rates in conjunction with logistic regression, naïve Bayes, and artificial neural networks. However, there are gaps in this existing body of work. Many studies, such as [12,13], focused on diagnosis without considering the vital role of biomedical markers. Furthermore, existing algorithms often come from standard libraries with little customization to the specific situation of heart disease prediction [18–20].

2.3.2 Our Contributions and Innovations

The main contributions of this work include the following:

- **Merging of Multiple Datasets**: Unlike other studies that primarily rely on the UCI Heart Disease dataset [15, 21], our work has taken a unique route by merging different datasets from Hungarian, Swiss, and American (Cleveland) sources. This merged dataset offers a more diverse and comprehensive view, enhancing the prediction's generality and robustness.

- **HeartGuard (A New Horizon)**: Our study introduces "HeartGuard", an ML-powered smart heart disease risk prediction system utilising biomedical markers. This innovative system not only aims to enhance accuracy but also emphasises identifying the most crucial biomedical markers [9]. It represents a significant leap in early detection and treatment.

- **Efficient Feature Selection and Utilization**: Whereas other studies have attempted to remove redundant features [19] or use PCA to speed up classification [20], our approach digs deeper. We focus on understanding the most valuable features for further study, recognising that all features are not equally important and that irrelevant or redundant features can decrease accuracy.

- **Achieving High Accuracy**: Our method's hallmark is the achievement of an impressive 97% accuracy after the 500th epoch in predicting the risk of heart disease. This surpasses the baseline methods on the same set of data, highlighting the effectiveness of our ensemble learning approach.

2.4 METHODOLOGY

The methodology for this study encompasses various stages, including data preparation, modelling, evaluation, and deployment to the cloud. The system architecture for our work, referred to as "HeartGuard" is as follows.

2.4.1 Dataset

The dataset is a compilation of heart disease data from three locations: Switzerland, Hungary, and Cleveland, obtained from the UCI Heart Disease dataset [13]. This composite dataset ensures a comprehensive and representative sample for developing and validating the models [22,23]. The explanation of dataset features is given as follows:

- **Age**: Represents the age of the individual in years. A continuous variable indicating the person's age.

- **Sex**: Categorises the gender of the individual. "0" denotes female, and "1" denotes male.

- **Chest Pain (CP)**: Specifies the level of chest pain the patient is suffering. Categorised into four types ranging from 0 to 3.

- **Resting Blood Pressure (RestBP)**: A continuous variable representing the resting blood pressure of the individual, measured in mm Hg.

- **Cholesterol (Chol)**: Represents the cholesterol levels in the individual's blood, measured in mg/dL.

- **Fasting Blood Sugar (FBS)**: Indicates the fasting blood sugar level of the person, categorised into two values to check if it is greater or lower than 120 mg/dL.

- **restECG**: Describes three different levels to display the waveforms as shown by an electrocardiogram (ECG) machine, ranging from 0 to 2.

- **HeartBeat**: Continuous attribute indicating the maximum heart rate achieved by the individual.

- **Exang (exercise-induced angina)**: A binary attribute, where "0" means no exercise-induced angina, and "1" means exercise-induced angina is present.

- **OldPeak**: A continuous attribute representing depression induced by exercise relative to rest. Values can range between 0 and 6.2.

- **Slope**: Describes the condition of the person during peak exercise. Categorised into three states representing the gradient of the tangent to the slope (increasing, decreasing, flat).

- **CA**: Indicates the number of blood vessels coloured by fluoroscopy, ranging from 0 to 4.

- **Thal**: Represents four different values as results of thallium tests, ranging from 0 to 3.

- **Target**: This is the label attribute signifying whether a person had heart disease or not. "0" represents a lack of heart disease, and "1" represents the presence of heart disease.

2.4.2 Preprocessing and Feature Engineering

Data preprocessing is performed to handle missing values, normalise features, and transform categorical attributes as shown in Figure 2.5. This stage ensures that the dataset is suitable for modelling.

2.4.3 Machine Learning Models

We have considered the following ML models:

- **Decision Tree Classifier**: Achieving 73% accuracy, this model provides a simple and interpretable way to identify key features. Figure 2.6 shows the feature importance according to the decision tree classifier.

#	Column	Non-Null Count	Dtype
0	age	920 non-null	int64
1	sex	920 non-null	int64
2	cp	920 non-null	int64
3	trestbps	920 non-null	object
4	chol	920 non-null	object
5	fbs	920 non-null	object
6	restecg	920 non-null	object
7	thalach	920 non-null	object
8	exang	920 non-null	object
9	oldpeak	920 non-null	object
10	slope	920 non-null	object
11	ca	920 non-null	object
12	thal	920 non-null	object
13	num	920 non-null	int64

FIGURE 2.5   After preprocessing.

```
Feature Importances According to Decision Trees:
cp: 0.28548
chol: 0.15828
age: 0.11110
thalach: 0.10519
trestbps: 0.09745
oldpeak: 0.08416
exang: 0.04145
sex: 0.04077
ca: 0.02901
slope: 0.01785
fbs: 0.01436
restecg: 0.01040
thal: 0.00451
```

FIGURE 2.6   Feature importance according to decision tree classifier.

```
                                     Feature
7                                st_depression
5                      max_heart_rate_achieved
3                                  cholesterol
8                            num_major_vessels
6                      exercise_induced_angina
1                                          sex
0                                          age
4                          fasting_blood_sugar
2                       resting_blood_pressure
9             thalassemia_type_fixed defect
```

FIGURE 2.7   Feature importance according to linear classifier.

- **Logistic Regression**: This model offers a 76.6% accuracy and is used for binary classification. Figure 2.7 shows the feature importance according to linear classifier.

- **Neural Networks**: With 97% accuracy after 500 epochs, this deep learning model demonstrates strong predictive capabilities. Figure 2.8 shows the feature importance according to neural networks.

2.5 MODEL EVALUATION AND COMPARISON

Models are evaluated using techniques like K-fold cross-validation, confusion matrices, and Receiver Operating Characteristic (ROC) curves. The performance is thoroughly compared to select the best-suited model for deployment. We deployed the neural network model for deployment, as its accuracy is 97%, as shown in Figure 2.9.

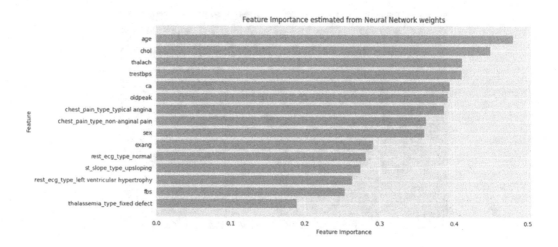

FIGURE 2.8   Feature importance according to neural networks.

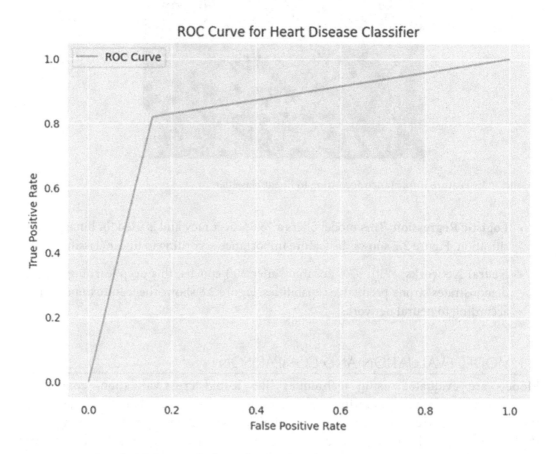

FIGURE 2.9   Sample ROC curve for heart disease classifier.

2.6 DEPLOYMENT TO GOOGLE CLOUD PLATFORM

The selected models are serialised using Pickle, and a Flask web application is developed to host the models. The application is then deployed to the GCP, allowing users to access the heart disease prediction service online. The cloud deployment benefits from scalable infrastructure and high availability:

- **Model Serialization**: Models are serialised using Pickle files, allowing them to be stored and loaded efficiently for deployment.

- **Flask Application**: A web application is created using Flask to serve the models, providing an Application Programming Interface (API) for accessing the heart disease prediction service.

- **Deployment on Google Cloud**: The Flask application, along with the serialised models, is deployed on GCP, leveraging its robust and scalable infrastructure.

Figure 2.10 shows an input form to predict heart disease in web interface, and Figure 2.11 shows the prediction result in web interface.

Input Details

Age:	63
Sex:	1
CP:	1
Trest BPS:	145
Cholestrol	233
FBS	1
Rest ECG	2
Thalach	150
Exang	0
Old Peak	2.3
Slope	3
CA	0.0
Thal	6.0

Submit

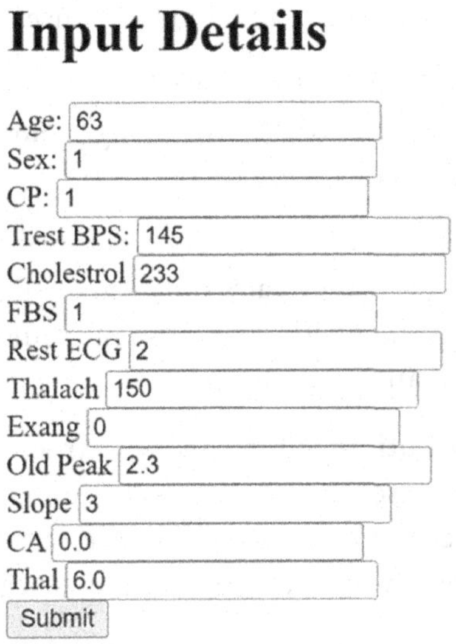

FIGURE 2.10   Input form to predict heart disease in web interface.

Prediction Result

There is Heart
Disease

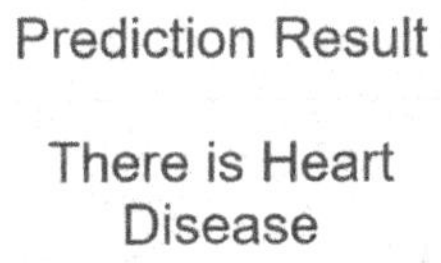

FIGURE 2.11   Prediction result in web interface.

2.7 CONCLUSIONS

Heart disease continues to be a formidable challenge worldwide, necessitating innovative approaches for early detection, prevention, and management. In this chapter, we have presented HeartGuard, an unprecedented solution that pushes the boundaries of heart disease prediction by leveraging advanced ML techniques and careful analysis of critical biomedical markers. Our study's contributions are manifold:

- **Development of a Novel Prediction System**: HeartGuard integrates decision trees, linear classifiers, and neural networks to achieve an impressive accuracy rate of 97% in heart disease risk prediction. This breakthrough system provides a remarkable improvement over existing methodologies.

- **Comprehensive Feature Importance Analysis**: We have embarked on an in-depth exploration of key biomedical markers like depression, age, sex, max heart rate achieved, and resting blood pressure. The identification of these markers and their hierarchical ranking provides a pioneering perspective in risk assessment and personalised healthcare.

- **Insightful Observations**: Our study elaborates on various facets of heart disease risk, from gender and age disparities to the role of chest pain intensity and specific physiological parameters. These insights lay the foundation for more multifaceted approaches to understanding and managing heart disease.

- **Cloud-Based Deployment**: By hosting HeartGuard on GCP, we have enabled global accessibility and real-time predictions, promoting prompt medical interventions and well-informed medical decisions.

- **Economic, Social Impact, and Privacy Considerations**: With potential fiscal benefits and an emphasis on patient privacy, our system aligns with both economic and ethical concerns. It complements the expertise of medical professionals, acting as a supplementary tool to enhance patient care.

- **Innovations and Contributions**: Our chapter introduces unique innovations like the merging of diverse datasets and the emphasis on efficient feature selection. The achievement of a 97% accuracy rate stands as a testament to our method's efficacy, representing a significant advancement in heart disease prediction.

2.8 FUTURE EXPLORATION: INCORPORATING ECG GRAPHICAL DATA

In our ongoing pursuit of developing an even more precise and adaptive system for heart disease prediction, a logical and potent next step is to incorporate ECG graphical data [24]. ECGs have been an essential diagnostic tool in cardiology, offering invaluable insights into the heart's electrical activities and underlying pathophysiological mechanisms. The following subsections detail the reasons behind this choice and the potential benefits it may bring.

- **Enhanced Diagnostic Capability**: ECG graphical data provide a continuous picture of the heart's electrical activity, revealing anomalies and irregular patterns that might be indicative of underlying heart conditions [18]. While the biomedical markers employed in the current study have significantly advanced the field, integrating ECG data add a dynamic and real-time aspect, enhancing the predictive model's sensitivity and specificity.

- **Detection of Subtle Abnormalities**: Heart diseases often present themselves through subtle changes in the ECG waveform. By analysing these graphical data, our future models could potentially identify early or latent cardiac conditions that might be missed through conventional biomedical markers. This can include rhythm abnormalities, ischemic changes, or other signs indicative of heart ailments.

- **Synergy with Existing Biomedical Markers**: Integrating ECG data does not negate the importance of the identified biomedical markers. Instead, it can act in synergy, combining the strength of static risk factors such as age, sex, and cholesterol levels with dynamic insights from the ECG [25]. This comprehensive approach might provide a fuller, more nuanced understanding of a patient's cardiovascular health, leading to more timely and accurate interventions [26].

- **Real-time Monitoring and Personalised Care**: The use of ECG data allows for continuous monitoring, opening the door to predictive analytics that can function in real time. This potential for real-time analysis would allow healthcare providers to respond to emergent situations more proactively, possibly even predicting events like heart attacks before they occur [19]. Such capabilities would indeed revolutionise personalised care and preventive strategies.

- **Challenges and Ethical Considerations**: While the integration of ECG graphical data presents enormous potential, it also brings unique challenges, especially concerning data quality, standardization, and privacy. Handling these complex and high-dimensional data requires sophisticated algorithms and robust methodologies [20]. Ethical considerations, such as informed consent and data protection, must be at the forefront of this endeavour.

The addition of ECG graphical data into our existing heart disease prediction system is a promising and logical progression. It represents an alignment with the broader trends in medicine towards more personalised, data-driven care, and leverages a well-established diagnostic tool in a novel way [27]. By melding static risk factors with dynamic, real-time data, we open the door to potentially groundbreaking advancements in heart disease prediction, early intervention, and patient care [28]. The careful handling of these data, with a keen eye on quality, ethics, and patient well-being, will be critical to realising this potential.

REFERENCES

[1] Golec, M., Gill, S. S., Parlikad, A. K. et al. (2023). HealthFaaS: AI based smart healthcare system for heart patients using serverless computing. *IEEE Internet of Things Journal*, 10 (21), 18469–18476.

[2] Hosseinzadeh, M., Koohpayehzadeh, J., Bali, A. O. et al. (2021). A diagnostic prediction model for chronic kidney disease in internet of things platform. *Multimedia Tools and Applications*, 80(11), 16933–16950.

[3] Goswami, P., Mukherjee, A., Sarkar, B. et al. (2021). Multi-agent-based smart power management for remote health monitoring. *Neural Computing and Applications*, 33, 1–10.

[4] Gill, S. S., Arya, R. C., Wander, G. S. et al. (2018). Fog-Based Smart Healthcare as a Big Data and Cloud Service for Heart Patients Using IoT. *In International Conference on Intelligent Data Communication Technologies and Internet of Things* (pp. 1376–1383). Springer, Cham.

[5] Health Europa. (2019). Avoidable Deficiencies in Heart Failure Cost NHS £21M. [online] Available at: ¡https://www.healtheuropa.eu/avoidable-deficiencies-in-heart-failure-cost-nhs-21m/98696/¿ (Accessed 6 August 2023).

[6] Tuli, S., Basumatary, N., Gill, S. S. et al. (2020). HealthFog: An ensemble deep learning based smart healthcare system for automatic diagnosis of heart diseases in integrated IoT and fog computing environments. *Future Generation Computer Systems*, 104, 187–200.

[7] Uyar, K., & Ilhan, A. (2017). Diagnosis of heart disease using genetic algorithm based trained recurrent fuzzy neural networks. *Procedia Computer Science*, 120, 588–593.

[8] Khourdifi, Y., & Bahaj, M. (2019). Heart disease prediction and classification using machine learning algorithms optimized by particle swarm optimization and ant colony optimization. *International Journal of Intelligent Engineering and Systems*, 12(1), 242–252.

[9] Amer, S. S., Wander, G., Singh, M. et al. (2022). BioLearner: A machine learning-powered smart heart disease risk prediction system utilizing biomedical markers. *Journal of Interconnection Networks*, 22(03), 2145003.

[10] Moqurrab, S. A., Tariq, N., Anjum, A. et al. (2022). A deep learning-based privacy-preserving model for smart healthcare in internet of medical things using fog computing. *Wireless Personal Communications*, 126(3), 2379–2401.

[11] Dhillon, A., Singh, A., Vohra, H. et al. (2022). IoTPulse: Machine learning-based Enterprise health information system to predict alcohol addiction in Punjab (India) using IoT and fog computing. *Enterprise Information Systems*, 16(7), 1820583.

[12] Iftikhar, S., Golec, M., Chowdhury, D. et al. (2022). FogDLearner: A Deep Learning-based Cardiac Health Diagnosis Framework Using Fog Computing. *In Proceedings of the 2022 Australasian Computer Science Week* (pp. 136–144).

[13] Desai, F., Chowdhury, D., Kaur, R. et al. (2022). HealthCloud: A system for monitoring health status of heart patients using machine learning and cloud computing. *Internet of Things*, 17, 100485.

[14] Tarawneh, M., & Embarak, O. (2019). Hybrid Approach for Heart Disease Prediction Using Data Mining Techniques. *In Advances in Internet, Data and Web Technologies* (pp. 447–454). Springer, Cham.

[15] Abdeldjouad, F., Brahami, M., & Matta, N. (2020). *A Hybrid Approach for Heart Disease Diagnosis and Prediction Using Machine Learning Techniques*. Lecture Notes in Computer Science (pp. 299–306). Springer, Cham.

[16] Gonsalves, A., Thabtah, F., Mohammad, R. M. A. et al. (2019). Prediction of Coronary Heart Disease using Machine Learning. *In Proceedings of the 2019 3rd International Conference on Deep Learning Technologies - ICDLT 2019*.

[17] Golec, M., Ozturac, R., Pooranian, Z. et al. (2021). iFaaSBus: A security and privacy based lightweight framework for serverless computing using IoT and machine learning. *IEEE Transactions on Industrial Informatics*, 18, 3522–3529.

[18] Gill, S. S., Xu, M., Ottaviani, C. et al. (2022). AI for next generation computing: Emerging trends and future directions. *Internet of Things*, 19, 100514.

[19] Gill, S. S., Wu, H., Patros, P. et al. (2024). Modern computing: Vision and challenges. *Telematics and Informatics Reports*, 13, 100116.

[20] Tuli, S., Tuli, S., Wander, G. et al. (2020). Next generation technologies for smart healthcare: Challenges, vision, model, trends and future directions. *Internet Technology Letters*, 3(2), e145.

[21] Archive.ics.uci.edu. (1988). UCI Machine Learning Repository: Heart Disease Data Set. [Online]. Available at: ¡https://archive.ics.uci.edu/ml/datasets/Heart+Disease¿ (Accessed 9 August 2020).

[22] Nikram, S., Shukla, P., & Shah, M. (2020). Cardiovascular Disease Prediction Using Genetic Algorithm and Neuro-Fuzzy System. [Online]. Available at: ¡https://www.ijltet.org/journal/149094578316.1568.pdf¿ (Accessed 7 August 2023).

[23] NHS.UK. (2016). Study Says There's No Link Between Cholesterol and Heart Disease. [Online]. Available at: ¡https://www.nhs.uk/news/heart-and-lungs/study-says-theres-no-link-between-cholesterol-and-heart-disease/¿ (Accessed 10 August 2023).

[24] Juan, A., Pazzi, R. W., & Boukerche, A. (2009). Using accuracy-based learning classifier systems for adaptable strategy generation in games and interactive virtual simulations. *Journal of Interconnection Networks*, 10(04), 365–390.

[25] Haq, A., Li, J., Memon, M. et al. (2018). A hybrid intelligent system framework for the prediction of heart disease using machine learning algorithms. *Mobile Information Systems*, 2018, 1–21.

[26] Gagliano, S., Ravji, R., Barnes et al. (2015). Smoking gun or circumstantial evidence? Comparison of statistical learning methods using functional annotations for prioritizing risk variants. *Scientific Reports*, 5(1), 13373.

[27] Singh, R., & Gill, S. S. (2023). Edge AI: A survey. *Internet of Things and Cyber-Physical Systems*, 3, 71–92.

[28] Gill, S. S., & Kaur, R. (2023). ChatGPT: Vision and challenges. *Internet of Things and Cyber-Physical Systems*, 3, 262–271.

CHAPTER 3

Deep Convolutional Neural Networks-Based Skin Lesion Classification for Cancer Prediction

Neelam Rathore and Sukhpal Singh Gill

3.1 INTRODUCTION

Skin cancer, one of the deadliest malignancies that has recently seen exponential development worldwide, is a hazardous and now common condition [1]. It significantly affects both the economy and public health. Skin cancers are mostly formed from cells in the epidermis and are categorised into melanoma skin cancer and non-melanoma skin cancer [2]. The most significant etiological cause of skin cancer is exposure to ultraviolet (UV) light [3]. Today, there are at least 1 million new infections identified yearly, and in the United Kingdom, the disease claims the lives of about 2500 individuals annually, or 7 people per day [4]. According to all of these views, cancer is curable if discovered in its earliest stages. In most situations, a straightforward biopsy can stop cancer from spreading. The most frequent cancer, both in men and women, is melanoma, which had around 300,000 new cases reported worldwide in 2018 [5]. A visual inspection of the suspected skin region is the first stage in a dermatologist's diagnosis of a malignant lesion. The similarity of symptoms necessitates a proper diagnosis of some of the forms of lesions.

Innovation in digital health does contribute to improving healthcare by expanding access to advanced knowledge [6]. The use of nanoscience in cancer treatment is tempting because it enables the safe and efficient delivery of medications and other biologically active materials to target tissues [7]. Medical image classification, especially for dermatology, has improved significantly in recent years and now includes the identification of skin cancers from dermoscopic images or macroscopic photos, among the countless other machine learning applications in the field of healthcare [8]. The classification of skin lesions has recently come under the attention of the machine learning community. Before 2016, most studies utilised the traditional machine learning methodology of preprocessing, segmentation, feature extraction, and classification. A modification in the study of

DOI: 10.1201/9781003467199-4

lesion classification methods took place in 2016. The approaches presented at the 2016 International Symposium on Biomedical Imaging (ISBI) provide evidence of this transformation [9]. The 25 participating teams all used convolutional neural networks (CNNs), a deep learning methodology, as opposed to the typical standard machine learning techniques [10]. To learn how to represent data hierarchically, deep learning uses numerous processing layers [11]. It provides a technique to harness a significant amount of information with only a few hands from feature engineers.

In the past few years, deep learning has evolved and made tremendous strides in healthcare [12]. The unique feature of deep CNN (DCNN) is that the last layers of the deep neural network learn concepts and strong features, whereas the initial layers typically learn relatively basic and "low-level" features of images [13]. Hence, DCNNs that have been finetuned and trained on a single dataset for image categorization tasks can be used again by others as a challenge for image categorization using many datasets. Deep learning and Python are employed and enable us to understand how they work as well as understand other techniques [14]. The work provides information at several levels, which aids in our understanding of the process in a very clear and exact way.

3.1.1 Motivation and Our Contributions

Skin cancer mortality rates have improved, and the number of fatalities associated with the condition is dropping steadily. Early detection is essential to lower fatalities. Various regression and classification models (including deep learning models) are advancements that can detect cancerous cells early. Skin cancer detection can be difficult, time-consuming, and expensive. For instance, Figures 3.2 and 3.3 depict two lesions that, on the surface, appear to be identical. However, the right image depicts a melanoma lesion, whereas the left image depicts a typical benign lesion. It is not unexpected that artificial intelligence (AI) technologies are being utilised to help diagnose skin cancer and recommend treatments as they get faster and smarter and take action.

This investigation aims to classify skin lesions using various DCNN layers. This research focuses on the presentation of a thorough approach to traditional deep learning algorithms for skin cancer diagnosis, including CNN, VGG16, ResNet, and DenseNet. The primary objective of the research is to comprehend how deep learning models can be used to categorise malignant cells using a DCNN model that has been trained on a sizeable batch of visual data. The processes go from a weak model to a strong model that provides great accuracy. In each method, neural network structures with various layer configurations are used. The main contributions to this work are the following:

- Fine-tune the DCNN for 10,000 dermoscopic images of 7 different types of skin lesions.

- VGG16, Inception V3, ResNet V2, and DenseNet performance for DCNN are compared. Every DCNN is adjusted from the top layers down. With Inception V3 and DenseNet 201, all layers are fine-tuned.

- Inception V3 and DenseNet 201 are combined, and all layers are adjusted.

3.2 RELATED WORK

This section will highlight some relevant work done in the past using a dataset on skin cancer using various deep learning techniques and systematic reviews. Here is a discussion of 16 prominent research journals that examine deep learning and computational analysis. Brinker et al. [15] conducted a systematic review of the CNN model that was applied to skin cancer studies and prospects. In this study, the researcher primarily focused on presenting the first systematic overview of the most recent studies on this classification of skin lesions using CNNs. We are just reviewing classifiers for skin lesions. Methods that use a CNN just for segmentation or to categorise dermoscopic patterns are specifically excluded from consideration. In addition, this study outlined the problems that need to be overcome going forward and why it is so difficult to compare the treatments that are now used. The study's information is pretty easy to understand and was shown using skin lesion datasets for CNN models from a number of papers, such as the current CNN-based classifier, CNN model training with transfer learning, and CNN as a feature extractor.

Wu et al. [9] also showed in their research paper a systematic skin cancer review classifier based on deep learning. Researchers provided a thorough summary of the latest deep learning-based skin cancer categorization algorithms in their research. A collection of the publicly available datasets that deal with skin cancer in this article, such as dermatological images, clinical images, and dermoscopy images, follows the introduction of three distinct classes of dermatological imaging. The effective uses of standard CNN for the skin cancer subclass are then reviewed. The highlights of this study include a summary of numerous frontier issues, such as data restriction, data imbalance, domain adaptability, model stability, and model effectiveness, and their associated solutions in the task of classifying skin cancer. The collection of publicly accessible datasets is as follows for the skin lesion study: PH2, MED-NODE, HAM10000, Derm7pt, BCN20000, and ISIC.

Popescu et al. [16] showed a new trend in melanoma detection using CNN; they also compared the classical method and the CNN approach. Examination of emerging methodologies in the field of automatic skin lesion detection is the primary goal of the researcher. The paper's primary objective is to show the expanding trend of applying neural network approaches to the creation of such a system. They selected 134 papers for review, showed the graph for the percentages dataset used between the years 2018 and 2021, and represented a highly used dataset with skin cancer classification. Their study showed approaches such as AlexNet, inception/LeNet, VGG16, ResNet, YOLO Network, Xception Net, MobileNet, EfficientNet, and DenseNet.

Palak and Bhumika [17] focused on practical approaches and processes that determine the detection of skin cancer for early scholars. In their study, they started with the basic approach of segmenting images, collecting features, using classifiers, and trend analysis. This area covers artificial neural networks (CNN), which are also a deep learning method. This article says that adaptive fuzzy inference neural network (AFINN) gives more accurate results than neural networks, fuzzy rule-based systems, and traditional biopsy methods. It also says that computer-aided diagnostics is better.

Manne et al. [18] performed a skin cancer analysis with opportunities and vulnerabilities. This research used transfer learning using CNN and achieved 89.3% accuracy for AlexNet. Their study was trying to determine whether a sample contains benign or malignant tissue, features that were collected and fed into the K-nearest neighbour (KNN), support vector machine (SVM), random forest (RF), and naïve Bayes (NB) classifiers. The classifiers were fed features, and the SVM classifier resulted in an accuracy of 85.19%. Experimental outcomes of feature extraction and classification techniques: SVM forecasts 85.19% accuracy, 50% recall, 45.62% precision, and a 46% F1 score using NB classification. Finally, CNNs have been demonstrated to be useful for classifying and assessing skin cancer diagnoses. However, CNN's design occasionally has limitations when it comes to image classification; serious repercussions may result from misclassifying skin cancer as benign.

Kumar et al. [19] had done a comparative experiment on the prediction of skin lesion cells using certain deep learning models. Their paper shows different approaches to deep learning, CNN, supervised learning, and transfer learning. The dataset should first be loaded and normalised. It employs ResNet 18, AlexNet, and ResNet 50 as part of its CNN network. Next, define the dataset's loss function, then train the network. The network in this case was trained using supervised learning. After that, divide the data into test and training data and proceed with testing and training. Finally, accuracy and loss are obtained after data validation. The proposed approaches in this article are ResNet, AlexNet, and transfer learning. Comparing the accuracy between these approaches, CNN achieved the lowest accuracy at 78%, followed by transfer learning with 96.12%, and AlexNet had similar accuracy of 98.32%. The ability of CNN to identify significant traits without human oversight is a major advantage. Moreover, various CNN layers provide findings that are more filtered.

Vijayalakshmi [20] researched a fully automated technique for identifying dermatological diseases from lesion photos. This machine intervention differs from traditional medical personnel-based identification. The four stages of our model's design are augmentation, information collection, model development, and forecasting. We optimised the structure and obtained a precision of 85% by integrating numerous AI approaches, such as CNN and SVM, with image-processing techniques.

Hosny et al. [21] categorised skin cancer using transfer learning and deep learning techniques. He suggested a system for automatically identifying skin lesions. This approach makes use of transfer learning and a deep learning network that has been trained before. By replacing the final layer with a softmax to categorise three different lesions, transfer learning is used in AlexNet in addition to fine-tuning and data augmentation (melanoma, common nevus, and atypical nevus). They used the PH2 dataset to train and evaluate the model. The performance of the technique is assessed using the well-known quantitative measures of accuracy, sensitivity, specificity, and precision, with achieved values of 98.61%, 98.33%, 98.93%, and 97.73%, respectively.

Kadampur and Al Riyaee [22] built a deep learning model for the classification of dermal cell images and finding skin cancer. In this research, deep learning system (DLS)-built networks performed pretty well when tested against the HAM10000 benchmark machine learning datasets. With a greater receiver operating characteristic (ROC) value, the classification algorithm has a higher chance of correctly classifying cancer as existent or not.

Among the pre-trained models, DenseNet, SqueezeNet, and Inception V3 models show higher ROCs than the ResNet model. These findings suggest that the models developed using DLS outperform many of the results from comparable studies. Model construction with DLS is fast and efficient. Researchers have developed a tool that enables people without programming experience to create sophisticated deep learning models. They implemented Deep Learning Studio, a model-driven architecture for deep learning. The characteristics of the DLS tool were discussed, along with instructions on how to utilise it to build a deep learning model.

Haggenmuller et al. [23] presented a review of trials employing human experts using CNNs for the categorization of skin cancer. This research is based on many papers, how they work, and which types of data were used to train the model. Peer-reviewed articles dealing with melanoma-based AI-based skin cancer classification that were published between 2017 and 2021 were searched in PubMed, Medline, and ScienceDirect. CNN, digital biomarkers, melanoma detection, histology, and entire slide images were integrated with search phrases for skin cancer categorization, deep learning, and CNN. Only studies with a meaningful correlation of AI outcomes with medical professionals and a diagnostic classification as its primary goal were included, according to the search results. Nineteen reader studies all met the requirements for inclusion, two dermatopathological studies used digitised histological full slide images, and six of them concentrated on the identification of imaging data. Of them, 11 CNN-based strategies focused on categorising dermoscopic data.

In 2022, Jones et al. [24] worked on community-based machine learning for skin cancer detection. This is a systematic review that contains a large number of paper sets. In this paper, they looked for publications that presented proof in Embase, Medline, Web of Science, and Scopus on employing AI/Machine Learning (ML) models for the initial diagnosis of skin cancer. The major outcomes demonstrated reasonable mean diagnosis accuracy for basal cell carcinoma (87.6%), squamous cell carcinoma (85.3%), and melanoma (89.5%). The secondary findings demonstrated the variability in AI/ML study design and techniques, as well as a significant amount of inadequate documentation.

Esteva et al. [25] categorised skin lesions by employing a single CNN trained end-to-end via images and only using pixels and disease labels as inputs. They trained a CNN on a sample of 129,450 clinical images, 2 orders of magnitude larger than previous datasets (12), and containing images of 2032 distinct illnesses. Using biopsy-validated clinical images, we compare its performance with 21 board-certified dermatologists. The first instance serves as an example of the most prevalent cancer, whereas the second case serves as an example of the deadliest skin cancer. In both tests, CNN performs on par with all evaluated expertise, demonstrating that AI is able to recognise skin cancer with an accuracy level comparable to that of dermatologists.

However, researchers in [26] worked on VGG16 and inception for skin cancer classification using deep learning models. After fine-tuning the model, the VGG16 model gets better accuracy compared with Inception V3, which is 73.33%. Similarly, the VGG16 model performed well on other skin cancer types. There is one comparison shown in the study between KNN, SVM, AlexNet, and VGG16. VGG16 scored the highest accuracy between these models. In actuality, taking into account the proposed VGG16 model, recall, precision, and F1 score values are equal to 51.35%, 95.00%, and 66.66%, respectively.

The research of Dildar et al. [27] gave a thorough analysis of deep learning methods to identify skin cancer at an early stage. The topic of cancer in skin diagnosis-related research and articles from reputable publications were examined. For easier understanding, the presentation of research results involves techniques, diagrams, tables, tools, and frameworks. The extensive discussion about deep learning methods for diagnosing skin cancer was the subject of the first quality assessment query. For the purpose of classifying images and identifying different forms of skin cancer, neural networks were developed. We looked into various learning methods, including artificial neural network (ANN), KNN, CNN, and generative adversarial network (GAN) for skin lesion identification systems. The author analysed these models using various datasets, including HAM10000, ISIC Archive, PH2, DermQuest, DermIS, AtlasDerm, and DermNet. In the photographs from the dataset, they discovered the variations. Because CNN has been more directly tied to computer vision, it is more effective at identifying image data.

3.2.1 Critical Analysis

Previous studies have shown that the accuracy of each technique varies depending on the investigation; for certain studies, CNN, SVM, transfer learning, and feature extraction had the highest accuracy [28,29]. According to research [30], AI is one of the simplest methods for spotting skin cancer, and as this technology is centred around algorithmic models, it is not dependent on actual clinical testing [14, 31]. We conclude that despite the positive accuracy findings of the constructed model, which ranged from 69.2% to 97.8%, it still requires significant holes to be filled before it can be used to identify large-scale projects.

3.3 PROPOSED TECHNIQUE

This study develops a deep learning model to categorise cancer tissue in skin lesions. Some of the built-in algorithms have limitations as outlined in Section 3.2. The diagnostic procedure known as dermoscopy improves the diagnosis of benign and malignant pigmented skin lesions compared with examination with the naked eye [32]. For the HAM10000 dataset, 10,015 dermoscopic pictures were gathered [33,34]. There are representative groups of basal cell carcinoma, benign keratosis-like lesions, dermatofibroma, melanoma, melanocytic nevi, and vascular lesions in the dataset. The proposed technique works on top layers as well as all the layers for this development.

3.3.1 Workflow Architecture

Figure 3.1 shows the basic workflow of neural networks. (1) Filtering and contrast-enhancing algorithms make up the preprocessing stage. (2) The lesion is to be found during the segmentation stage. (3) The feature extraction phase, which is based on the computation of the four parameters (asymmetry, border irregularity, colour, and diameter) is the third step. (4) The classification stage, which adds the four extracted parameters and their weights, produces the total dermoscopy value.

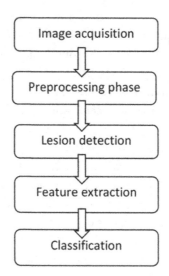

FIGURE 3.1   The workflow of neural network working.

3.3.2 Modelling

The following models have been used: Basic DCNN, VGG16, Inception V3, DenseNet, and ResNet.

3.4 IMPLEMENTATION

In this section, we discuss the implementation of various models along with a dataset description [28, 32].

3.4.1 Dataset

This process involves both studying the data and getting it ready for neural network training. We can see the images of the dataset from HAM10000 [33] in Figures 3.2 and 3.3. The five skin lesions included in the dataset include actinic keratoses, dermatofibroma, benign keratosis-like lesions, basal cell carcinoma, and melanocytic nevi. The majority of skin lesions are benign, with the exception of deadly basal cell carcinoma, melanoma, and actinic keratoses. In the dataset, 8000 samples are benign and 2000 are malignant. Melanocytic nevi, which includes about 7000 cases, are also overrepresented in the sample. The accuracy of our neural network model should therefore be greater than 60%, even in the worst-case situation. We resize the data from its excessively large original size of 450 × 600 to 64 × 64 RGB images for baseline models and 192 × 256 images for fine-tuning models. The dataset is divided into 7210 training examples, 1803 validation examples, and 1002 test examples after being normalised by dividing by 255. Five samples of each type of skin lesion are shown in Figure 3.2. It is incredibly challenging for non-experts to tell which type is which. Figure 3.3 shows the graph for male and female patients with skin cancer.

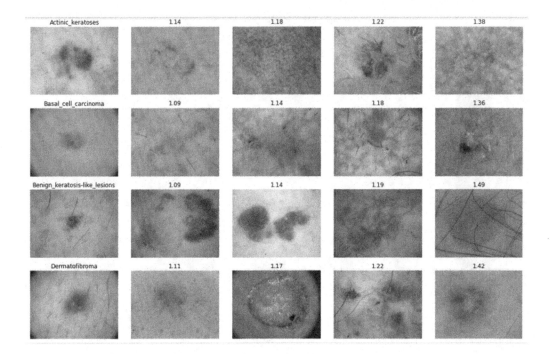

FIGURE 3.2   Five samples of each type of skin lesion.

A typical selection of significant diagnostic categories for pigmented lesions is available in the dataset, including basal cell carcinoma, benign keratosis-like lesions, actinic keratoses, intraepithelial carcinoma/disease, Bowen's dermatofibroma, melanoma, melanocytic nevi, and vascular lesions. This cancer type is displayed in Figure 3.4. Also, Figure 3.5 shows the number of male and female patients in the dataset.

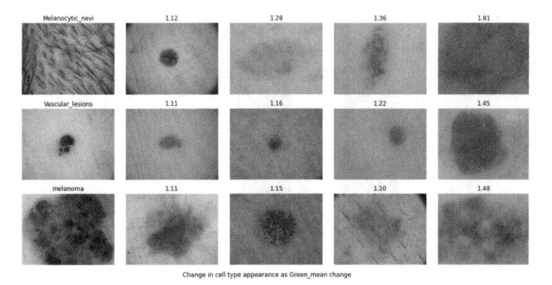

Change in cell type appearance as Green_mean change

FIGURE 3.3   Gender comparison in skin cancer patients.

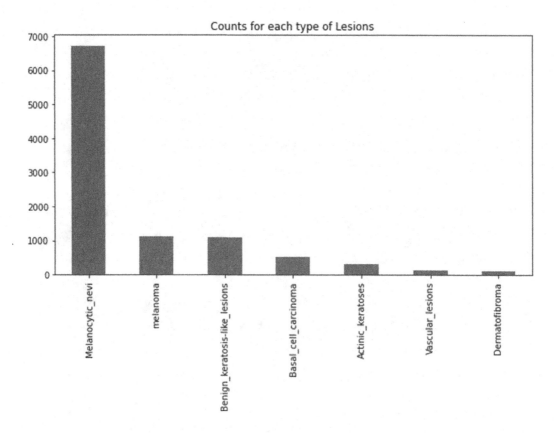

FIGURE 3.4   Cancer types.

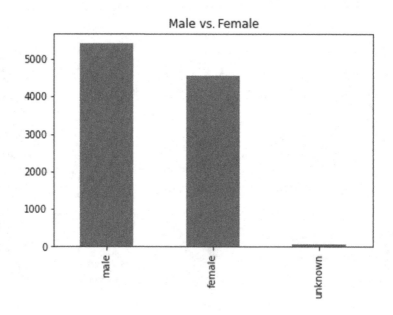

FIGURE 3.5   Number of male and female cancer patients.

3.4.2 CNN

To assess the challenge of categorising skin lesions before fine-tuning DCNNs, we first developed a simple CNN. The first step is a convolutional layer using 16, 3-size kernels that each have padding to maintain the size of the image. Following that comes a 2 × 2 window of a max pooling layer. As a result, feature maps have two times less spatial activation. The next layer is a convolutional layer that has 32, 3-size kernels per layer with padding to maintain the size. The next convolutional layer has padding to preserve the same size and 64 kernels, each of size 3. The final layer has max pools with a window of 2 × 2. The resultant feature maps have spatial activation sizes that are two times smaller than before. This model is trained via data augmentation. To provide some variation and verify that the model never sees the same image multiple times, the main idea behind this approach is to slightly change the training dataset at the start of each epoch. Adam optimiser is employed, with the learning rate set to 0.01 initially. Additionally, once the validation accuracy achieves a 3-epoch plateau, learning rate loss is used to induce the learning rate to decrease by half. We train the baseline model across a total of 30 epochs after training the model with 64 batch sizes and getting a validation accuracy of 73.76% and a test accuracy of 73.05%.

3.4.3 Inception V3

Inception V3 performed much better on ImageNet, with a 30-epoch accuracy of 79.9% and a 3-epoch accuracy of 70.1%. The Inception modules used by Inception V3 bear the same name; they are essentially miniature versions of the main model. The idea that you must choose what kind of convolution to make at each layer served as the inspiration for this study. The notion is that you do not have to know in advance which course of action would be preferable. Additionally, this design enables the model to recover high abstraction features using larger convolutions while also recovering local features using smaller convolutions. Because larger convolutions need more processing, it is recommended that you perform a 1 × 1 convolution to reduce the dimensionality of your feature map, then run the resulting feature map through a ReLU before performing the larger convolution. Using the 1 × 1 convolution will make its feature map less dimensional, which is essential. After that, we had to make final adjustments to all of Inception V3's layers as well as the top two Inception blocks, with all of the batch normalization layers in the model set to trainable. Thirty epochs were used in this experiment. It took 30 epochs to perfect the entirety of Inception V3.

3.4.4 DenseNet

DenseNet, a newly released DCNN architecture, ranks among the top performers on ImageNet with a top 1 ranking of 93.6% and a top 5 ranking of 77.3%. Although DenseNet has fewer parameters, it performs similarly to Inception V3 in terms of performance. The model figure shows the general layout of a dense block, one of the four dense blocks that make up DenseNet 201. The feature maps from all previous convolutional blocks are the *lth* layer's inputs in a dense block, and their feature maps are handed on to all following layers L through l. Every layer writes to the layer after it and reads the state from the layer before it. It alters the situation while transmitting important information. By concatenating features rather than summing them as in ResNet, DenseNet design explicitly distinguishes between information that is contributed to the network and information that is kept.

3.4.5 ResNet

Inception-ResNet is another variation of Inception that excels on ImageNet. Since its Inception, ResNet has included residual connections, which have been demonstrated to be indispensable for training extremely deep convolutional networks. The general architecture of this model is shown in Figure 3.6, and the architecture of the Inception ResNet module, which will be adjusted, is shown in Figure 3.7. Inception V3, Inception-ResNet V2, and VGG16 were tuned using the same training method. Inception-ResNet V2's top layers were adjusted for 30 epochs.

3.4.6 Merged Model

A merged model is an ensemble of the model. In this, Inception V3 and DenseNet are merged. This is fine-tuned with all the layers; thus, the accuracy is the highest among all the models.

3.5 PERFORMANCE AND EVALUATION

Tables 3.1–3.6 show the performance of each learning model that was trained for epochs 3 and 30. It shows how accuracy improves based on an increasing number of epochs. Table 3.1 metrics are for basic CNN with epoch 3. It has the lowest accuracy among all the models. After increasing the epochs, accuracy has improved for the CNN model and achieved 0.7376 accuracies. Similarly, the remaining tables show accuracy and loss for the testing and validation datasets. Table 3.2 depicts the metrics for the Inception V3 model, in which accuracy improved from the previous model and reached 0.7993. Table 3.3 represents the efficiency of the VGG16 model, and the efficiency ratio was like the model trained before. Accuracy and loss for ResNet and DenseNet are shown in Tables 3.4 and 3.5, respectively. Overall accuracy for these models is better compared with the VGG16 and bath sic CNN models, which show significant improvement. After training and fine-tuning, the model ResNet achieved 0.8082 accuracy, and DenseNet achieved .8580 accuracy with 30-fold on the validation dataset.

Better results are obtained when all layers are fine-tuned rather than just the top layers; applying fine tuning to all layers takes less time overall, as shown in Table 3.6 (ensemble model). We only performed about 30 iterations when fine-tuning all of the layers, and we ran for 30 epochs when doing so, which is why this is the case. The findings would not be as nice if we merely adjusted the top layers for a period shorter than 30 epochs. This finding suggests that, in contrast to fine-tuning the top layers only, fine-tuning the entire model yields superior results and speeds up convergence. DenseNet provides the best single outcome in all scenarios, which is amazing considering that this model has even fewer parameters than Inception V3. Thick Net is a very dense, deep model with few parameters, as stated in [27]. The fact that DenseNet worked well in this experiment shows that it can be used for transfer learning in a totally different domain dataset after it has been trained on ImageNet. We used ensemble learning to generate an ensemble of the previously fully tuned Inception V3 and DenseNet 201 models, and we got the best results with 88.8% accuracy on the validation set and 88.52% accuracy on the test set. Using the following performance metrics, the classification efficiency of the five models and the suggested ensemble models has been assessed. The true class of the objects must be known to evaluate a classifier. The class that the classifier assigns is compared with the real class to assess the quality of the classification.

3.5.1 Accuracy

Accuracy is a measure that generally indicates how the model performs across all classes. When every class is equally important, it is useful. It is determined by dividing the overall number of predictions by the total number of accurate predictions. Accuracy demonstrates how well learning models can categorise the image data samples.

$$Accuracy = \frac{TP + FP}{TP + FP + TN + FN}$$

where:
  TP = true positive
  FP = false positive
  TN = true negative
  FN = false negative

3.5.2 Precision

Precision, a performance measure, is calculated by dividing the total number of positive samples that were correctly classified by the total number of positive samples that might have been correctly or wrongly classified. Accuracy measures how accurately the model classifies a sample as positive.

$$Precision = \frac{TP}{TP + FP}$$

3.5.3 Recall

The recall is calculated by dividing the total count of positively identified positive samples by the total number of positive samples. The recall increases with the number of positive samples discovered.

$$Recall = \frac{TP}{TP + FN}$$

3.5.4 F1 Score

The F1 score is computed using recall and precision. This can also be viewed as the weighted average of recall and precision. The value range for it is [0, 1]. F1 scores range from 0 to 1, with 1 being the best.

$$F1\ Score = 2 * \frac{Precision * Recall}{Precision + Recall}$$

3.5.5 Performance Metrics

Using the following performance metrics, the classification efficiency of the five models and the suggested ensemble models has been assessed.

TABLE 3.1   For CNN Performance Metrics

Epoch	Train Accuracy	Train Loss	Val Accuracy	Val Loss
3	0.6637	1.0094	0.6766	0.8980
30	0.7305	0.7410	0.7376	0.7246

TABLE 3.2   For Inception V3 Performance Metrics

Epoch	Train Accuracy	Train Loss	Val Accuracy	Val Loss
3	0.6674	1.036	0.7014	0.9118
30	0.7994	0.7482	0.7993	0.6765

TABLE 3.3   For VGG16 Performance Metrics

Epoch	Train Accuracy	Train Loss	Val Accuracy	Val Loss
3	0.6686	1.0268	0.6588	1.0094
30	0.7964	0.7080	0.7982	0.6501

TABLE 3.4   For ResNet Performance Metrics

Epoch	Train Accuracy	Train Loss	Val Accuracy	Val Loss
3	0.6736	1.0015	0.7062	0.9083
30	0.8253	0.6401	0.8082	0.6691

TABLE 3.5   For DenseNet Performance Metrics

Epoch	Train Accuracy	Train Loss	Val Accuracy	Val Loss
3	0.7108	0.8189	0.7023	0.7769
30	0.8393	0.6912	0.8580	0.6012

TABLE 3.6   For Ensemble Performance Metrics

Epoch	Train Accuracy	Train Loss	Val Accuracy	Val Loss
30	0.8852	0.4115	0.8880	0.3998

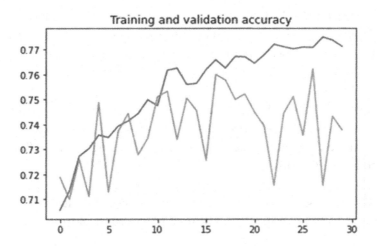

FIGURE 3.6   CNN accuracy.

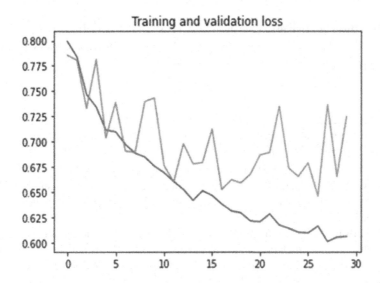

FIGURE 3.7   CNN loss.

Figures 3.6 and 3.7 show the curve of accuracy and loss for the Basic CNN model. Both figures display the line for the training and validation datasets.

3.6 CONCLUSION AND FUTURE WORK

Numerous studies have been conducted on the classification of skin cancer, but the majority of them were not effective in extending their research to the high-performance classification of various classes of skin cancer. By using the techniques of transfer learning and ensemble learning, we were able to assemble a fine-tuned version of Inception V3 with DenseNet that produced an accuracy for HAM10000 of 88.52% on the test set and 88.8% on the validation set. Through testing, we have discovered that fine-tuning the entire model for this dataset not only produces better results overall but also hastens the model's convergence. Furthermore, for the classification of many classes of skin cancer, the suggested ensemble models are better than the recently reported deep learning techniques.

3.6.1 Future Work

Overfitting is one severe issue that has been noted throughout training. All of the experiments have a 10–13% overfit to the training set. Many techniques are employed to reduce overfitting, but we were unable to reduce the level of overfitting anymore. The future scope of this research is the following:

- **Reduce Overfitting**: In the future, various techniques like data augmentation, regularisation, and adding dropouts can be used to reduce overfitting.

- **Web application**: This is the model that can be implemented as a web application using edge AI [27]. So, it looks beautiful, and it also contains information that will help users become more aware of skin cancer disease.

- **Chatbot**: Additional features, such as a robot system that, when given a picture's path, can identify the type of cancer and offer a cure for the sickness, can be added to the web application [35].

REFERENCES

[1] Lambert, P. F., Münger, K., Rösl, F. et al. (2020). Beta human papillomaviruses and skin cancer. *Nature*, 588(7838), E20–E21.

[2] Lacy, K., & Alwan, W. (2013). Skin cancer. *Medicine*, 41(7), 402–405.

[3] Mattiuzzi, C., & Lippi, G. (2020). Cancer statistics: A comparison between world health organization (WHO) and global burden of disease (GBD). *European Journal of Public Health*, 30(5), 1026–1027.

[4] Keith, D. J., Bray, A. P., Brain, A. et al. (2020). British association of dermatologists (BAD) national audit on non-melanoma skin cancer excision 2016 in collaboration with the royal college of pathologists. *Clinical and Experimental Dermatology*, 45(1), 48–55.

[5] Kaur, G., & Yusuf, N. (2021). The Epidemiology of Skin Cancer Worldwide. *In Skin Cancer: Pathogenesis and Diagnosis* (pp. 69–77). Springer.

[6] Desai, F., Chowdhury, D., Kaur, R. et al. (2022). HealthCloud: A system for monitoring health status of heart patients using machine learning and cloud computing. *Internet of Things*, 17, 100485.

[7] Abu Owida, H. (2022). Biomimetic nanoscale materials for skin cancer therapy and detection. *Journal of Skin Cancer*, 2022, 2961996.

[8] Tuli, S., Tuli, S., Wander, G. et al. (2019). Next generation technologies for smart healthcare: Challenges, vision, model, trends and future directions. *Internet Technology Letters*, 3(2), e145.

[9] Wu, Y., Chen, B., Zeng, A. et al. (2022). Skin cancer classification with deep learning: A systematic review. *Frontiers in Oncology*. 12, 893972.

[10] Haenssle, H. A., Fink, C., Schneiderbauer, R. et al. (2018). Man against machine: Diagnostic performance of a deep learning convolutional neural network for dermoscopic melanoma recognition in comparison to 58 dermatologists. *Annals of Oncology*, 29(8), 1836–1842.

[11] Gill, S. S., Xu, M., Ottaviani, C. et al. (2022). AI for next generation computing: Emerging trends and future directions. *Internet of Things*, 19, 100514.

[12] Gill, S. S., Wu, H., Patros, P. et al. (2024). Modern computing: Vision and challenges. *Telematics and Informatics Reports*, 13, 1–46.

[13] Moqurrab, S. A., Tariq, N., Anjum, A. et al. (2022). A deep learning-based privacy-preserving model for smart healthcare in internet of medical things using fog computing. *Wireless Personal Communications*, 126(3), 2379–2401.

[14] Singh, R., & Gill, S. S. (2023). Edge AI: A survey. *Internet of Things and Cyber-Physical Systems*, 3, 71–92.

[15] Brinker, T. J., Achim, H., Jochen, U. S. et al. (2018). Skin cancer classification using convolutional neural networks: Systematic review. *Journal of Medical Internet Research*, 20(10), e11936.

[16] Popescu, D., Mohamed, E., Hassan, E. et al. (2022). New trends in melanoma detection using neural networks: A systematic review. *Sensors*, 22(2), 496.

[17] Palak, M., & Bhumika, S. (2016). Review on techniques and steps of computer aided skin cancer diagnosis. *Procedia Computer Science*, 85, 309–316.

[18] Manne, R., Kantheti, S., & Kantheti, S. (2020). Classification of skin cancer using deep learning, convolutional neural networks - opportunities and vulnerabilities – a systematic review. *International Journal for Modern Trends in Science and Technology*, 6(11), 101–108.

[19] Kumar, S. S., & Dhanesh, M. S. (2020). A comparative study on the diagnosis of skin cancer using different models in deep learning. *International Journal of Science and Research*, 9(6).

[20] Vijayalakshmi, M. M. (2019). Melanoma skin cancer detection using image processing and machine learning. *International Journal of Trend in Scientific Research and Development (IJTSRD)*, 3(4), 780–784.

[21] Hosny, K. M., Kassem, M. A., & Foaud, M. M. (2018). Skin Cancer Classification using Deep Learning and Transfer Learning. *2018 9th Cairo International Biomedical Engineering Conference*, IEEE.

[22] Kadampur, M. A., & Al Riyaee, S. (2020). Skin cancer detection: Applying a deep learning based model driven architecture in the cloud for classifying dermal cell images. *Informatics in Medicine Unlocked*, 18, 100282.

[23] Haggenmuller, S., Maron, R. C., Heckler, A. et al. (2022). Skin cancer classification via convolutional neural networks: Systematic review of studies involving human experts. *European Journal of Cancer*, 156, 202–216.

[24] Jones, O. T., Matin, R. N., van der Schaar, M. et al. (2022). Artificial intelligence and machine learning algorithms for early detection of skin cancer in community and primary care settings: A systematic review. *The Lancet Digital Health*, 4(6), e466–e476.

[25] Esteva, A., Kuprel, B., Novoa, R. A. et al. (2017). Dermatologist-level classification of skin cancer with deep neural networks. *Nature*, 542(7639), 115–118.

[26] Kahia, M., Echtioui, A., Fathi, K. et al. (2022). Skin cancer classification using deep learning models. *International Conference on Agents and Artificial Intelligence*, Springer (ICAART'2022).

[27] Dildar, M., Akram, S., Irfan, M. et al. (2021). Skin cancer detection: A review using deep learning techniques. *International Journal of Environmental Research and Public Health*, 18(10), 5479.

[28] Dhillon, A., Singh, A., Vohra, H. et al. (2022). IoTPulse: Machine learning-based Enterprise health information system to predict alcohol addiction in Punjab (India) using IoT and fog computing. *Enterprise Information Systems*, 16(7), 1820583.

[29] Murugesan, S. S., Velu, S., Golec, M. et al. (2024). Neural Networks based Smart e-Health Application for the Prediction of Tuberculosis using Serverless Computing. *IEEE Journal of Biomedical and Health Informatics*. 1–12.

[30] Iftikhar, S., Golec, M., Chowdhury, D. et al. (2022). FogDLearner: A deep learning-based cardiac health diagnosis framework using fog computing. *In Proceedings of the 2022 Australasian Computer Science Week* (pp. 136–144). ACM.

[31] Golec, M., Gill, S. S., Parlikad, A. K. et al. (2023). HealthFaaS: AI based smart healthcare system for heart patients using serverless computing. *IEEE Internet of Things Journal*, 10(21), 18469–18476.

[32] Sarker, I. H. (2021). Deep learning: A comprehensive overview on techniques, taxonomy, applications and research directions. *SN Computer Science*, 2(6), 420.

[33] Aamodt, E. (2022). *Combating class imbalances in image classification-a deep neural network-based method for skin disease classification* (Master's thesis, University of Agder).

[34] Marchetti, M. A., Codella, N. C. F., Dusza, W. S. et al. (2018). Results of the 2016 international skin imaging collaboration international symposium on biomedical imaging challenge: Comparison of the accuracy of computer algorithms to dermatologists for the diagnosis of melanoma from dermoscopic images. *Journal of the American Academy of Dermatology*, 78(2), 270–277.

[35] Gill, S. S., & Kaur, R. (2023). ChatGPT: Vision and challenges. *Internet of Things and Cyber-Physical Systems*, 3, 262–271.

CHAPTER 4

Explainable AI for Cancer Prediction

A Model Analysis

Aswin Kumar Govindan and Sukhpal Singh Gill

4.1 INTRODUCTION

According to a report issued in 2023 by Siegel and colleagues, there are around 1,958,310 new cancer cases and 609,820 cancer deaths in 2023. Due to particular risk factors (smoking, poor nutrition, etc.), 480,000 people have died every year in the United States, according to a 2018 data report [1]. Many medical problems and fatal illnesses can be detected at earlier stages if the person is subjected to a annual checkup. A tumour is a group of abnormal cells with the potential to invade or spread to other parts of the body. They are considered cancer cells, which are often thought to be an untreatable, unbearably painful disease with no cure. Cancer is one of the main causes of death throughout the world.

The National Cancer Institute [2] defined cancer as "an abnormal mass of tissue that results when cells divide more than they should or do not die when they should". In a healthy body, cells grow, divide, and replace each other in the body. As new cells form, the old ones die. When a person has cancer, new cells form when the body does not need them. If there are too many new cells, a group of cells, or tumour, can develop. Certain signs, symptoms, or screening tests can detect cancer. Medical imaging and a biopsy follow to further investigate for the disease. Currently, 15% of cancers are due to major infections such as *Helicobacter pylori*, hepatitis B, hepatitis C, human papillomavirus infection, Epstein-Barr virus, and human immunodeficiency virus (HIV). Typically, many genetic changes happen before cancer develops. Approximately 5–10% of cancers are due to inherited genetic defects.

4.1.1 Classification of Tumour

According to an article on tumour classification by Han and colleagues [3], tumours are considered benign and consist of noncancerous cells, whereas those with cancerous cells

DOI: 10.1201/9781003467199-5

are malignant. Malignant tumours are cancerous, and the cells can spread to other parts of the body. There are three main types of tumours:

1. **Benign**: These tumours are not cancerous. They either cannot spread or grow, or they do so very slowly. It does not recur once it is cured.

2. **Premalignant**: In these tumours, the cells are not yet cancerous, but they have the potential to become malignant.

3. **Malignant**: These tumours are cancerous. The cells can grow and spread to other parts of the body.

4.1.2 Causes of Cancer

About 95% of cancer cases are due to genetic mutations from environmental and lifestyle factors, and the remaining cases are due to inherited genetics, according to a 2016 research article by Blackadar [4]. Anything that might lead to an abnormal development of a normal body cell could potentially lead to cancer. Many things can cause cell abnormalities and have been linked to cancer development. Some cancer causes remain unknown, whereas other cancers have environmental or lifestyle triggers or may develop from more than one known cause. A person's genetic makeup might have an impact on some. Many patients develop cancer due to a combination of these factors. Although it is often difficult or impossible to determine the initiating event(s) that cause cancer to develop in a specific person, research has provided clinicians with a number of likely causes that, alone or in concert with other causes, are the likely candidates for initiating cancer. The following is a listing of major causes and is not all inclusive, as specific causes are routinely added as research advances:

1. Chemical or toxic compound exposures

2. Ionising radiation

3. Heredity

4.1.3 Explainable Artificial Intelligence (XAI)

Explainable artificial intelligence (XAI) is a set of procedures and techniques that enables consumers to comprehend and believe the output produced by machine learning (ML) algorithms used in AI [5]. Users, operators, or developers may be the target audience for the explanations that go along with AI/ML output. These explanations are meant to solve issues and problems with user adoption, governance, and system development, among other things [6]. This "explainability" is essential to AI's capacity to win over the trust and confidence required in the market to promote widespread AI use and benefit [7]. Trustworthy AI and responsible AI are two further connected and developing initiatives [8].

4.1.4 How is explainable AI implemented?

According to an article by Phillips and colleges [9], there are four principles that drive XAI:

1. **Explanation**: Systems deliver accompanying evidence or reason(s) for all outputs.

2. **Meaningful**: Systems provide explanations that are understandable to individual users.

3. **Explanation accuracy**: The explanation correctly reflects the system's process for generating the output.

4. **Knowledge limits**: The system operates only under conditions for which it was designed or when its output has achieved sufficient confidence levels.

The National Institute of Standards and Technology (NIST) noted that explanations may range from simple to complex and that they depend on the consumer in question. The agency illustrates some explanation types using the following five non-exhaustive sample explainability categories:

1. User benefit

2. Societal acceptance

3. Regulatory and compliance

4. System development

5. Owner benefit

4.1.5 Motivation and Contributions

Cancer prediction using XAI with "Deep SHapley Additive exPlanations" (DeepSHAP), offers several motivations and contributions to the field of medical research and AI. DeepSHAP is a technique used to provide interpretability and insights into the decisions made by complex machines and deep learning models. However, these models are often considered black boxes due to their intricate architecture, making it challenging to understand the rationale behind their predictions. In the medical field, it is crucial to have a clear understanding of the factors contributing to a prediction. Clinicians, researchers, and patients need to know why a particular prediction was made to build trust in the AI system and to make informed decisions. Transparency and accountability are vital for medical AI systems. Regulatory bodies and ethical guidelines demand explanations for AI-driven medical decisions to ensure patient safety, prevent biases, and maintain fairness [10]. The main contributions of this research article are as follows:

- **Interpretability**: DeepSHAP contributes by providing interpretability to deep learning models [11]. It helps explain the predictions made by these models in terms of feature contributions, showing which input features influenced the prediction and how much.

- **Feature Importance**: DeepSHAP quantifies the importance of each input feature in influencing the model's output. In the context of cancer prediction, it can reveal which features (e.g., specific genetic markers, image regions) play a significant role in the model's decision-making process [12].

- **Clinical Insights**: DeepSHAP's explanations provide valuable insights into clinicians and researchers [13]. By understanding the reasons behind a prediction, medical professionals can refine treatment plans, conduct further investigations, and improve patient outcomes.

- **Building Trust**: DeepSHAP's transparency aids in fostering trust between stakeholders and AI systems. Patients and clinicians are more likely to embrace AI-based predictions when they have a clear understanding of how the predictions are generated.

- **Research Validation**: The insights provided by DeepSHAP can guide future research endeavours. Researchers can validate the model's predictions against known medical knowledge and uncover new patterns or associations that were not previously recognised.

4.2 RELATED WORKS

The related works in the areas of cancer prediction and XAI, along with some of their applications, are discussed in this section. It also includes a detailed analysis of the previously proposed works by different authors and highlights some defective areas that are required to be filled up in this regard. Alkassar et al. [14] stated that brain tumour segmentation is a challenging issue due to the heterogeneous appearance, shape, and intensity of tumours. In this chapter, the author presents an automatic method for brain tumour segmentation in magnetic resonance (MR) brain image using deep neural networks (DNNs). Transfer learning (TL) and a fully convolutional network (FCN) have been utilised to achieve robust tumour segmentation using the VGG16 network. The proposed architecture of the VGG16 network includes the encoder and decoder networks with a classification layer to generate the pixel-wise classification. Comparison results demonstrate that the proposed method achieved state-of-the-art results with a global accuracy of 0.97785 and a 0.89 dice score in terms of whole tumour segmentation on images from the BRATS2015 database.

Hirahara [15] proposed that the brain tumour is one of the most detrimental diseases. MR imaging (MRI) has been used for the diagnosis of brain tumours; however, manual tumour diagnosis in MRIs is a time-consuming process, necessitating the development of an automatic brain tumour diagnosis system. This study applied a novel architecture, named Xception, which enabled both high-performance and reduced size and computational cost of convolutional neural networks (CNNs) using depthwise separable convolution to develop a high-performance computer-aided diagnosis (CADe) system for brain tumour detection from MRI. Preliminary assessment for the Xception model utilising TL demonstrated good performance with high accuracy and prediction probability. Interestingly, prediction probabilities were different when different layers were learned. The prediction probability values were highest in both normal and tumour cases when the

109th layer and after (i.e., the exit flow) were relearned, indicating the importance of re-learning for the exit flow. The study results suggest that a high-performance CADe system for brain tumours in MRIs could be developed with relatively cheap small-scale learning utilising TL in the Xception model.

Agrawal & Aurelia [16] described that the precise identification of skin disease is an exigent process, even for more experienced doctors and dermatologists, because there is a small variation between surrounding skin and lesions, a visual affinity between different skin diseases. TL is an approach that stores acquired knowledge while solving one problem and applies that knowledge to similar problems. It is a type of ML task where a model proposed for a task can be used again. TL is used in various areas, like image processing and gaming simulation. Image processing is an evolving field in the diagnosis of various kinds of skin diseases. Here, TL is used to identify three skin diseases, such as melanoma, vitiligo, and vascular tumours. The Inception V3 model was used as a base model. Networks were pre-trained and then fine-tuned. Considerable growth in training accuracy and testing accuracy was achieved.

Westerlund and colleagues [17] explored the fact that cardiovascular diseases (CVDs) annually take about 18 million lives worldwide. Most lethal events occur months or years after the initial presentation. Indeed, many patients experience repeated complications or require multiple interventions (recurrent events). Apart from affecting the individual, this leads to high medical costs for society. Personalised treatment strategies aimed at prediction and prevention of recurrent events rely on early diagnosis and precise prognosis. In addition to the usual environmental and clinical risk factors, multi-omics data give a full picture of the patient and the disease's progression. This lets studies look at risk stratification from new angles. Specifically, predictive molecular markers allow insights into regulatory networks, pathways, and mechanisms underlying disease. Moreover, AI represents a powerful, yet adaptive, framework able to recognise complex patterns in large-scale clinical and molecular data with the potential to improve risk prediction. Here, we review the most recent advances in risk prediction for recurrent cardiovascular events and discuss the value of molecular data and biomarkers for understanding patient risk in a systems biology context. Finally, we introduce explainable AI, which may improve clinical decision systems by making predictions transparent to the medical practitioner.

Sanjana et al. [18] explained that the electrocardiogram (ECG) signal is one of the most reliable methods to analyse the cardiovascular system. In the literature, there are different deep learning architectures proposed to detect various types of tachycardia diseases, such as atrial fibrillation, ventricular fibrillation, and sinus tachycardia. Even though all types of tachycardia diseases have fast beat rhythm as a common characteristic feature, existing deep learning architectures are trained with the corresponding disease-specific features. Most of the proposed works lack interpretation and understanding of the results obtained. Hence, the objective of this letter is to explore the features learned by the deep learning models. For the detection of different types of tachycardia diseases, the authors used a TL approach. In this method, the model is trained with one of the tachycardia diseases, atrial fibrillation, and tested with other tachycardia diseases, such as ventricular

TABLE 4.1   Comparison of Proposed Work with Existing Works

Work/Study	Models Used	Importance of Features	Implementation of XAI
Alkassar et al.[9]	DNN	X	X
Hirahara [10]	CNN	X	X
Agrawal & Aurelia (2021) [11]	TL-CNN	X	X
Westerlund [12]	KNN (K-nearest neighbour)	X	✓
Sanjana [13]	RNN	X	✓
Proposed Work	RFC, LR, XGBoost	✓	✓

fibrillation and sinus tachycardia. The analysis was done using a deep learning model, such as recurrent neural networks (RNNs). The RNN was able to correctly identify 96.47% of cases of atrial fibrillation and 90.88% of cases of CU ventricular tachycardia. It was also able to correctly identify 94.71% of cases of malignant ventricular ectopy in ECG lead I and 94.18% of cases in lead II. The RNN model could only achieve an accuracy of 23.73% for the sinus tachycardia dataset. Other models exhibit a similar trend. From the analysis, it was evident that even though tachycardia diseases have a fast beat rhythm as their common feature, the model was not able to detect different types of tachycardia diseases. The deep learning model could only detect atrial and ventricular fibrillation and failed in the case of sinus tachycardia. From the analysis, they were able to interpret that, along with the fast beat rhythm, the model has learned the absence of a P wave, which is a common feature for ventricular fibrillation and atrial fibrillation, but sinus tachycardia disease has an upright positive P wave. The time-based analysis is conducted to find the time complexity of the models. The analysis conveyed that RNN and remote-sensing CNN (RSCNN) models could achieve better performance with less time complexity. Table 4.1 shows the comparison of proposed work with existing work.

4.3 METHODOLOGY

This section presents a detailed description of the proposed system architecture for predicting cancer using XAI and various ML algorithms. Especially in this article, this is the question is being answered: Which feature plays the most important role in confirming whether the model is trustworthy or not [19]?

4.3.1 Dataset

The dataset (Figure 4.1) used in this research article is available at the Breast Cancer Wisconsin (Diagnostic) dataset: https://archive.ics.uci.edu/dataset/17/breast+cancer+wisconsin+diagnostic.

This dataset is commonly used in ML and pattern recognition for breast cancer classification tasks. It was obtained from the University of Wisconsin Hospitals, Madison, by Dr William H. Wolberg. The dataset contains features computed from a digitised image of a fine-needle aspirate (FNA) of a breast mass. These features are computed for each cell nucleus present in the image, and they describe various characteristics of the cell nuclei [20]. The main aim of using this dataset is to distinguish between

	id	diagnosis	radius_mean	texture_mean	perimeter_mean	area_mean	smoothness_mean	compactness_mean	concavity_mean
0	842302	M	17.99	10.38	122.80	1001.0	0.11840	0.27760	0.3001
1	842517	M	20.57	17.77	132.90	1326.0	0.08474	0.07864	0.0869
2	84300903	M	19.69	21.25	130.00	1203.0	0.10960	0.15990	0.1974
3	84348301	M	11.42	20.38	77.58	386.1	0.14250	0.28390	0.2414
4	84358402	M	20.29	14.34	135.10	1297.0	0.10030	0.13280	0.1980

FIGURE 4.1 The sample of the dataset.

benign and malignant breast tumours based on these features. Here are some details about the dataset:

- **Number of Instances**: 569

- **Number of Features**: 30 numeric features computed from the cell nuclei characteristics

- **Target Variable**: Binary class label (Malignant or Benign)

The features include information about the radius, texture, smoothness, compactness, concavity, symmetry, fractal dimension, and other properties of the cell nuclei. These features are calculated both for the mean, standard error, and "worst" or largest values found in the image. Researchers often use this dataset to develop and evaluate ML algorithms for breast cancer classification [21]. Common tasks include building models to predict whether a tumour is malignant or benign based on the provided features. Algorithms like logistic regression, decision trees, random forest, support vector machines, and more advanced methods like XGBoost and neural networks can be applied to this dataset to achieve accurate classification results [22].

4.3.2 Proposed Technique

Figure 4.2 presents the proposed system architecture of the interpretability system for cancer prediction. The architecture consists of six processes: (1) loading the cancer dataset, (2) data preprocessing, (3) feature selection, (4) training and testing of the models, (5) ranking the features, and (6) interpretability using DeepSHAP. The dataset is obtained from the UCI Machine Learning Repository, which is real-life science data that has 30 attributes and 569 instances.

Features are computed from a digitised image of FNA of a breast mass. The data preprocessing process includes data cleaning and statistical analysis of the data. Then the features are selected using a correlation plot, and the features that have relatability with each other are selected [23]. Features are dropped, and the other features are used for training and testing purposes.

The training and testing section of the system first splits the dataset into 70-30 splits and then into train and test splits, where the train data are parsed to the models (random forest classifier, logistic regression, XGBoost), and their classification report for the test data is provided. Then the features are ranked according to their importance in the models and plotted as bar graphs.

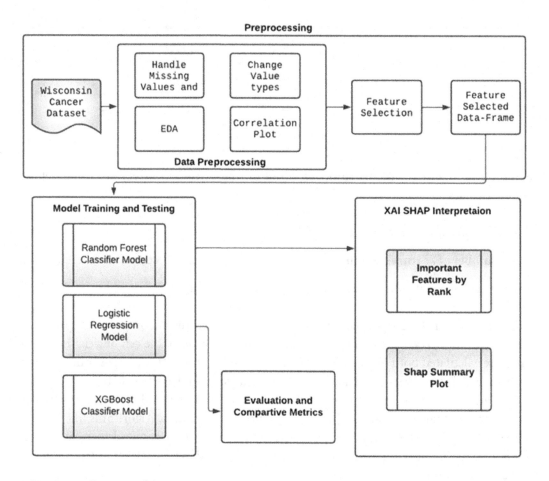

FIGURE 4.2   System architecture.

DeepSHAP is a technique that analyses the ML models and helps us understand, interpret, and make a decision on which feature has the most significant impact on confirming whether the patient has cancer or not. This decision-making quality helps to confirm whether the model is trustworthy or not.

4.3.3 Machine Learning Models and Operating Mechanism

Algorithm 1 shows an operating mechanism of the proposed system. We have used the following ML models in this proposed system:

- **Random forest classification**: Random forest is a popular ML algorithm used for both classification and regression tasks [24]. It is an ensemble learning method that combines multiple individual decision trees to create a more accurate and robust model. It does this by training multiple decision trees on different subsets of the data and features, and then combining their individual predictions through a voting mechanism to arrive at a final classification. This ensemble approach improves the model's accuracy, reduces overfitting, and makes it robust to noisy data. Random forest classification is used in various domains for tasks like image recognition, medical diagnosis, and customer behaviour prediction.

- **Logistic regression**: Logistic regression is a statistical and ML algorithm used for binary classification tasks [25]. It predicts the probability that a given input belongs to a specific class, typically 0 or 1. Despite its name, logistic regression is used for classification, not regression. It models the relationship between the input features and the probability of the binary outcome using the logistic function. The algorithm estimates coefficients for each feature to determine their influence on the outcome probability. It is a simple yet widely used method for tasks like spam detection, medical diagnosis, and credit risk assessment.

Algorithm 1: Operating mechanism of the proposed system

1) Begin
2) Input = Cancer Dataset
3) Output = Analysis using DeepSHAP of the ML Models
4) Clean and prepare data using statistical methods
5) Visualize data with diagnosis
6) Generate heatmap to compare and select features using correlation plot
7) Split dataset into test and train data by 70/30 split.
8) Train Models:
    1) Random Forest Classifier
        Train model
        Obtain classification report and heatmap
        Rank the important features and plot
        Summary plot of model using SHAP
    2) Logistic Regression Classifier
        Train model
        Obtain classification report and heatmap
        Rank the important features and plot
        Summary plot of model using SHAP
    3) XGBoost Classifier
        Train model
        Obtain classification report and heatmap
        Rank the important features and plot
        Summary plot of model using SHAP
9) End

- **XGBoost classification**: XGBoost (extreme gradient boosting) classification is an advanced ML algorithm designed for both classification and regression tasks. It belongs to the gradient boosting family of algorithms, which iteratively combine weak learners (usually decision trees) to create a strong predictive model. XGBoost enhances traditional gradient boosting by incorporating regularization techniques, handling missing values, and optimising computation efficiency [26]. It focuses on minimising the loss function by adding trees that correct the errors made by the previous ones. XGBoost is known for its exceptional performance on structured data, winning numerous ML competitions, and being widely used in various applications due to its accuracy and robustness.

- **DeepSHAP**: DeepSHAP is a method used in ML and specifically in the field of interpretability for DNNs. SHAP is a framework for explaining the output of ML models by attributing the contributions of each feature to the final prediction [27]. DeepSHAP extends the SHAP framework to work with deep learning models, which are complex and often considered as "black boxes" due to their intricate internal workings. DeepSHAP aims to provide more transparent insights into how these models make predictions by calculating the SHAP values for individual features in the context of DNN [28]. This allows practitioners to understand the importance of various input features in influencing the model's output. In essence, DeepSHAP helps in interpreting and explaining the decision-making process of deep learning models, enhancing transparency and enabling users to have more confidence in the reliability and fairness of these models.

4.4 PERFORMANCE EVALUATION

To show the practicality of the proposed strategy, this section uses a dataset to predict whether the patient has cancer using real-time values. The dataset is obtained from Kaggle and the platform used is Google Colaboratory.

4.4.1 System Configuration

The proposed system runs on a PC laptop with the following configurations as described in the following:

- **Processor**: Intel Core i7-CPU@ 2.6 GHz

- **RAM**: 16 GB 2400 MHz DDR4

- **System Type**: Macintosh-macOS 13.4 64-bit

4.4.2 Experimental Results and Performance Comparison

The proposed system is developed using Jupyter Notebook (.ipynb) in Google Colaboratory. The proposed system architecture involves the following components:

- Data Loading and Preprocessing

- Exploratory Data Analysis (EDA)

- Feature Selection

- Model Training and Evaluation

- Interpretability using SHAP

	diagnosis	radius_mean	texture_mean	perimeter_mean	area_mean	smoothness_mean	compactness_mean	concavity_mean
count	569.000000	569.000000	569.000000	569.000000	569.000000	569.000000	569.000000	569.000000
mean	0.372583	14.127292	19.289649	91.969033	654.889104	0.096360	0.104341	0.088799
std	0.483918	3.524049	4.301036	24.298981	351.914129	0.014064	0.052813	0.079720
min	0.000000	6.981000	9.710000	43.790000	143.500000	0.052630	0.019380	0.000000
25%	0.000000	11.700000	16.170000	75.170000	420.300000	0.086370	0.064920	0.029560
50%	0.000000	13.370000	18.840000	86.240000	551.100000	0.095870	0.092630	0.061540
75%	1.000000	15.780000	21.800000	104.100000	782.700000	0.105300	0.130400	0.130700
max	1.000000	28.110000	39.280000	188.500000	2501.000000	0.163400	0.345400	0.426800

8 rows × 31 columns

FIGURE 4.3   Statistical summary of the dataset.

The following are the important details related to the experimental setup and results:

- **Import Libraries and Dependencies**: The necessary libraries and packages are imported, including data manipulation (NumPy, pandas), visualization (Matplotlib, Seaborn), ML: models (random forest, logistic regression, XGBoost), and SHAP (SHapley Additive exPlanations) for model interpretability [29].

- **Data Loading and Preprocessing**: The dataset is loaded from a CSV file named "data. csv". The data are viewed and the data is preprocessed using preprocessing tools [30].

- **EDA**: Summary statistics of the dataset are displayed in Figure 4.3. Visualizations are created to understand the distribution of diagnoses (malignant vs. benign) and are displayed in Figure 4.4. The features are analysed with the diagnosis and are displayed in Figure 4.5.

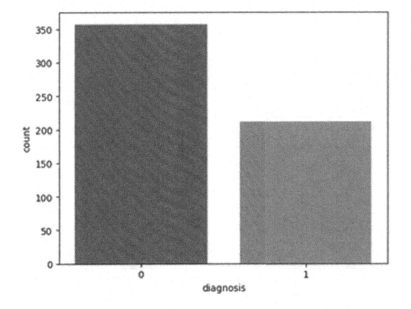

FIGURE 4.4   Count of diagnosis.

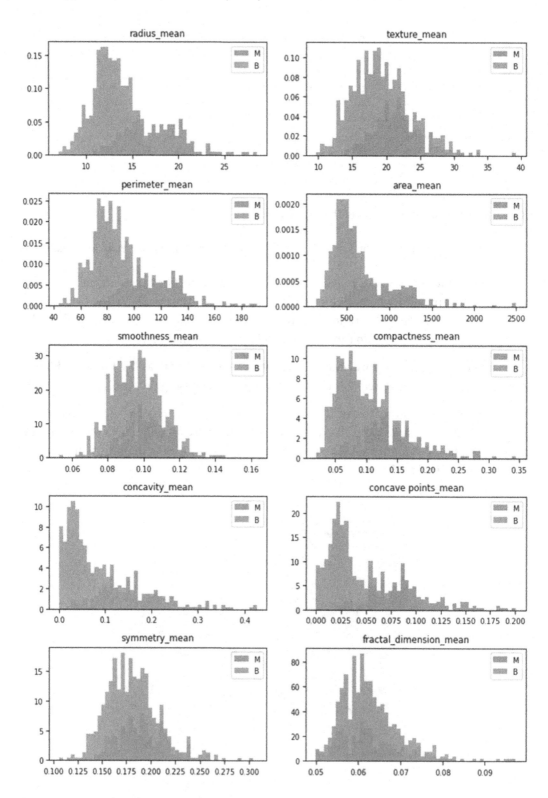

FIGURE 4.5   Nucleus features vs. diagnosis.

TABLE 4.2   Comparison of Machine Learning Models

Model	Accuracy	Precision		Recall		F1 Score	
		0	1	0	1	0	1
Random forest classifier	0.96	0.96	0.97	0.98	0.94	0.97	0.95
Logistic regression classifier	0.95	0.96	0.96	0.95	0.94	0.96	0.93
XGBoost classifier	0.98	0.98	0.97	0.98	0.97	0.98	0.97

- **Feature Selection and Data Preparation**: Features that are correlated with other features are dropped from the dataset. The dataset is split into features and the target variable. Data are split into training and testing sets using a 70-30 ratio.

- **Model Training and Evaluation**: Using the training data the ML models, random forest classifier, logistic regression and XGBoost, are trained and tested [31, 32]. The model is evaluated using accuracy, classification report, and a confusion matrix, which are shown in Table 4.2.

4.5 CONCLUSIONS AND FUTURE WORK

This system falls under XAI, which is now an advanced technique. ML algorithms like support vector machine, logistic regression, etc. are more suitable for numerical processing, especially in medical classification. We conclude that the experimental result we are getting from the developed system is more than 90% accurate. XAI is employed to make AI decisions both understandable and interpretable by humans. This leaves them open to significant risk without a human looped into the development process. The system takes a dataset containing medical features as input and goes through a series of steps to preprocess the data, analyse it, select relevant features, train multiple classification models, evaluate their performance, and provide interpretability using SHAP values. This architecture can be further improved by including hyperparameter tuning, cross-validation, and ensemble methods to enhance the predictive performance of the models [33]. Additionally, incorporating a user interface or deploying the model as a service could make the system more accessible and user-friendly. By incorporating deep learning techniques, better interpretability can be achieved to build the trustworthiness of the model [34].

REFERENCES

[1] Siegel, R. L., Miller, K. D., Wagle, N. S. et al. (2023). Cancer statistics, 2023. *CA: A Cancer Journal for Clinicians*, 73(1), 17–48.

[2] National Cancer Institute (2007). *What Is Cancer? - National Cancer Institute*. [Online]. Available at: https://www.cancer.gov/about-cancer/understanding/what-is-cancer#:~:text=When%20 cells%20grow%20old%20or

[3] Han, S. S., Kim, M. S., Lim, W. et al. (2018). Classification of the clinical images for benign and malignant cutaneous tumors using a deep learning algorithm. *Journal of Investigative Dermatology*, 138(7), 1529–1538. doi: 10.1016/j.jid.2018.01.028.

[4] Blackadar, C. B. (2016). Historical review of the causes of cancer. *World Journal of Clinical Oncology*, 7(1), 54–86. doi: https://doi.org/10.5306/wjco.v7.i1.54.

[5] Turri, V. (2022). What Is Explainable AI?. In *Carnegie Mellon University, Software Engineering Institute's Insights (Blog)*. Carnegie Mellon's Software Engineering Institute. Available at: https://insights.sei.cmu.edu/blog/what-is-explainable-ai/. (Accessed: 22-Aug-2023).

[6] Gill, S. S., Xu, M., Ottaviani, C. et al. (2022). AI for next generation computing: Emerging trends and future directions. *Internet of Things*, 19, 100514.

[7] Gill, S. S., Wu, H., Patros, P. et al. (2024). Modern computing: Vision and challenges. *Telematics and Informatics Reports*, 13, 100116.

[8] Singh, R., & Gill, S. S. (2023). Edge AI: A survey. *Internet of Things and Cyber-Physical Systems*, 3, 71–92.

[9] Phillips, P. J., Hahn, C. A., Fontana, P. C. et al. (2021). *Four Principles of Explainable Artificial Intelligence* (p. 18). National Institute of Standards and Technology, Gaithersburg, Maryland: U.S. Department of Commerce.

[10] Gill, S. S., & Kaur, R. (2023). ChatGPT: Vision and challenges. *Internet of Things and Cyber-Physical Systems*, 3, 262–271.

[11] Deepak, S., & Ameer, P. M. (2019). Brain tumour classification using deep CNN features via transfer learning. *Computers in Biology and Medicine*, 111, 103345.

[12] Zhou, L., Zhang, Z., Chen, Y. C. et al. (2019). A deep learning-based radionics model for differentiating benign and malignant renal tumours. *Translational, Oncology*, 12(2), 292–300.

[13] Hemanth, G., Janardhan, M., & Sujihelen, L. (2019). Design and implementing brain tumour detection using machine learning approach. *International Conference on Trends in Electronics and Informatics (ICOEI)*, pp. 1289–1294, IEEE.

[14] Alkassar, S., Abdullah, M. A. M., & Jebur, B. A. (2019). Automatic brain tumour segmentation using fully convolution network and transfer learning. *2nd International Conference on Electrical, Communication, Computer, Power and Control Engineering (ICECCPCE)*, pp. 188–192. IEEE.

[15] Hirahara, D. (2019). Preliminary assessment for the development of CADe system for brain tumor in MRI images utilizing transfer learning in Xception model. *2019 IEEE 8th Global Conference on Consumer Electronics (GCCE)*, pp. 922–924. IEEE.

[16] Agrawal, N., & Aurelia, S. (2021). Corroboration of skin diseases: melanoma, vitiligo & vascular tumor using transfer learning. *2021 7th International Conference on Electrical Energy Systems (ICEES)*, pp. 590–592. IEEE

[17] Westerlund, A. M., Hawe, J. S., Heinig, M. et al. (2021). Risk prediction of cardiovascular events by exploration of molecular data with explainable artificial intelligence. *International Journal of Molecular Sciences*, 22(19), 10291.

[18] Sanjana, K., Sowmya, V., Gopalakrishnan, E. A. et al. (2020). Explainable artificial intelligence for heart rate variability in ECG signal. *Healthcare Technology Letters*, 7(6), 146–154.

[19] Dhillon, A., Singh, A., Vohra, H. et al. (2022). IoTPulse: Machine learning-based enterprise health information system to predict alcohol addiction in Punjab (India) using IoT and fog computing. *Enterprise Information Systems*, 16(7), 1820583.

[20] Wu, S., Zhong, S., & Liu, Y. (2018). Deep residual learning for image steganalysis. *Multimedia Tools and Applications*, 77(9), 10437–10453.

[21] Moqurrab, S. A., Tariq, N., Anjum, A. et al. (2022). A deep learning-based privacy-preserving model for smart healthcare in internet of medical things using fog computing. *Wireless Personal Communications*, 126(3), 2379–2401.

[22] Iftikhar, S., Golec, M., Chowdhury, D. et al. (2022). FogDLearner: A deep learning-based cardiac health diagnosis framework using fog computing. *In Proceedings of the 2022 Australasian Computer Science Week*, pp. 136–144.

[23] Bernal, J., Kushibar, K., Asfaw, D. S. et al. (2019). Deep convolutional neural networks for brain image analysis on magnetic resonance imaging: A review. *Artificial Intelligence in Medicine*, 95, 64–81.

[24] Holzinger, A., Langs, G., Denk, H. et al. (2019). Causability and explainability of artificial intelligence in medicine. *Wiley Interdisciplinary Reviews: Data Mining and Knowledge Discovery*, 9(4), e1312. doi: https://doi.org/10.1002/widm.1312.

[25] Novakovsky, G., Dexter, N., Libbrecht, M. W. et al. (2023). Obtaining genetics insights from deep learning via explainable artificial intelligence. *Nature Reviews Genetics*, 24(2), 125–137.

[26] Došilović, F. K., Brčić, M., & Hlupić, N. (2018). Explainable artificial intelligence: A survey. *2018 41st International Convention on Information and Communication Technology, Electronics and Microelectronics (MIPRO)*, pp. 0210–0215, doi: 10.23919/MIPRO.2018.8400040.

[27] Albahri, A. S., Duhaim, A. M., Fadhel, M. A. et al. (2023). A systematic review of trustworthy and explainable artificial intelligence in healthcare: Assessment of quality, bias risk, and data fusion. *Information Fusion*, 96, 156–191.

[28] Saranya, A., & Subhashini, R. (2023). A systematic review of explainable artificial intelligence models and applications: Recent developments and future trends. *Decision Analytics Journal*, 7, 100230.

[29] Zhang, Y., Teoh, B. K., Wu, M. et al. (2023). Data-driven estimation of building energy consumption and GHG emissions using explainable artificial intelligence. *Energy*, 262, 125468.

[30] Jaiswal, V., Saurabh, P., Lilhore, U. K. et al. (2023). A breast cancer risk predication and classification model with ensemble learning and big data fusion. *Decision Analytics Journal*, 8, 100298.

[31] Botlagunta, M., Botlagunta, M. D., Myneni, M. D. et al. (2023). Classification and diagnostic prediction of breast cancer metastasis on clinical data using machine learning algorithms. *Scientific Reports*, 13(1), 485.

[32] Ebrahim, M., Sedky, A. A. H., & Mesbah, S. (2023). Accuracy assessment of machine learning algorithms used to predict breast cancer. *Data*, 8(2), 35.

[33] Desai, F., Chowdhury, D., Kaur, R. et al. (2022). HealthCloud: A system for monitoring health status of heart patients using machine learning and cloud computing. *Internet of Things*, 17, 100485.

[34] Golec, M., Gill, S. S., Parlikad, A. K. et al. (2023). HealthFaaS: AI based smart healthcare system for heart patients using serverless computing. *IEEE Internet of Things Journal*, 10(21), 18469–18476.

CHAPTER 5

Machine Learning-Based Web Application for Breast Cancer Prediction

Shabnam Manjuri and Sukhpal Singh Gill

5.1 INTRODUCTION

Breast cancer occurs in both men and women, but it is more common in women when compared with men. According to breastcancer.org, about 43,600 women in the United States are expected to die in 2021 from carcinoma [1]. Death rates have been steady for women below 50 since 2007, but they have continued to rise in women over the age of 50. The general death rate from carcinoma decreased by one chromosome annually from 2013 to 2018 [2]. These decreases are thought to be the result of treatment advances and earlier detection through screening [3]. Signs and symptoms of breast cancer include a breast lump or thickening that feels different from the surrounding tissue and a change in the size, shape, or appearance of the breast as well as changes to the skin over the breast. A newly inverted nipple, peeling, scaling, crusting, or flaking of the pigmented area of skin surrounding the nipple or breast skin can also be signs and symptoms of cancer [4]. These factors and more information, such as the perimeter (mean size of the tumour), radius, area, and smoothness, would give a good insight into how the cancer correlates with these factors and how we can estimate the type of cancer with good accuracy.

5.1.1 Motivation and Our Contributions

Breast cancer survival rates have increased, and the number of deaths associated with this disease is steadily declining, largely due to factors such as earlier detection. One such advancement that can easily detect the tumour beforehand is using various regression and classification models (sometimes including deep neural networks) [4]. Understanding the type of cancer is a difficult task for medical use cases, and there are chances of wrong detection. The main aim of this research is to identify breast cancer and detect the patient's breast tissues as being one of the two categories of cancer: malignant or benign. The web portal can be accessed by a doctor or even a patient by registering once through the welcome page and then logging in whenever they want to check the class of the cancer.

DOI: 10.1201/9781003467199-6

The patient or the doctor will input the feature values for the various measurements of the breasts and their properties, and the machine learning (ML) model in the backend will predict the class of tumour tissues.

In this chapter, the main aim is to develop an end-to-end system that uses state-of-the-art ML techniques to detect breast cancer through a user-friendly web portal deployed on the cloud [5]. The main research work consists of understanding the use case of artificial intelligence (AI) in predicting the class of cancerous tumours based on training an ML model on a cleaned dataset consisting of 569 varying data points with 32 features measuring the various properties of breasts [4]. The processes involved training the classification models such as logistic regression (LR), support vector machine (SVM), K-nearest neighbour (KNN), Gaussian naïve Bayes, decision tree (DT), random forest, hybrid model 1 (KNN, DT), hybrid model 2 (random forest, gradient boosting [GB] machine), and hybrid model 3 (LR, SVMs) and measuring their performance using various performance metrics, mainly accuracy on training and validation datasets based on F1 score [6]. After the training phase, the best-performing model was stored on the servers, and based on its performance, it was used on the production server to predict cancerous tumours for real-time patients and doctors and to help understand whether the cancer was malignant or benign.

5.2 RELATED WORKS

In this section, some of the related work that has been done previously on the breast cancer dataset will be discussed, including where researchers used different kinds of ML approaches. To explore ML and computational methods, 20 recent research papers are reviewed here.

Yue et al. [7] researched ML techniques that are applied in breast cancer analysis and prospects. The researcher focused on various ML models such as KNNs, DTs, artificial neural networks (ANNs), SVMs, and the Wisconsin Breast Cancer dataset (WBCD). These ML models did show significant results by improving accuracy in prediction and classification. The paper contains very intuitive and clear information that was shown in a table format with supporting elements such as algorithms, classification accuracy, and sample strategies. According to researchers, although many algorithms performed very well with high accuracy, further experimentation is still needed to improve algorithms. The researchers intend to study the Friedreich's ataxia (FRDA) dataset using ML in depth in the future to develop a smart FRDA healthcare system.

Chaurasia et al. [8] also used the WBCD and built cancer prediction models that predict malignant or benign breast cancer. Waikato Environment analysed the research for knowledge analysis (Weka). The researchers used three popular data mining algorithms, such as radial basis function (RBF) network, J48, and naïve Bayes, to build their cancer prediction models. To ration the unbiased estimate of the three built prediction models for performance comparison purposes, the researchers used ten-fold cross-validation techniques. Based on the method's accuracy and effectiveness, the model's performance evaluation was obtained. For this experiment, all three models achieved high accuracy. For example, the RBF network achieved an accuracy of 96.77% and J48 achieved a classification accuracy of 93.41%, but naïve Bayes performed the best and achieved a classification accuracy of 97.36%. To comprehend the relative contributions of the independent variables to predicting breast cancer survival, the researchers also conducted specificity and sensitivity analyses. According to the sensitivity result, the prognostic factor "class" was the most important predictor.

Banu and Thirumalaikolundusubramanian [9] used different classifier techniques to predict breast cancer. The researchers focused on Bayes classifiers like boosted augmented naïve Bayes (BAN), Bayesian belief network (BBN), and tree augmented naïve Bayes (TAN), and according to them, the techniques could be used to improve accuracy and classification. WDBC was used for this research, which has 569 instances and 32 features. Here, with the GB model, all classifiers were combined to improve the classification accuracy. The combined GB result was improved compared with the other three models, which achieved an almost similar accuracy of 90%. Depending on the sensitivity, specificity, and prediction of accuracy, the classifier's performance evaluation was done. The achieved results proved that in breast cancer classification, using TAN was clearly beneficial as it enhanced the results. In their research, Ahmad et al. [10] compared the performance of a few ML algorithms, such as ANN, DT, and SVM. The breast cancer dataset was collected from an Iranian centre. The result showed that among those three classifier models, SVM performed the best.

Nematzadeh et al. [11] did comparative research on neural networks (NNs), DT, NB, and SVM to classify Wisconsin Breast Cancer (WBC) and Wisconsin Prognostic Breast Cancer data (WPBC) with three different kernel functions as classifiers. The results show that the NN (10-fold) (98.09%) achieved the highest accuracy in the WBC dataset, and SVM-RBF (10-fold) achieved the highest classification accuracy in the WPBC dataset, at 98.32%.

Mirajkar and Lakshmi [12] used the naïve Bayes classification model to predict the cancer type. The researchers aimed to predict the risk of specific types of cancer through their proposed technique. Breast and ovarian cancer symptoms were classified to identify the risk of them based on the naïve Bayes algorithm.

Mandal [13] conducted a study using the WDBC breast cancer dataset that was collected from the UCI Machine Learning Repository. It has 569 instances and 32 attributes, of which 70% were used for training and 30% for test purposes. The researcher applied three ML classification models, such as LR, DTs, and naïve Bayes, to distinguish if the tumour is malignant or benign. The LR model performed with the highest accuracy among all, and its time complexity is lower than the other models as well.

Oskouei et al. [14] performed a broad investigation on 45 articles that applied ML and data mining methods to breast cancer detection, cure, and prognosis. The researcher divided those articles and categorised them into four sections based on their research topic. This study shows that 11 articles focused on the development of a prediction model for early breast cancer detection, 21 articles investigated the classification accuracy of the models, 12 articles researched the detection of breast cancer, and 1 article studied and applied a regression model to diagnose the first stage of breast cancer. The results show there are no tools that can detect breast cancer automatically and propose an appropriate treatment for the patient. Therefore, the researchers felt a need to develop an advanced tool that would automate the diagnosis process and recommend necessary treatments.

Abed et al. [15] aimed to help doctors in the early prediction of breast cancer and build a hybrid classification model that uses the KNN and genetic algorithm (GA). They used

GA to improve the existing techniques. For example, the KNN algorithm was used for classification, but GA was used to select the best features of KNN along with the optimisation of the k value to enhance the accuracy. The WBCD was used for this study, which was collected from the UCI Repository of ML. This particular WBCD dataset has 10 attributes and 699 instances compared with the WDBC dataset, which has 31 attributes and 569 instances. The researchers achieved 99% accuracy with the proposed hybrid model, which is higher than other existing classifier models.

Chidambaranathan [16] developed a hybrid breast cancer prediction model by using extreme learning machine (ELM) and k_means algorithms. The k_means algorithm precisely extracts features based on those cluster tumours. An individual cluster signifies a definite tumour pattern. Single hidden layer feedforward neural networks (SLFNs) are an extended version of ELMs that is faster and more accurate with cancer detection. After the SVM sorts the images into groups, the k_means and ELM hybrid algorithms take the extracted columns as input and use them to find things like sensitivity, specificity, accuracy, and the distance between features. According to the results, the proposed hybrid system performed with better accuracy than the others.

Akinsola et al. [17] developed a breast cancer prediction app to help doctors diagnose the tumour as malignant or benign based on the patient's medical data. The dataset was collected from the Lagos Federal Government Hospital. The researchers used three supervised learning algorithms in the Weka toolkit to classify the dataset, such as multilayer perceptron (MLP), C4.5, and naïve Bayes. The researchers did the performance evaluation based on the prediction accuracy, and building time was measured. The C4.5 model performed faster and better than the rest of the models. It took 0.28 seconds and achieved an accuracy of 93.9%. For future work, it was suggested to add more functionality to enhance the patient's usability.

Majal et al. [18] performed classification and association techniques by using the Wisconsin dataset to build the cancer prediction system. This particular dataset has 699 data points and 9 features. To find the frequent patterns of the cancer, the frequent pattern growth (FP) algorithm was applied with the association of rule mining methodology. A tree-based algorithm DT was also used to make the prediction based on a few predictor features, which were gender, age, and intensity of the symptoms. The researchers claim that the approach model attained a high level of accuracy that is acceptable and suitable for use by medical professionals.

Azmi and Cob [19] presented a breast cancer classifier system that was developed by using a backpropagation algorithm for training feedforward NNs. The WBCD was used for this study, which was collected from the UCI repository. The final result showed that NN with a hidden seven-layer model achieved the highest accuracy among the others at 93.63%. Ojha and Goel [20] worked with different ML models such as DTs, SVMs, and fuzzy c-means on the WPBC dataset. The researchers found that DT and SVM are better predictors with 81% than fuzzy c-means, which achieved the lowest accuracy of 37%.

In [21], the scientist also created a Computer-Aided Diagnosis (CAD) scheme for detecting breast cancer using a deep belief network unsupervised path and a backpropagation supervised path. The scheme was constructed based on a backpropagation NN with the learning function of Liebenberg Marquardt, and the weights were initialised from the deep belief network path (DBNNN). Their technique was tested using the WBCD, and their classifier complex gave an accuracy of 99.68%.

In their study, Tafish and El-Halees [22] presented several ML algorithms benchmarked to differentiate breast cancer patients as sick or healthy. With an accuracy rate of 84%, their results show that the ANN model is better than SVM, KNN, or DT for finding out the severity of the breast cancer. This was found after comparing and evaluating results using different parameters. A model was proposed to help in resolving the difficulty of determining the level of risk of the disease and to obtain best practices, longevity, and effect objectives of advance well-being based on data collected from hospitals in the Gaza Strip by the authors in [10]. The model applied classification techniques such as SVM, ANN, and KNN to the collected breast cancer data, which in turn determined the severity of breast cancer. After evaluating and testing the model using the previously mentioned classification techniques on the breast cancer dataset, its accuracy was 77%.

However, researchers [20] engaged in eight different data mining techniques for predicting breast cancer. The dataset for the experiment was WPBC [7]. The experiments were done on the four classification algorithms: SVM, DT C5.0, Bayes network (BN), and KNN, and the clustering algorithms: K-means, and fuzzy c-means. The experiment was run using the programming language R, and the results showed that classifying algorithms work better than clustering algorithms. SVM and DT (C5.0) had the best accuracy of 81%, whereas fuzzy c-means had the lowest accuracy of 37%. In [23], researchers talked about how they used three data mining techniques to decide whether breast cancer was malignant or benign. The techniques conducted on the WBDC dataset are, namely, LR, naïve Bayes, and DT. From their results, it showed their classification accuracy is 97.90% between the other two tested classifiers compared with the accuracy of our study, which gives a higher predictive accuracy.

Khanom et al. [24] engaged in 12 different techniques for diagnosing breast cancer. The techniques used were BN, Lady IBK, multilayer perceptron, decision table, J-Rip, AdaBoost M1, J48, J-Rip, LR, Lazy K-star, multiclass classifier, Random Forest (RF) and Random Tree (RT). The WBCD dataset was used to train the model; a larger percentage of the applied methods gave more than 94% accuracy. Gaussian naïve Bayes underperformed compared with the other models, with an accuracy of 73.21%. The RT and lazy classifier algorithms outperformed the others with an accuracy close to 99%.

Although the authors in [25] engaged in six different data mining techniques: ANN, LR, SVM, BN, ANN, KNN, and DT (C4.5), the experiment was carried out on the WBCD dataset using the Weka tool. Gaussian naïve Bayes and SVM showed the algorithms with the highest accuracy of 97.28%, even though the BN classifier produced minimal time compared with SVM.

Sivakami [26] concatenated SVM and DT algorithms and developed a hybrid model. This hybrid model was applied to classify tumours into two categories: malignant and benign. The WBCD was used, which contains 11 features and 699 instances. The dataset was taken from the UCL ML repository. This dataset was not clean, as it had many missing values. Weka software was used to compare the results. The outcome shows that the hybrid model (DT+SVM) performed well (91% accuracy, low error rate of 2.58%) in breast cancer data classification compared with other ML algorithms.

5.2.1 Critical Analysis

Past research shows that each of the techniques has varied accuracies according to each study; in some studies, Gaussian naïve Bayes had the highest accuracy, followed by SVM, DT (C5.0), LR, and J48 classifiers, and vice versa [27]. Research shows that AI is one of the easiest ways to detect breast cancer, and it has been concentrated around algorithmic models, which makes this innovation independent of real-world clinical evaluation [28]. Our conclusion is that despite the encouraging performance of the accuracy results of the developed model, which range from 69.2% to 97.8%, there are still some gaps that need to be addressed before it can be transferred to detecting large-scale projects [20].

5.3 PROPOSED TECHNIQUE

In this study, an application is created using ML learning algorithms to develop an ML model that can detect the type of cancer tissue in breast cancer [29]. In the works cited in this review, there have been limitations to some of the algorithms built [30]. This study did experiments on a few techniques testing nine different algorithms after preprocessing differently, and carefully selecting the features on which the model would be built, which makes it preferable and reliable for developing our web portal.

5.3.1 Hybrid Modelling

- Hybrid model 1 (KNN+DTree)
- Hybrid model 2 (RForest+GBN)
- Hybrid model 3 (LR+SVM)

5.3.2 Application

This is a fully functional breast cancer detection app that detects the tumour as malignant or benign based on the given patient's information that offers easy navigation and interaction.

5.4 PERFORMANCE EVALUATION

In this section, we discuss the dataset and experimental results.

5.4.1 Dataset

The initial testing dataset was collected from various sources, but the final dataset was chosen from the UCI Machine Learning Repository, which consists of 569 data points. The major features in the dataset help in the understanding of the breast measurements for an individual patient and contain the following features [31]: radius, texture, perimeter, area, smoothness, compactness, concavity, and concave points with their mean (μ), standard error (σ), and worst (α) calculated values. The detailed explanation of each feature with its calculation metrics is mentioned in the following:

- **Radius**: The distances from the centre to points on the perimeter with μ, σ, and α values as individual features.

- **Texture**: Standard deviation of grey-scale values. With μ, σ, and α values as individual features.

- **Perimeter_mean**: Size of the core tumour with μ, σ, and α values as individual features.

- **Smoothness_mean**: Local variations in radius lengths with μ, σ, and α values as individual features.

- **Compactness_mean**: The perimeter^2/area −1.0 with μ, σ, and α values as individual features.

- **Concavity_mean**: Severity of concave portions of the contour with μ, σ, and α values as individual features.

- **Concave points**: Number of concave portions of the contour with μ, σ, and α values as individual features.

The dataset was clean, with no missing values in any column, and the features were clean. There were no duplicates in the complete dataset, and it was free from repetitive user entries. The data consisted of 32 columns, and each column defied one property about the breasts of the patient. The data spread was not equally distributed for both categories of tumours, with malignant tumours having 37.7% of the data points whereas benign tumours had 62.7% of the data points, as shown in Figure 5.1.

After analysing the plot in Figure 5.2, we can say that perimeter radius and area have a straight, direct correlation with the linear line of scattered points. Using this understanding,

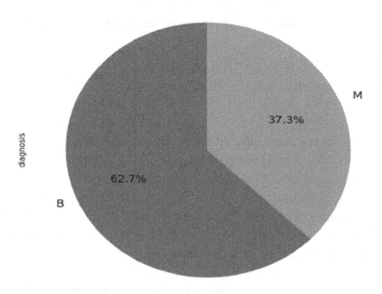

FIGURE 5.1   The categories of tumour.

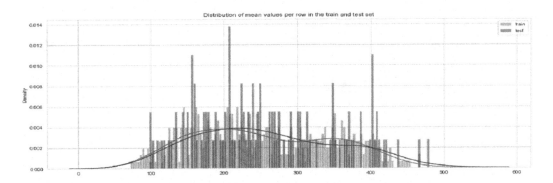

FIGURE 5.2   The distribution plot for the Shepherd data split of training and testing data.

it can be inferred that these three columns will have very similar behaviour for training the model [32]. To eliminate any kind of bias in training the models, the complete dataset is split into the training as well as the testing datasets, with 80% of the data points (455 points) in the training data and 20% of the data points (114 points) in the testing data (validation data). Figure 5.2 shows the distribution plot for the Shepherd data split of training and testing data, giving a clear idea about this fact.

5.4.2 Understanding the Features and Correlations

Although there were 32 curated features in the complete data, as shown in Figure 5.3, some of them did not contribute to developing the best model, whereas others showed a high

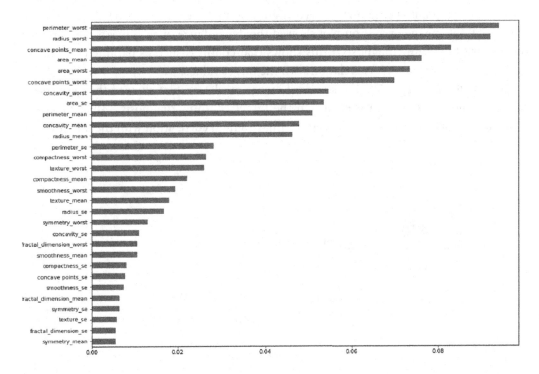

FIGURE 5.3   The curated features in the complete data.

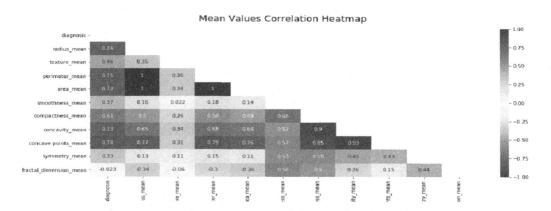

FIGURE 5.4   Mean values correlation heatmap.

correlation with the prediction of the tumour class and showed good feature importance. As a result, only 30 features are displayed in Figure 5.3. The feature importance was calculated based on the ensemble extra tree classifier, and the top 90% of features that contributed to the model performance were used in the final predictions. This helped in not only reducing the time of execution of the prediction by a significant amount but also helped in developing a more optimum model with better accuracy and F1 score values by avoiding the biases generated due to the useless features.

Before the modelling phase started, all the features were tested to see their correlation with each other, as well as the predicting column "diagnosis", which classifies the cancer as M (malignant, a tumour) or B (benign, not a dangerous tumour). As depicted in Figure 5.4, the mean correlation plot showed the dependence of each mean measurement on the target column "diagnosis". This shows that columns such as parameter, area, and concave points have a high correlation with the target values.

As depicted in Figure 5.5, the standard error correlation plot showed the dependence of each standard error measurement on the target column "diagnosis". This shows that columns such as radius, area, and perimeter have a high correlation with the target values.

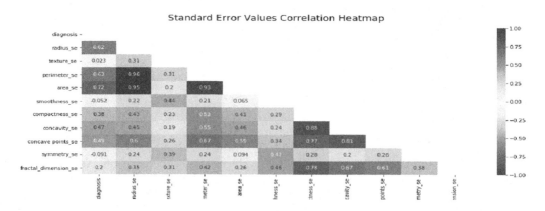

FIGURE 5.5   Standard error values correlation heatmap.

5.4.3 Training and Machine Learning

The final features were chosen based on their importance using the extra tree classifier. All the selected features were encoded to avoid any data discrepancy using label encoders, and the encoded values were used for training and testing purposes [28]. For the web portal, the encoder was also stored as pickle files along with the model that was used to inverse transform the columns that were initially transformed before the training phase. Thus, it will implement the same feature engineering on the new data points that were processed on the training data. During the experiments, various state-of-the-art classification ML algorithms were used with techniques to detect carcinogenic tumours in tissues.

Along with these algorithms, some hybrid custom models were created to understand the performance when multiple classical models are assembled and stacked together to develop new hybrid variants. These three hybrid models were used to train on 80% of the dataset and are used to predict performance using both training accuracy and the F1 score on the validation dataset. All nine ML models were used to protect performance, and the final performance of each model is mentioned in Table 5.1.

Based on Table 5.1, it can be inferred that the SVM has good training and testing accuracy as well as a good F1 score. All three hybrid models have a decent F1 score but are not as comparable to the individual scores of SVMs. However, models suggest that the DT and random forest models have 100% training accuracy, less test accuracy, and one school, which signifies that these models are overfit on the data and require some hyperparameter tuning [33]. Based on the performance of the SVM, it can be used as a final model for predicting the diagnosis of patients on the live web portal for real-time cancer predictions. SVM with hinge loss is used for training the final chosen model for predictions on real-time queries. It will be minimised to get the optimum support vectors for the data spread.

5.4.4 Justification for Using SVM for This Prediction System

The study describes a model that is developed to predict the class of tumour tissue in breast cancer using a single algorithm in place of the hybrid model after the training and testing of the ML model. After testing, the SVM algorithm appears to be able to classify breast cancer tumours into classes of tumour tissue with a higher overall performance accuracy compared with the three hybrid models that we came up with. The SVM algorithm tells if

TABLE 5.1   Performance Comparison of ML Models

ML Models	Train Accuracy	Test Accuracy	F1 Score
LR	93.85	88.60	0.878
SVM	98.90	98.25	0.981
KNN	98.68	92.98	0.925
Gaussian NB	92.97	96.49	0.963
Decision Tree	100.00	93.86	0.935
Random Forest	100.00	96.49	0.962
Hybrid1: KNN, D Tree	98.90	94.74	0.943
Hybrid2: RForest, GBN	97.14	95.61	0.953
Hybrid3L LR, SVM	97.14	93.86	0.932

it is benign or malignant, and its performance outweighs that of the three hybrid models. Its outcome as an algorithm also consists of accuracy and precision. It is used for classification that trains the model to show cancer according to the diagnosis. Generalisation performance is an important feature of SVM and has a great impact on our model [34]. Structural risk minimisation (SRM) is a feature of the SVM model that attempts to tackle the problem of overfitting by not taking into consideration empirical risk minimisation [35]. The upper bound of the generalisation error is minimised rather than the training error, as in the case of some models used in previous work, such as ANN.

5.4.5 Implementing Website-Based Interface

Once the experiments were completed with all the chosen models as well as the transformers stored as pickle files, a web portal was created using HTML, CSS, JavaScript, and Bootstrap to detect cancer in real time. The web portal is fully functional and includes a home page, register, login, feedback, and prediction pages.

- **Welcome page**: The landing page where a user first interacts with the website has information about breast cancer, as shown in Figure 5.6.

- **Register page**: On this web page, a new user visiting the website for the first time can enter their email and site password to register for the first time, after which we can login to their portal, as shown in Figure 5.7.

- **Login page**: This is a web page where an existing user can enter their email ID and password to login to their portal, as shown in Figure 5.8.

- **Feedback page**: On this web page, any user can provide their feedback after using the web portal to help others get information about the portal and its use cases, as shown in Figure 5.9.

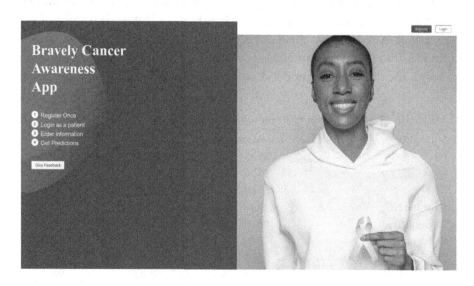

FIGURE 5.6 Welcome page.

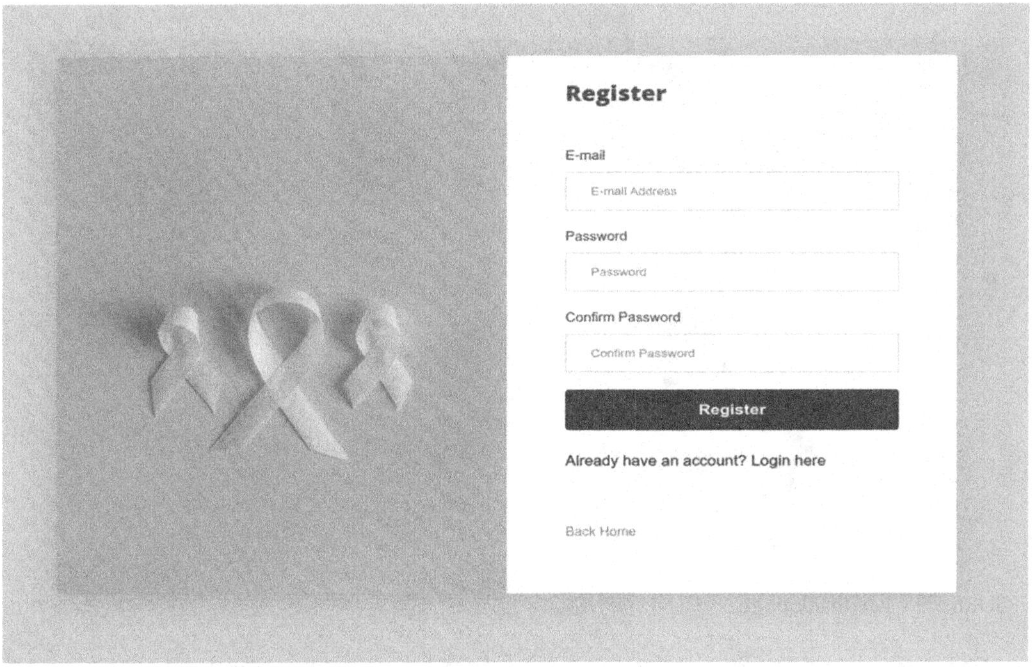

FIGURE 5.7 Registration page.

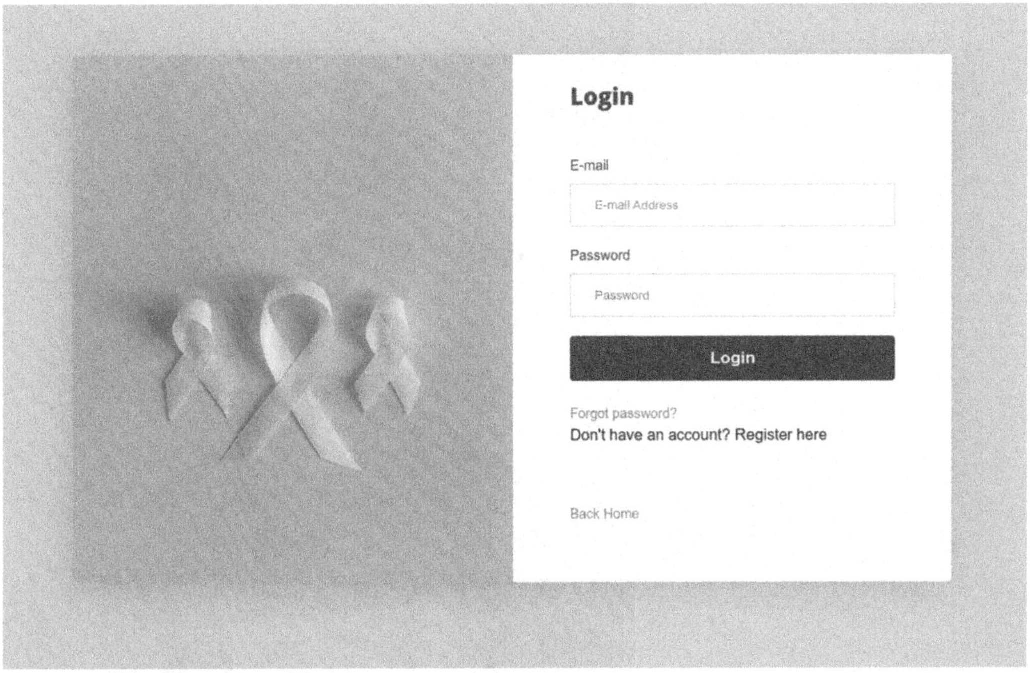

FIGURE 5.8 Login page.

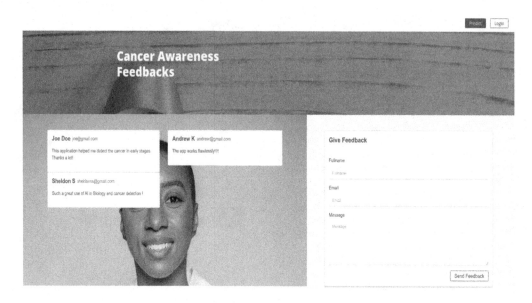

FIGURE 5.9   Feedback page.

- **Home page**: Once the user has successfully logged in, they will land on the home page, as shown in Figure 5.10. On this page, they can see information about their profile as well as enter all the information about the patient, including the mean standard error and the worst measurements of each feature. Once they click the predict button, they will land on the prediction page.

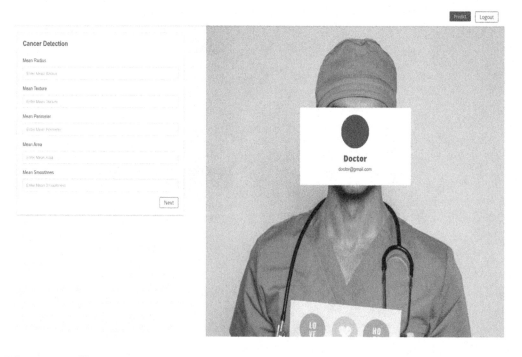

FIGURE 5.10   Home page.

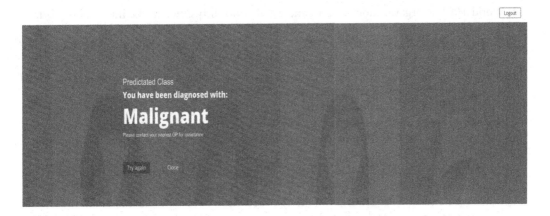

FIGURE 5.11   Prediction page.

- **Prediction page**: Figure 5.11 shows the prediction page. On the prediction, every user who tried to predict their cancer tumour type will get a specific class, malignant or benign, for the data they entered. The value of the class is protected using the locally stored ML model, and the features are transformed using the transformer encoders.

5.5 CONCLUSIONS AND FUTURE WORK

The application was created using state-of-the-art ML algorithms to develop an ML model that predicts the type of cancer tissue in breast cancer. Various ML algorithms were tested based on their performance on the training data, and the finally chosen SVM performed the best compared with the other models used in developing the web portal. The website for doctors and patients consists of a cancer awareness home page, an easy-to-guide simple process for registration and login, and a home page to predict the type of cancer for the new user who enters the platform for the first time. The complete research work ends up predicting the model's performance with 98.25% accuracy.

However, the proposed experimental hybrid algorithms achieved good train accuracy, test accuracy, and F1 score, but they could be improved on a larger sample that is unbiased. For future work, these hybrid algorithms can be applied to other health datasets to measure their performance and into a potential practical environment for clinical help to physicians with fast additional outlook [27]. Although the developed application is visually pleasing, it can be more interactive if its usability is improved [28]. More functionalities can be added to the web application, such as the ability to send an automated greeting email to customers after registering [29]. The reset password page can be completed, which was left due to time constraints. Adding additional pages to the website that will contain more information and raise awareness about breast cancer will be beneficial to the users.

REFERENCES

[1] World Health Organization. (June 2023). WHO: Prevention and control; report 2020. World Health Organization. Cardiovascular diseases (CVDs). https://www.who.int/cardiovascular_diseases/en/. [Accessed 3rd June 2023].

[2] World Health Organization Breast cancer (who.int). https://www.who.int/news-room/fact-sheets/detail/breast-cancer. [Accessed 3rd June 2023].

[3] Breast Cancer Wisconsin (Diagnostic) Data Set | Kaggle. https://www.kaggle.com/uciml/breast-cancer-wisconsin-data. [Accessed 28th may 2023].

[4] Alaa, A. M., Gurdasani, D., Harris, A. L. et al. (2021). Machine learning to guide the use of adjuvant therapies for breast cancer. *Nature Machine Intelligence*, 3(8), 716–726.

[5] Gill, S. S., Xu, M., Ottaviani, C. et al. (2022). AI for next generation computing: Emerging trends and future directions. *Internet of Things*, 19, 100514.

[6] Gill, S. S., Wu, H., Patros, P. et al. (2024). Modern computing: Vision and challenges. *Telematics and Informatics Reports*, 13, 100116.

[7] Yue, W., Wang, Z., Chen, H. et al. (2018). Machine learning with applications in breast cancer diagnosis and prognosis. *Designs*, 2(2), 13.

[8] Chaurasia, V., Pal, S., & Tiwari, B. B. (2018). Prediction of benign and malignant breast cancer using data mining techniques. *Journal of Algorithms & Computational Technology*, 12(2), 119–126. https://doi.org/10.1177/1748301818756225

[9] Banu, B., & Thirumalaikolundusubramanian, P. (2018). Comparison of bayes classifiers for breast cancer classification. *Asian Pacific Journal of Cancer Prevention (APJCP)*, 19(10), 2917–2920. https://doi.org/10.22034/APJCP.2018.19.10.2917

[10] Ahmad, L. G., Eshlaghy, A. T., Poorebrahimi, A. et al. (2013). Using three machine learning techniques for predicting breast cancer recurrence. *Journal of Health & Medical Informatics*, 4, 124. https://doi.org/10.4172/2157-7420.1000124

[11] Nematzadeh, Z., Ibrahim, R., & Selamat, A. (2015). Comparative studies on breast cancer classifications with k-fold cross validations using machine learning techniques. *Proceeding in 2015 10th Asian Control Conference (ASCC)*, pp. 1–6. IEEE.

[12] Mirajkar, P., & Lakshmi, P. (2017). Prediction of cancer risk in perspective of symptoms using naïve bayes classifier. *International Journal of Engineering Research in Computer Science and Engineering*, 4(9), 145–149.

[13] Mandal, S. K. (2017). Performance analysis of data mining algorithms for breast cancer cell detection using naïve bayes, logistic regression and decision tree. *International Journal of Engineering and Computer Science*, 6(2), 20388–20391.

[14] Oskouei, R. J., Kor, N. M., & Maleki, S. A. (2017). Data mining and medical world: Breast cancers diagnosis, treatment, prognosis and challenges. *American Journal of Cancer Research*, 7(3), 610–627.

[15] Abed, B. M., Shaker, K., Jalab, H. A. et al. (2016). A hybrid classification algorithm approach for breast cancer diagnosis. *2016 IEEE Industrial Electronics and Applications Conference (IEACon)*, pp. 269–274.

[16] Chidambaranathan, S. (2016). Breast cancer diagnosis based on feature extraction by hybrid of k-means and extreme learning machine algorithms. *ARPN Journal of Engineering and Applied Sciences*, 11(7), 4581–4586.

[17] Akinsola, A. F., Sokunbi, M. A., & Onadokun, I. O. (2017). Data mining for breast cancer classification. *International Journal of Engineering And Computer Science*, 6(8), 22250–22258.

[18] Majali, J., Niranjan, R., Phatak, V. et al. (2015). Data mining techniques for diagnosis and prognosis of cancer. *International Journal of Advanced Research in Computer and Communication Engineering*, 4(3), 613–616. https://doi.org/10.17148/IJARCCE.2015.43147

[19] Mohd Azmi, M. S. B., & Cob, Z. C. (13–14 Dec 2010). Breast cancer prediction based on backpropagation algorithm. *Proceedings of 2010 IEEE Student Conference on Research and Development (SCOReD 2010)*, pp. 164–168, Putrajaya, Malaysia.

[20] Ojha, U., & Goel, S. (2017). A study on prediction of breast cancer recurrence using data mining techniques. *2017 7th Int. Conf. on Cloud Computing, Data Science & Engineering – Confluence*, pp. 527–530. IEEE.

[21] Abdel-Zaher, A. M., & Eldeib, A. M. (2016). Breast cancer classification using deep belief networks. *Expert Systems With Applications*, 46, 139–144.

[22] Tafish, M. H., & El-Halees, A. M. (2018). Breast Cancer Severity Degree Predication Using Data Mining Techniques in the Gaza Strip. *2018 International Conference on Promising Electronic Technologies (ICPET)*, Deir El-Balah, pp. 124–128.

[23] Khanom, N. N., Nihar, F., Hassan, S. S. et al. (2020). Algorithms for breast cancer cell detection using naïve bayes, logistic regression and decision tree. *international journal of engineering and computer science"* 6(2): 20388–20391. *Journal of Physics: Conference Series*, 1577, 012051.

[24] Saoud, H., Ghadi, A., Ghailani, M. et al. (2018). Application of data mining classification algorithms for breast cancer diagnosis. *ACM International Conference Proceeding Series*.

[25] Maity, N. G. Dr., & Das, S. (2017). Machine learning for improved diagnosis and prognosis in healthcare. *2017 IEEE Aerospace Conference*. IEEE.

[26] Sivakami, K. (2015). Mining big data: Breast cancer prediction using DT-SVM hybrid model. *International Journal of Scientific Engineering and Applied Science (IJSEAS)*, 1(5), 418–429.

[27] Singh, R. & Gill, S. S. (2023). Edge AI: A survey. *Internet of Things and Cyber-Physical Systems*, 3, 71–92.

[28] Gill, S. S., & Kaur, R. (2023). ChatGPT: Vision and challenges. *Internet of Things and Cyber-Physical Systems*, 3, 262–271.

[29] Dhillon, A., Singh, A., Vohra, H. et al. (2022). IoTPulse: Machine learning-based Enterprise health information system to predict alcohol addiction in Punjab (India) using IoT and fog computing. *Enterprise Information Systems*, 16(7), 1820583.

[30] Moqurrab, S. A., Tariq, N., Anjum, A. et al. (2022). A deep learning-based privacy-preserving model for smart healthcare in internet of medical things using fog computing. *Wireless Personal Communications*, 126(3), 2379–2401.

[31] Purnami, S. W., Rahayu, S. P., & Embong, A. (2008). Feature selection and classification of breast cancer diagnosis based on support vector machines. *2008 International Symposium on Information Technology*, 1

[32] Iftikhar, S., Golec, M., Chowdhury, D. et al. (2022). FogDLearner: A deep learning-based cardiac health diagnosis framework using fog computing. *Proceedings of the 2022 Australasian Computer Science Week*, pp. 136–144.

[33] Golec, M., Gill, S. S., Parlikad, A. K. et al. (2023). HealthFaaS: AI based smart healthcare system for heart patients using serverless computing. *IEEE Internet of Things Journal*, 10(21), 18469–18476.

[34] Desai, F., Chowdhury, D., Kaur, R. et al. (2022). HealthCloud: A system for monitoring health status of heart patients using machine learning and cloud computing. *Internet of Things*, 17, 100485.

[35] Al-Musaylh, M. S., Deo, R. C., Adamowski, J. F. et al. (2018). Short-term electricity demand forecasting with MARS, SVR and ARIMA models using aggregated demand data in Queensland, Australia. *Advanced Engineering Informatics*, 35, 1–16.

II

Natural Language Programming (NLP)

CHAPTER 6

Machine Learning-Based Opinion Mining and Visualization of News RSS Feeds for Efficient Information Gain

Jairaj Patil and Sukhpal Singh Gill

6.1 INTRODUCTION

The COVID-19 pandemic has unavoidably led to an increase in the use of digital gadgets because of social norms that promote social isolation and extensive lockdowns. Worldwide, individuals and organisations have had to adapt to new ways of living and working. Most individuals are now using the Internet and Internet-based services to communicate, engage, and carry out their work duties from home because of the lockdown [1]. Compared with pre-lockdown levels, utilisation of Internet services has increased from 40% to 100% [2]. The major sources of information continue to be news and online media, even though governments, epidemiologists, school administrators, business owners, and families around the world are already preparing for the next steps.

The world's largest source of information is the Internet. The web's ability to instantly display news from around the globe via Really Simple Syndication (RSS) feeds is one of its key features [3]. In addition to passive media consumption, Web 2.0 technology enables an increasing number of users to actively contribute to this priceless information source by easily creating content [4, 5]. There are several ways to participate actively on the Internet, including blogs, reviews, and other commenting methods. For many people and organisations, it is crucial to analyse news articles and user-generated material. Economic analysts, for example, would like to find consumer and public opinions on their products and services. Similarly, prospective buyers look for user reviews before learning about a product's flaws or praising its functioning. Additionally, they look for changes in government, rules and regulations, political disputes and much more. Brute forcing and processing the huge

DOI: 10.1201/9781003467199-8

amount of data by a human eye is very inefficient and much more time-consuming [6]. Because conducting public opinion surveys is an expensive and time-consuming endeavour, our goal is to provide a semi-automatic method by searching the web for specific news feeds, analysing the text to determine how positive or negative a particular news article is, comparing sentiment trends followed by different newspapers, and then presenting the results in an effective visual format [7, 8]. While the lack of precision makes our approach unsuitable to totally replace a thoroughly performed opinion poll, it does have some special benefits, such as inexpensive costs and the ability to continuously monitor a feed in real time and accumulate data for future analysis.

In this chapter, we describe an innovative approach to combining a visual representation and text analytic techniques. On the one hand, this technology automatically assesses a news article's emotional content. The visual interface, on the other hand, enables the human expert to reach meaningful conclusions, to selectively read a few news articles with strong emotional content, to identify patterns, and to get a general sense of how a given issue is developing in the media.

6.1.1 Motivation and Our Contributions

The fundamental driving force behind this effort is to get the most information possible out of the enormous textual data. The user can choose the category they would like to spend their time on because the news feeds are divided into positive, negative, and neutral categories. Furthermore, the work visualizes a few features of the news (such as common terms, word polarity, and live feed analysis) for further human analysis. A self-updating model runs a significant risk of experiencing slower processing times and memory problems. A few pre-existing problems with opinion mining include the tone problem, the polarity problem, sarcasm, the use of idioms, and others are few of the challenges faced in this work. As the approach is unsupervised learning, it is difficult to determine the accuracy metric.

6.2 RELATED WORKS

Significant efforts have been made in recent years to foresee the future pattern of specific subjectivity analysis on social issues in the form of news, postings, blogs, feeds, etc. In [9], the authors demonstrated a very niche implementation of opinion mining on stock news and its influence on the stock market. To forecast sentiment around stock news, this study develops a predictive algorithm. First, pertinent real-time RSS stock news from Arab Bank (ARBK) Company was examined to determine whether the sentiment score values were favourable, negative, or neutral. The suggested approach can prove to be a useful tool for investors in helping them make the best stock-related decisions. Finally, sentiment polarity news gives those in the stock market a useful indication of when to purchase or sell their stocks. The key differentiator in this work is the availability of labelled data from the ARBK public domain, allowing them to incorporate a machine learning approach, generate a future prediction for the stocks, and test its accuracy.

In [10], the authors proposed a case study using two separate open-source online sentiment analysis technologies in RSS news feeds that have an impact on broadcast ratings for sports.

In this study, sentiment analysis is employed on the description of 500 RSS feeds containing text and phrases to perform various text analytics on five distinct sports group RSS feeds gathered from different news sources. Two tools used were Voyant tools, a web-based text reading and analysis platform used to learn the scalable computer-aided analysis functions, and Linguistic Inquiry and Word Count (LIWC) to classify RSS feeds on each sport as positive and negative to identify the significant influence of news feeds about different sports on users and readers. The study lacked solutions to the limited dataset and the possibility of misclassification of RSS feed text such as humour, irony, or sarcasm terms or phrases due to dependency on available online tools. Another research work [11] presented a comparative analysis of the Valence Aware Dictionary for Sentiment Reasoning (VADER) sentiment lexicon to seven other well-established sentiment analysis lexicons: LIWC, General Inquirer (GI), Affective Norms for English Words (ANEW), SentiWordNet (SWN), SenticNet (SCN), Word-Sense Disambiguation (WSD) using WordNet, and the Hu-Liu04 opinion lexicon. Their results are not only encouraging but also astonishing; VADER outperformed 11 other well-regarded sentiment analysis tools in most of the cases.

6.3 PROPOSED TECHNIQUE

Sentiment analysis, also known as opinion mining, is the process of automatically determining a sentiment (such as a positive or negative sentiment) from a collection of words, such as a sentence or document. Most of the time, newspapers try to portray the news objectively, but textual affect analysis of news documents reveals that many words have either a positive or negative emotional charge. There are three major steps used for opinion mining. They are shown in Figure 6.1 and will be covered in detail further.

6.3.1 RSS Feeds and Data Mining

An Extensible Markup Language (XML) document called Really Simple Syndication (RSS), or Rich Site Summary (RSS) makes it easier to distribute content. It is a quick, efficient way to read news-related websites, Weblogs, and other online publishers who republish their information as an RSS feed for anyone who requests it. RSS pulls the most recent headlines from many news websites and pushes them to the computer for easy perusal. It is an easy technique to transfer data between websites that mostly use XML. RSS feeds are often tiny and load quickly. In contrast to email, an RSS feed requires no upkeep and never has any messages censored or banned. Users can now distinguish between needed and unwanted content using RSS feeds. Along with a link and a description, RSS news feeds also provide the author, title, and date. Figure 6.2 depicts popular tags extracted from the RSS feeds.

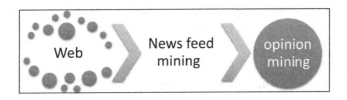

FIGURE 6.1   Proposed steps.

```
<? xml version="1.0" encoding="ISO-8859-1"?>
<rss version="2.0">
  <channel>
    <title>BBC Home Page</title>
    <link>http://www.BBC.co.uk/news/</link>
    <description>BBC News Home</description>
    <item>
      <title>News Tutorial</title>
      <link>http://www.BBC.co.uk/news/uk/link>
      <description>New Web tutorial
      </description>
    </item>
    <item>
      <title>Politics Tutorial</title>
      <link>http://www.BBC.co.uk/news/</link>
      <description>New Politics tutorial
      </description>
    </item>
  </channel>
```

FIGURE 6.2   Components of RSS feed.

The XML declaration appears on the first line of the RSS news stream. The RSS declaration, which states that this is an RSS document, appears on the next line (in this case, RSS version 2.0). Each feed only has one <channel> tag. It provides an overview of an RSS feed. Each <item> on news websites corresponds to a single recent news article. Three child elements are necessary for the <channel> element. The title of the channel is specified by the <title> element (e.g., BBC Home Page). The <link> element follows the <title> element and specifies the channel's hyperlink (e.g., http://www.BBC.co.uk/news/). The following element, known as "description", describes a succinct overview or, occasionally, the entire material (e.g., News Tutorial). There may be one or more "item" elements for each "channel" element. The item's title is specified using the <title> tag (e.g., News Tutorial). The next tag is <link>, which specifies the item's hyperlink (http://www.BBC.co.uk/news/uk/news/). The last tag, "description", provides a definition for the item (such as New Web tutorial).

The RSS feed reader pulls the necessary news content from web pages, such as title, description, date, author, link, etc. and reads it as an XML document. This uses the most recent headlines from the different news channels every time the application is run. This RSS feed is useful for compiling a dataset of recent news feeds. The corpus for this system is built using three different websites (i.e., Time of India, BBC News, and New York Times News). Text mining is performed to extract valuable information and sentiment, and static analysis is performed in fields that consist of words.

6.3.2 Sentiment Analysis

Sentiment analysis is a technique for determining whether unstructured data can infer the polarity of a piece of content [12]. The content's tone, polarity, and sentiment might be either positive, neutral, or negative.

1. **Level of analysis**: This has been divided into three types: document, sentence, and entity.

    a. **Document level**: The aim at this document level is to ascertain the general impression of the document. It is founded on the notion that sentiment analysis at the document level communicates ideas about a single entity [13].

    b. **Sentence level**: Identifying if each statement represented a good, negative, or neutral viewpoint.

    c. **Entity level**: Also known as feature-level analysis, it is a detailed level of analysis that discovers like or dislike of individuals [14].

2. **Sentiment detection**: There are two techniques for sentiment analysis, supervised learning and unsupervised learning. Supervised learning is carried out on labelled data and can be performed using algorithms such as naïve Bayes, support vector machine (SVM), regression, etc.; whereas unsupervised learning is carried out using lexicon-based, dictionary, or corpus-based methods as shown in Figure 6.3 [15]. For our model, we are using a sentence level, unsupervised, lexicon-based approach. Details will be covered in the architecture of the model in Section 6.4.

3. **Architecture**: A novel methodology for assessing sentiment trend on different news channels and creating a database for extensive analysis and visualization for effective information gain as shown in Figure 6.4.

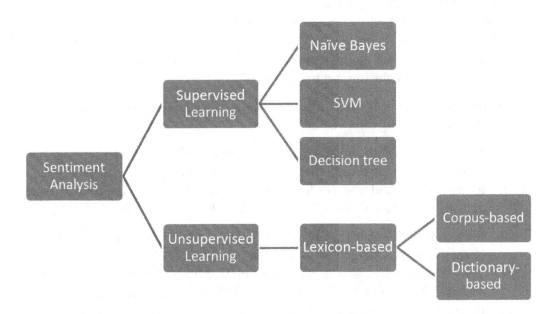

FIGURE 6.3   Taxonomy of sentiment analysis.

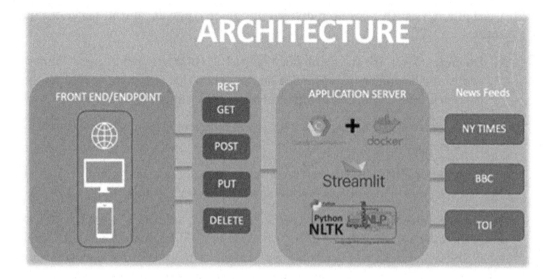

FIGURE 6.4   Application architecture.

The major components of the architecture are considered as follows:

a. **Front end/endpoint**: Front end or endpoint refers to clients or devices that will be using the service [16]. As a cloud application, the service will be available across all devices and platforms.

b. **REST APIs**: Application Programming Interfaces (APIs), are a collection of guidelines that specify how devices and software can connect to and communicate with one another [17]. An API that adheres to the representational state transfer (REST) design principles is known as a REST API. REST APIs are sometimes referred to as RESTful APIs as a result [18]. Two computer systems can communicate safely over the Internet using the RESTful API interface. A RESTful API's fundamental purpose is the same as using the Internet to browse [19].

c. **Application server**: It can be thought of as the brain of the system and can be further divided into following components:

1. **Front end**: The front end is developed using Streamlit. An open-source Python toolkit makes it simple to develop and distribute stunning, personalized web apps for data science and machine learning. The front end displays the polarity score and other analytical findings in efficient visual forms.

2. **Back end**: To calculate the polarity of the news, the system utilizes the Python Natural Language Toolkit (NLTK) toolkit and NLTK VADERVADER package. VADERVADER is a gold-standard sentiment lexicon with a focus on content resembling those of microblogs [11]. The NLTK VADER evaluates the text's sentiment and assigns scores in three categories—negative, neutral, and positive—based on the results. Additionally, for each text supplied to the NLTK VADER

function, the compound is calculated. The result of the three categories' scores are basically summed in the compound attribute [20]. Compound values range from −1 (most extreme negative) to +1 (most extreme positive). This number has been standardized to aid in analysis and future use.

3. **Application server**: The application is launched as a container on Google Cloud using the Google Apps Engine (GAE) [21]. For creating and hosting apps, Google offers the service, scalable environment, and cloud computing technology known as GAE [22]. It provides a safe execution environment in addition to several services that make it easier to create scalable and quick web applications [23]. This solves our problem of growing memory as the database increases and slow processing time. Another advantage is version control as the app progresses its development phase.

4. **Information source/RSS feeds**: An information source can be referred to news channels or the RSS feed of those from which the data will be retrieved.

6.4 PERFORMANCE EVALUATION

Automatic sentiment analyses are notorious for not being completely accurate for a variety of reasons (ambiguity, implicitness, etc.). To allow analysts to assess the level of confidence in the analysis results, we tested VADER and other sentiment analysis algorithms with the dataset sentiment140 [24]. This common dataset combines 160,000 tweets that have already had their emoticons removed and mimics RSS feed data. Table 6.1 shows the accuracy of various algorithms on the dataset. Table 6.2 shows the comparison of various opinion mining algorithms and their sentiment and Table 6.3 shows the comparison of various opinion mining algorithms and their polarity.

6.4.1 VADER

The NLTK VADER evaluates the text's sentiment and assigns scores in three categories—negative, neutral, and positive—based on the results. The advantages of VADER including the following. (1) Texts obtained from social media and texts in general perform better when using VADER sentiment analysis. It is based on lexicons of words with subjective implications. (2) NLTK VADER is able to comprehend how emoticons, slang, capitalization, and other factors can modify the meaning of a statement. (3) If we run into NLTK VADER-related problems, we can anticipate receiving a lot more support from our colleagues thanks to the NLTK's large community and well-organized documentation.

TABLE 6.1 Performance
Evaluation on Sentimental Dataset

Algorithm	Accuracy
VADER	96.5%
TextBlob	77.2%
Pattern	75%
Transformer	72%

TABLE 6.2   Comparison of Various Opinion Mining Algorithms and Their Sentiment

Sentence	The GeoSolutions technology will leverage Benefon's GPS solutions by providing location-based search technology, a Communities Platform, location relevant multimedia content, and a new and powerful commercial model.	For the last quarter of 2010, Componeta's net sales doubled to 131 m euros from 76 m euros for the same period a year earlier, while it moved to a zero pre-tax profit from a pre-tax loss of 7 m euros.	According to the Finnish-Russian Chamber of Commerce, all the major construction companies of Finland are operating in Russia.	Circulation revenue by 5% in Finland and 4% in Sweden in 2008.
Ground Truth	Positive	Positive	Neutral	Positive
VADER	Positive	Positive	Neutral	Positive
TextBlob	Positive	Neutral	Positive	Neutral
Pattern	Positive	Neutral	Positive	Neutral
Transformer	Positive	Negative	Positive	Positive

TABLE 6.3   Comparison of Various Opinion Mining Algorithms and Their Polarity

Sentence	The GeoSolutions technology will leverage Benefon's GPS solutions by providing location-based search technology, a Communities Platform, location relevant multimedia content, and a new and powerful commercial model.	For the last quarter of 2010, Componeta's net sales doubled to 131 m euros from 76 m euros for the same period a year earlier, while it moved to a zero pre-tax profit from a pre-tax loss of 7 m euros.	According to the Finnish-Russian Chamber of Commerce, all the major construction companies of Finland are operating in Russia.	Circulation revenue by 5% in Finland and 4% in Sweden in 2008.
Ground Truth	Positive	Positive	Neutral	Positive
VADER	0.5423	0.1531	0	0.2732
TextBlob	0.2090	0	0.625	0
Pattern	0.2090	0	0.0625	0
Transformer	0.9992	0.994	0.9969	0.9964

The disadvantages of VADER include the following. (1) Compared with other libraries, it is slow. (2) Due to its high learning requirements, this library is difficult for beginners to use. (3) NLTK VADER needs extra libraries and might not be the best option for use in production.

6.4.2 TextBlob

The Python NLP package TextBlob offers high-level, straightforward APIs for fundamental NLP functionality. Beginners or those without a deep understanding of Python will find it quite helpful. It is not surprising that TextBlob includes user-friendly functions to carry out sentiment analysis with ease, given its design and purpose. The advantages of

TextBlob are as follows: (1) it is capable of optimising memory and can handle massive text corpora. (2) TextBlob processes information more quickly. (3) Because TextBlob offers features that are simpler to use, it is suggested as an excellent starting library for beginners. They can learn about fundamental tasks like sentiment analysis, Part-of-speech (POS) tagging, lemmatization, etc. with this library. The disadvantages of TextBlob include the following: (1) because of its limited feature set, users must rely on other libraries to complete more complex tasks. (2) Because TextBlob was created using NLTK, it has some of NLTK's shortcomings, which is why it is not recommended for tasks involving production.

6.4.3 Pattern

As a multifunctional library, the pattern library can be used for network analysis, data mining, machine learning, and visualization. It can download and parse PDF files and includes modules for data mining from Wikipedia, social networks, and search engines. The pattern library has a feature that allows you to extract emotion from a text string. The sentiment object in pattern is used to determine a text's polarity (positivity or negativity) as well as its subjectivity. Subjectivity values range from 0 to 1. Subjectivity measures how much information and subjective opinion are present in the text. The content contains opinion rather than information due to the text's heightened subjectivity. The advantages of pattern include the following. (1) For projects involving web mining, pattern is excellent. (2) Through pattern, we can access a variety of APIs, including those from Twitter and Facebook, which may then be used to scrape social media content. The disadvantages of Pattern include the following. (1) Pattern is still in the planning stages. (2) Changes to pattern occur once every 3–4 months and are inadequately documented, whereas updates to NLTK occur every 3–4 days. (3) Pattern also has a limited peer network.

6.4.4 Transformer

Hugging Face published a library titled Transformers. Pre-trained models are downloaded from this library for Natural Language Generation (NLG) tasks like adding additional text to a prompt or translating it into a different language, as well as Natural Language Understanding (NLU) tasks like assessing a text's sentiment. The opinionated library Transformers was created for hands-on practitioners who want to hone those models and/or serve them in production, engineers who just want to download a pre-trained model and use it to complete a specific NLP task [25], and NLP academics and educators interested in using, studying, and extending large-scale Transformer models. The advantages of Transformer are (1) decent accuracy, (2) code that is brief and simple to use, (3) simple preprocessing is sufficient, and (4) there is no tinkering with threshold levels. The disadvantages of Transformer are (1) significantly slower and (2) only employs two classes by default.

6.5 EXPERIMENTAL RESULTS

Table 6.4 shows the news feeds that were collected from three different channels for experiments: The Times of India (TOI), an Indian newspaper; BBC News, a British news outlet; and New York Times (NYT), an American news channel. The key aim of the study is

TABLE 6.4   Number of Records in the Database

News Feeds Source	Number of Records
BBC	1059+
TOI	434+
NY Times	426+

to find sentiment trends, classify them into three categories (i.e., positive, negative, and neutral), and provide effective visualisation to increase information gain based on those classifications.

The records contain details such as title, description, and publishing date and a link to the News. However, every time the app is used it retrieves and stores the most recent feeds, which means the number of records will keep increasing; this is a Cloud application to avoid scalability issues. Moreover, this data can be further used to perform in-depth analysis or even be implemented as a time-series problem. The application is divided into two parts: first it provides a quick overview of recent trends, and second, it provides an in-depth analysis and visualisation using some popular tools. Figure 6.4. depicts the sentiment and polarity score for a recent feed pulled from the TOI RSS feeds.

The left side reflects the title and description, while the right side shows its sentiment and polarity score, respectively. "Negative" refers to a compound negative score, which is reflected just below it. Negative and positive are determined based on whether the compound is less than or greater than zero. The compound score of a sentence is between −1 and +1. The higher the score, the greater the strength of the sentence being either positive or negative. This helps to get a quick overview of the news and decide whether to spend time on it or not. This is similarly done for the rest of the news channels in the study. Moreover, Figure 6.5 represents an area graph of the polarity score of the most recent feeds.

Many inferences can be made from Figure 6.5, such as the NYT most often shows a negative description trend, whereas the BBC description has the highest positive polarity.

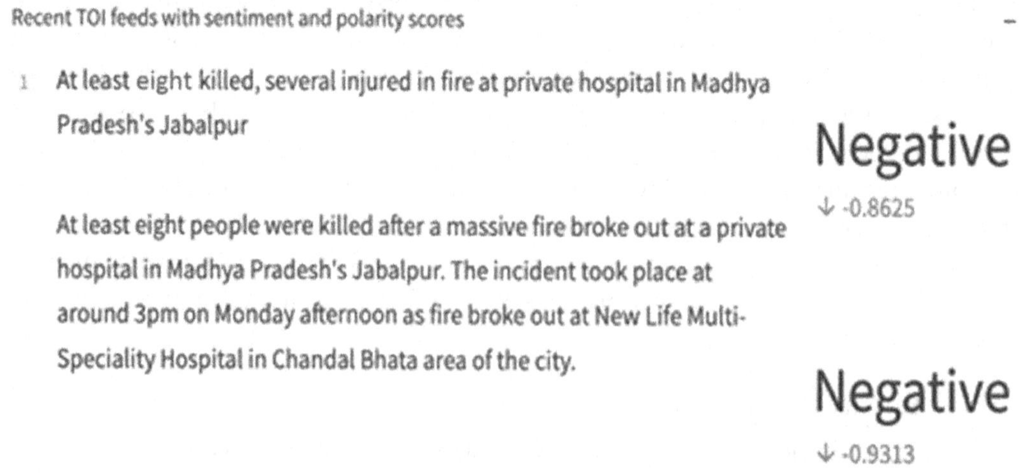

Recent TOI feeds with sentiment and polarity scores   −

1   At least eight killed, several injured in fire at private hospital in Madhya
    Pradesh's Jabalpur

Negative

↓ -0.8625

At least eight people were killed after a massive fire broke out at a private
hospital in Madhya Pradesh's Jabalpur. The incident took place at
around 3pm on Monday afternoon as fire broke out at New Life Multi-
Speciality Hospital in Chandal Bhata area of the city.

Negative

↓ -0.9313

FIGURE 6.5   TOI recent feed with its sentiment and polarity score.

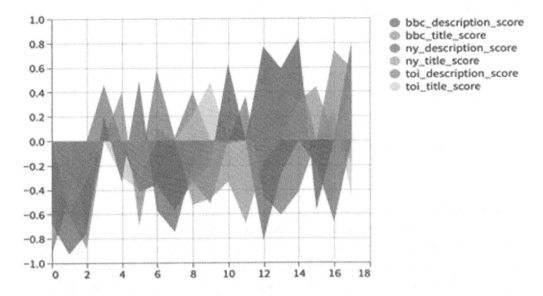

FIGURE 6.6   Area graph of news feed polarity scores.

Overall, BBC News and the NYT seem to cover most of the area, whereas TOI has the least area coverage, which suggests that TOI has a neutral polarity trend. However, this kind of inference can be easily seen on the average polarity widget on the app shown in Figure 6.6.

Figure 6.6 is a snapshot of the widget that reflects the ongoing polarity trends of the most recent data pulled from the RSS feeds (red indicates negative and green indicates positive). We can see that TOI has a strong negative polarity. Meanwhile, BBC has a polarity of –0.02, which, if rounded off, could be considered neutral. Moving on to the second part of the app, Table 6.5 shows the classification of the entire news feed dataset in terms of percentage (the database was accumulated over the period from June 2022 to July 2022). Comparing the area graph in Figure 6.5 with the percent distribution in Table 6.5, they both tell a different story. This is one of the main reasons for dividing the app into two parts, as news changes in hours and even minutes on various occasions, which allows us to carry out current trend analysis as well as historic trend analysis. According to Table 6.5, the BBC depicts an overall negative trend, whereas the NYT has a negative description and a neutral title trend. Meanwhile, TOI has a positive description and neutral title trend.

TABLE 6.5   Percentage Distribution of Sentiment-Wise Classification

Feeds	Title/Description	Positive	Negative	Neutral
BBC	Description	35.6%	37%	27.4%
	Title	25%	37.5%	36.5%
TOI	Description	38.2%	28.1%	33.6%
	Title	23.2%	31.7%	44.9%
NYT	Description	35.6%	40.8%	23.4%
	Title	24.8%	33.8%	41.3%

Average NY Times Trend
↓ -0.61005

Average TOI Trend
↓ -0.0975611111111111

Average BBC News Trend
↓ -0.02872777777777...

FIGURE 6.7 Polarity widget of ongoing polarity trend.

The percentage distribution is split into two parts, i.e., title and description, because headlines and actual news are sometimes misleading. These insights can be useful in various ways. (In making investments or business decisions, a quick overview for millennials who do not spend time reading news, etc.). Similarly, we can also use a word cloud with sentiment classification to highlight the key words in the news feeds. In the word cloud, the more particular and frequent words appear bigger and bolder in the source of the corpus. Word clouds are also known as tag clouds or text clouds [26]. Word clouds are used to identify patterns and examples that would be difficult or impossible to find in a tabular arrangement and make frequent keywords more visible. Basic terms that might be overlooked in a tabular structure are highlighted in larger text and stand out when displayed as a word cloud, as shown in Figures 6.7–6.10.

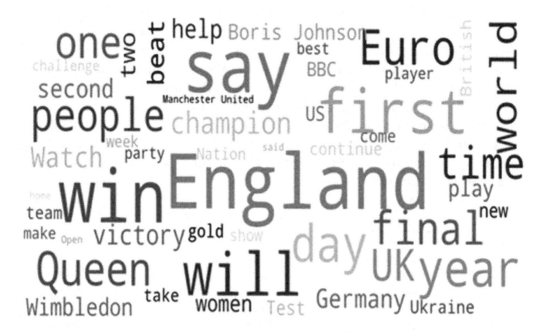

FIGURE 6.8 Prevalent words used by the BBC with positive sentiment

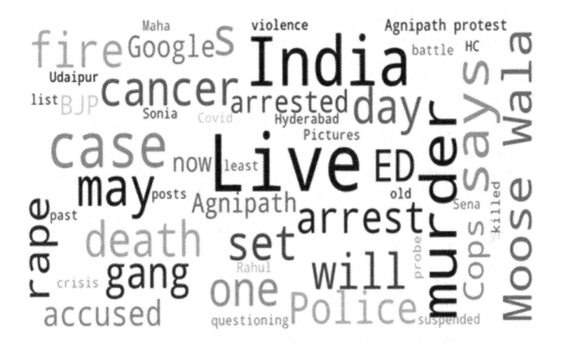

FIGURE 6.9   Prevalent words in titles used by the TOI with negative sentiment.

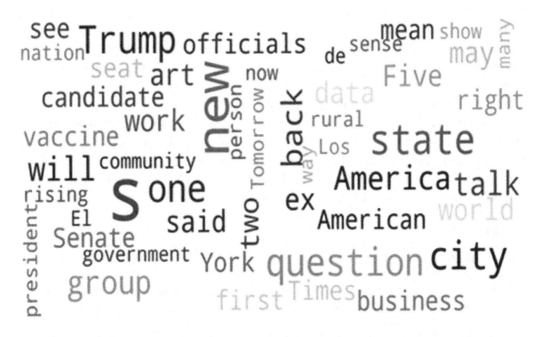

FIGURE 6.10   Prevalent words used in the NYT with neutral sentiment.

6.6 CONCLUSIONS AND FUTURE WORK

Numerous applications that could benefit from the results of sentiment analysis include news inspection, showcasing, question answering, readers' behaviour, and user behaviour. For some firms and institutions, the essential experiences from perspectives expressed online, especially through social media, are crucial, whether it concerns product feedback, open-mindedness, or the sentiments of financial experts and sentiment trends. Our novel approach creates the sentiments of day-to-day news and categorises them into three subclasses, providing a polarity score with comparison, visual analytics, and information visualization. This is done for the user's convenience, in contrast to standard supervised stock market prediction systems and Twitter data analysis. Moreover, the model uses and collects the data from the most recent RSS feeds, which, in turn, requires no training for the model. The data collected can be used to see various insights, such as feed trends followed by different news channels and overall polarity trends over time.

As covered in Section 6.4, an exhaustive study of algorithms and their accuracy, the choice of algorithm (VADER) clearly outperforms other existing algorithms and shows promising results for an unsupervised learning model. However, further research is needed to address the ambiguity and complexity of language that make automatic analysis uncertain. Moreover, thorough feature coverage and visual inspection are required because it is not always evident in advance what kinds of intriguing temporal patterns might be present in the data. The major goal of this study is to improve communication by offering a web-based RSS system that will automate the manual process. However, this can be further developed for the medical sector to track mental health on various levels [1], such as tracking the mental health of employees or kids based on texts, emails, web searches, and Internet activities. Moreover, it can also be used to filter social content to avoid cyberbullying, although this is subject to human limitations and ethical implications [16].

Most businesses typically employ sentiment analysis to learn more about their products from the perspective of their customers [21]. With the aid of this knowledge, they can adjust their marketing tactics or product lines to better appeal to consumers. However, the current use of sentiment analysis during this pandemic crisis can be to examine a person's coping methods, and this information can be used to filter out the fear sentiment and give the public information aimed at motivation and awareness [27].

REFERENCES

[1] Desklib (2022). The Internet and The Pandemic. [Online]. Available at: https://desklib.com/2022/7/20/the-internet-and-the-pandemic/

[2] De, R., Pandey, N., & Abhipsa, P. (2020). Impact of digital surge during COVID-19 pandemic: A viewpoint on research and practice. *International Journal of Information Management*, 55, 102171.

[3] Morente-Molinera, J. A., Kou, G., & Peng, Y. (2018). Analysing discussions in social networks using group decision making methods and sentiment analysis. *Information Sciences*, 447, 157–168.

[4] Haribhakta, K. D. Y. (2017). Categorization of news articles using sentiment analysis. *International Journal of Scientific Research in Computer Science, Engineering and Information Technology*, 2(5), 52–60.

[5] ChandraKala, S., & Sekharan, S. C. (2012). Opinion mining and sentiment classification: A survey. *ICTACT Journal on Soft Computing*, 3(1), 420–425.

[6] D'Andrea, A., Ferri, F., & Grifoni, P. (2015). Approaches, tools and applications for sentiment analysis implementation. *International Journal of Computer Applications*, 125(3), 26–33.

[7] Haddi, E., Liu, X., & Shi, Y. (2013). The role of text preprocessing in sentiment analysis. *Procedia Computer Science*, 17, 26–32.

[8] Miner, A. S., Chow, A., Adler, S. et al. (2016). Conversational Agents and Mental Health: Theory-Informed Assessment of Language and Affect. *Proceedings of the Fourth International Conference on Human Agent Interaction*, pp. 123–130.

[9] Bharathi, S., & Geetha, A. (2019). Sentiment analysis for online stock market news using RSS feeds. *International Journal of Current Engineering and Scientific Research*, 4(4), 58–63.

[10] Mahboob, K., Ali, F., & Nizami, H. (2019). Sentiment analysis of RSS feeds on sports news – A case study. *International Journal of Information Technology and Computer Science (IJITCS)*, 11(12), 19–29.

[11] Hutto, C., & Gilbert, E. (2014). VADER: A Parsimonious Rule-Based Model for Sentiment Analysis of Social Media Text. *Proceedings of the Eighth International AAAI Conference on Weblogs and Social Media*.

[12] Khasnis, N. S., Sen, S., & Khasnis, S. S. (2021). A machine learning approach for sentiment analysis to nurture mental health amidst COVID-19. *1st International Conference on Data Science, Machine Learning and Artificial Intelligence*, pp. 248–289.

[13] Bahrainian, S.-A., & Dengel, A. (2013). Sentiment analysis using sentiment features. *IEEE/WIC/ACM International Joint Conferences on Web Intelligence (WI) and Intelligent Agent Technologies (IAT)*, pp. 26–29.

[14] Behdenna, S., Barigou, F., & Belalem, G. (2018). Document level sentiment analysis: A survey. *EAI Endorsed Transactions on Context-Aware Systems and Applications*, 4(13), e2.

[15] Mittal, S. P. A. (2019). Sentiment Analysis on Twitter Data: A Survey. *Proceedings of the 2019 7th International Conference on Computer and Communications Management*.

[16] Gill, S. S., & Kaur, R. (2023). ChatGPT: Vision and challenges. *Internet of Things and Cyber-Physical Systems*, 3, 262–271.

[17] Nandhakumar, A. R., Baranwal, A. et al. (2024). Edgeaisim: A toolkit for simulation and modelling of AI models in edge computing environments. *Measurement: Sensors*, 31, 100939.

[18] I. C. Education, 6 April 2021. [Online]. Available at: https://www.ibm.com/uk-en/cloud/learn/rest-apis

[19] Gill, S. S. (2024). Quantum and blockchain based serverless edge computing: A vision, model, new trends and future directions. *Internet Technology Letters*, 7(1), e275.

[20] Sharma, T. Sentiment Analysis Using Pre-trained models and Transformer. (25 1 2023). [Online]. Available at: https://medium.com/@sharma.tanish096/sentiment-analysis-using-pre-trained-models-and-transformer-28e9b9486641

[21] Gill, S. S., Wu, H., Patros, P., Ottaviani, C.,. et al. (2024). Modern computing: Vision and challenges. *Telematics and Informatics Reports*, 13, 100116.

[22] Gill, S. S., Xu, M., Ottaviani, C. et al. (2022). AI for next generation computing: Emerging trends and future directions. *Internet of Things*, 19, 100514.

[23] Singh, R & Gill, S. S. (2023). Edge AI: A survey. *Internet of Things and Cyber-Physical Systems*, 3, 71–92.

[24] Go, A., Bhayani, R., & Huang, L. (2009). Twitter sentiment classification using distant supervision. *CS224N Project Report, Stanford*, 1(12), 1–6.

[25] Hugging Face. Philosophy - Hugging Face. [Online]. Available at: https://huggingface.co/docs/transformers/philosophy

[26] Gamon, M., Aue, A., & Corston-Oliver, S. (2005). Mining customer opinions from free text. *Advances in Intelligent Data Analysis*, 6, 121–132.

[27] Vanga, L. K. R., Kumar, A. et al. (2022). Machine Learning Models for Sentiment Analysis of Tweets: Comparisons and Evaluations. *In Transforming Management With AI, Big-Data, and IoT* (pp. 273–292). Springer International Publishing.

III

Economics and Finance

CHAPTER 7

Advanced Machine Learning Models for Real Estate Price Prediction

Satyam Sharma and Sukhpal Singh Gill

7.1 INTRODUCTION

The intricate nature of the real estate market, especially in the United Kingdom, serves as a testament to the myriad complexities and nuances inherent in property valuation. Recent data reveal that the UK housing market faced an unprecedented drop in August 2023, marking its most substantial dip in 5 years. This 1.9% decrease, translating to over £7,000, is attributed to rapidly escalating mortgage rates [1]. Are these complexities and economic nuances hinting at an imminent shift in the housing market?

Traditional real estate valuation was predominantly based on tangible attributes, focusing on factors like property location and size. However, the evolving era showcases a myriad of advanced techniques, from vision-based methodologies [2, 3] to the application of neural networks [4], adding depth to property assessments. Recent studies, such as those by Zhao et al. [5] and Fu et al. [6], have highlighted that while geographical attributes still play a pivotal role, emerging intangible metrics—like traffic patterns [7] and sentiments derived from social media [8]—are increasingly influencing property valuations.

7.1.1 Motivation and Our Contributions

The ever-shifting dynamics of the real estate market, compounded by broader socioeconomic factors, emphasise the significance of accurate property valuation. An oversight or miscalculation in such valuations can have far-reaching financial ramifications, affecting homeowners and the larger economic framework alike. By tapping into the potential of machine learning (ML) and artificial intelligence (AI), fused with comprehensive datasets [9], we aspire to offer improved accuracy in property valuations, acting as a bulwark against uninformed financial decisions. Our research brings forth:

- **A Comprehensive Analysis**: Drawing from the H4M "heterogeneous, multi-source, multi-modal, multi-view and multi-distributional" dataset, we conduct a comparative study of seven vital ML techniques, demonstrating their potential in predicting real estate prices.

DOI: 10.1201/9781003467199-10

- **Diverse Metric Consideration**: Utilising the comprehensive H4M dataset, our study spans 26 diverse features, from traditional property characteristics to contemporary metrics like traffic conditions and emotional sentiments, with "price" as the target.

- **Robustness in Prediction**: The random forest model, with its remarkable accuracy, underscores its dominance in real estate price prediction.

- **Macroeconomic Influences**: Our analysis, especially in the realm of ML-based predictions, provides stakeholders with an advanced toolset to anticipate and navigate the challenges posed by macroeconomic factors like inflation. By enhancing prediction accuracy and reliability, stakeholders can better prepare and strategise in the face of economic adversity.

7.2 RELATED WORKS

In the expanding world of real estate valuation and analysis, Zhao et al. [5] delivered the pioneering work "PATE" for real estate price prediction using the H4M dataset. They employed linear regression and XGBoost to forecast property prices, setting the stage for future research. Their technique skilfully combined property details, neighbourhood features, traffic data, and public emotions, highlighting the multilayered factors behind property pricing. There have been many studies shedding light on the nuances of property valuation. For instance, You et al. [2] explored how images can help determine the visual appeal of properties. Similarly, neural networks have been brought into play by McGreal et al. [4] emphasising their utility in predicting residential values. A pivotal dimension of real estate analysis revolves around geographical dependencies, as noted by Fu et al. [6], who combined ranking and clustering to harness these dependencies. Studies by Wardrip [10] about public transport's effect on property prices and research by Cortright [11] and Hamilton & Dourado [12] about walkability's economic impact show the variety of elements influencing property prices. Urban charm and cultural significance are also pivotal, as highlighted by Wang et al. [13] and Hristova et al. [14]. De Nadai and Lepri [15] discussed how urban surroundings impact property values. With the advent of novel datasets like H4M, researchers, including [16], have heralded a new era in socioeconomic analytics, magnifying the lens through which urban real estate is assessed. This evolving area promises exciting breakthroughs and in-depth studies, as our research aims to demonstrate [17]. To further elucidate the methodologies employed in a recent study on the H4M dataset, Table 7.1 summarises the comparison of methodologies on the H4M dataset.

TABLE 7.1 Comparison of Methodologies on the H4M Dataset

Study	Methodologies Used for Price Prediction
Zhao et al. [6]	Linear regression, XGBoost
This study	Linear regression, XGBoost, AdaBoost, CatBoost, random forest, KNN regressor, MLP neural network

7.3 DATA EXPLORATION AND PREPROCESSING

In the section, we discuss about dataset and its preprocessing.

7.3.1 Dataset Description and Refinement

Our study leverages data from the H4M dataset, an exhaustive compilation encapsulating information on 28,550 houses located in Beijing, China. Available for public access at H4M dataset, this dataset originally consisted of 29 columns. To enhance clarity and improve model performance, certain modifications were made. Specifically, we dropped the "id" column, as it served only as a unique identifier and held no intrinsic predictive value. Simultaneously, we excluded the "TtlPrc" column to circumvent multicollinearity concerns, recognising that this variable could be inferred from "Unit Price" and other attributes—thus risking data leakage and model destabilisation. The "UntPrc" label was subsequently renamed "Price" for improved interpretability. The final dataset encapsulates 27 features that span properties, amenities, traffic, and emotional metrics, with "Price" as the target variable. Table 7.2 offers a concise description of each feature, its category, and its role within the dataset.

TABLE 7.2   Dataset Descriptions (H4M Dataset)

Feature ID	Category	Feature Name	Description
0	Property	Year	Year when the building was constructed
1	Property	Elvt	Indicates if the building contains an elevator
2	Property	RmNum	Total bedrooms in the residence
3	Property	H11Num	Count of living and dining areas in the residence
4	Property	KchNum	Total kitchens inside the residence
5	Property	BthNum	Total bathroom within the residence
6	Property	Lat	Geographical latitude of the residence
7	Property	Lng	Geographical longitude of the residence
8	Amenity	TspNum	Count of nearby transportation facilities
9	Amenity	TspDst	Average proximity to nearby transportation facilities
10	Amenity	AtrNum	Count of tourist spots in the vicinity
11	Amenity	AtrDst	Mean distant to nearby tourist spots
12	Amenity	EdcNum	Count of educational institutions in the vicinity
13	Amenity	EdcDst	Mean distance to nearby educational institutions
14	Amenity	HthNum	Count of healthcare facilities around the residence
15	Amenity	HthDst	Average distance to these healthcare facilities
16	Amenity	RstNum	Count of restaurants in the vicinity
17	Amenity	RstDst	Average distance to these restaurants
18	Amenity	RtlNum	Count of retail outlets in the vicinity
19	Amenity	RtlDst	Mean distance to these retail outlets
20	Traffic	Trfv	Daily average traffic speed
21	Amenity	AgrPct	Portion of anger emotions from total
22	Amenity	DstPct	Portion of aversion emotions from total
23	Amenity	HppPct	Portion of joy emotions from total
24	Amenity	SadPct	Portion of sorrow emotions from total
25	Amenity	FeaPct	Portion of fear emotions from total
26	Property	Price	Cost per square meter of the residence in the Renminbi (RMBa)

7.3.2 Preprocessing and Model Preparation

Initial inspection revealed an absence of missing values across all data columns, negating the need for imputation. For consistency and to ensure optimal model compatibility, each data element underwent type conversion to float [18]. A correlation matrix, computing the pairwise correlation between the features using Pearson's method, was subsequently plotted as shown in Figure 7.1. This matrix provided insights into feature interrelations and their associations with our target variable, "Price". We visualised this correlation matrix using a heatmap, masking the redundant upper triangle, making it straightforward to identify the relationships between features at a glance.

From our correlation matrix, we observed that the correlation coefficients (denoted as "r") between "Price" and other variables were confined within the range of [−0.2, 0.4]. Such observations underscore the importance of not relying on just a few features for predicting real estate prices. Rather than focusing solely on select attributes, a comprehensive evaluation of all features is crucial because every attribute can jointly enhance prediction accuracy and resilience.

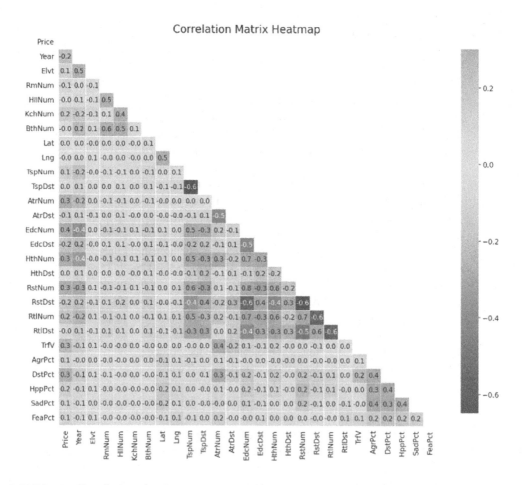

FIGURE 7.1   Correlation matrix.

TABLE 7.3   Outlier Distribution Across Variables

Column_1	Number of Outliers	Column_2	Number of Outliers
Price	236	EdcDst	239.0
Year	236	HthNum	263.0
Elvt	0	HthDst	827.0
RmNum	368	RstNum	614.0
HllNum	240	RstDst	421.0
KchNum	1132	RtlNum	0.0
BthNum	210	RtlDst	207.0
Lat	30	TrfV	83.0
Lng	25	AgrPct	353.0
TspNum	0	DstPct	251.0
TspDst	233	HppPct	1425.0
AtrNum	76	SadPct	1493.0
AtrDst	5	FeaPct	168.0
EdcNum	0	-	-

Subsequently, we determined the presence of outliers through the application of the z-score technique. While conducting outlier detection (Table 7.3), we made a deliberate choice to retain these data points in our analysis, aligning with the methodology adopted in [5]. The decision to keep outliers was grounded in several considerations:

- **Nature of Real Estate Data**: Given the intrinsic variability of real estate, some outliers may be emblematic of unique properties, providing crucial insights into distinct price ranges.

- **Influential Data Points**: Within the real estate sphere, outliers often serve as pivotal data points. Their exclusion could jeopardise the model's ability to generalise effectively to diverse real-world scenarios.

- **Commitment to Comprehensive Analysis**: To ensure fidelity to both the dataset's inherent character and the referenced paper's approach, it is vital to incorporate every data point, facilitating a thorough examination.

- **Revelatory Potential of Outliers**: Outliers are not merely anomalies; they can spotlight patterns or tendencies that would otherwise remain obscured. Such outliers might correspond to luxury residences, heritage properties, or other singular listings that enrich the analysis.

In summary, our decision to preserve outliers stems from a desire to capture the full spectrum of data variations, thereby creating a predictive model that is both robust and versatile, echoing the rationale presented by Zhao et al. [5].

Finally, to facilitate ML applications, the dataset was partitioned into training and testing subsets following a 7:3 ratio. Additionally, we introduced an empty "model_metrics" DataFrame, architecture to document and compare the performance of diverse ML models throughout our study.

7.4 MODELLING TECHNIQUES AND ARCHITECTURES

In the section, we discuss ML models utilised in this research work.

7.4.1 Linear Regression

The linear regression model, a stalwart in statistical analytics, seeks to delineate the relationship between a target variable and its predictors through a linear equation [19]. It is predicated on the minimisation of the sum of squared differences between actual and estimated outcomes. We used the "LinearRegression" module from the "scikit-learn" library in this research. The model was trained using our partitioned training data, and predictions were subsequently made on both training and testing sets. For assessing the effectiveness of our model on the training dataset, we considered a range of evaluation criteria, namely R^2 (Equation 7.1), its adjusted version (Equation 7.2), the average absolute error (mean absolute error [MAE]) (Equation 7.3), squared average error (mean squared error [MSE]) (Equation 7.4), and the square root of the latter (root-mean squared error [RMSE]) (Equation 7.5). Similar metrics were determined for the test set, ensuring a robust evaluation of the model's efficacy on unseen data. To gauge the effectiveness of our linear regression model, we plotted the test data's actual prices against the predicted ones (see Figure 7.5). The dashed line represents the ideal line of best fit. If the predictions were spot on, all points would align along this line. This visualisation provides a clear view of how our predictions measure up against the actual prices.

7.4.2 XGBoost Regressor

Extreme gradient boosting, often termed XGBoost, operates as an optimised distributed gradient boosting algorithm designed to enhance computational speed and forecast precision. By integrating decision trees in a sequential manner where subsequent trees aim to rectify errors made by prior ones, XGBoost showcases a robust mechanism against overfitting, rendering it an ideal choice for diverse regression problems [20]. For our endeavour, the XGBRegressor from the XGBoost suite was harnessed. Once we instantiated the regressor, it was then trained using our earmarked training subset. Post training, predictions were solicited from both the training and testing datasets. Analytical metrics, encompassing R^2, Adjusted R^2, MAE, MSE, and RMSE, were computed to appraise the model's performance on the training data. An analogous assessment was carried out for the test dataset, thereby ensuring a rigorous scrutiny of the model's predictive prowess on unexplored data. One of the salient offerings of the XGBoost framework is its ability to rank features based on their importance. To that end, we derived the importance scores from our trained model. These scores offer insight into the influence each feature exerts on the model's predictions. To vividly portray this, we arranged the features in descending order of their importance scores and encapsulated them in a bar chart (Figure 7.6). Each bar colour from the "viridis" palette captures the gradient of importance, while annotated percentages, affixed adjacent to the bars, quantify the degree of influence.

7.4.3 AdaBoost Regressor

The AdaBoost (Adaptive Boosting) approach serves as a dynamic ensemble method, meticulously designed to fortify the performance of ML models. It operates by orchestrating a cavalcade of weak learners, typically decision trees, in an effort to cumulatively enhance their predictive capabilities [21]. At its core, AdaBoost thrives by attributing emphasis on instances that are habitually misclassified, compelling subsequent models in the ensemble to address these missteps with heightened precision. In the context of our investigative foray, the "AdaBoostRegressor" derived from the "sklearn.ensemble" suite was enlisted. The regressor was instantiated with specific hyperparameters: "n_estimators" set to 100, "learning_rate" at 0.1, and a fixed "random_state" of 42. Upon this configuration, the model was then trained with our designated training dataset. Subsequent to this indoctrination, we beckoned predictions from the model for both training and testing subsets. To ensure a holistic evaluation of the model's prowess, we calculated an array of evaluative metrics, which encompassed R^2, Adjusted R^2, MAE, MSE, and RMSE, for the training dataset. A symmetrical assessment was executed for the test data, thereby facilitating a comprehensive appraisal of the model's generalisation capabilities on untapped data segments.

7.4.4 CatBoost Regressor

CatBoost ("Categorical Boosting"), is a state-of-the-art gradient boosting algorithm. Its intricate design boosts computational efficiency and prediction accuracy [22]. When building decision trees in a sequential fashion, each tree is tasked with mending the mistakes of its predecessors. This approach ensures that CatBoost offers a strong resilience against overfitting, positioning it as a premier tool for various regression tasks.

For our analytical venture, we employed the CatBoostRegressor from the CatBoost library. The regressor was instantiated with specific hyperparameters: iterations set to 1000, learning_rate at 0.1, depth calibrated to 6, verbosity set to 0 for silent operation, and a fixed random_seed of 42. Rigorously trained using our demarcated training ensemble, the model's predictions were derived from both our training and test datasets. A suite of metrics, including R^2, Adjusted R^2, MAE, MSE, and RMSE, were used to critically evaluate its performance on the training samples. A parallel appraisal was executed on the test data, serving as a comprehensive review of the model's predictive capabilities on fresh data.

Another key facet of our exploration was feature importance. Using CatBoost's built-in capabilities, we fetched importance scores, shedding light on each feature's predictive influence. These were neatly arranged in a descending order and portrayed in a bar chart, with the "viridis" palette highlighting the gradation of significance (Figure 7.7). Alongside, annotated percentages quantified their influence, serving as a tangible guide for future feature selection strategies.

7.4.5 Random Forest Regressor

Random forest, emblematic of its name, is a paradigmatic ensemble learning approach that establishes a multitude of decision trees at the time of training and yields the mean prediction of the individual trees for regression problems [18]. Characterised by its intricate architecture, random forest not only minimises overfitting, often encountered with individual decision trees, but also augments generalisation. The inherent randomness, as inferred from its nomenclature, offers a blend of diverse models, ensuring a robust and comprehensive predictive framework.

During our analytical journey, we employed the "RandomForestRegressor" from the sklearn.ensemble package. For accuracy and consistency, we set specific hyperparameters for the regressor: n_estimators were fixed at 100, and random_state was chosen as 42. Based on these settings, we trained the model with our selected training data. After training, the model made predictions on both the training and testing sets. To evaluate its performance, we measured a range of metrics, including R^2, Adjusted R^2, MAE, MSE, and RMSE, for the training data. Similarly, we analysed the test data to understand the model's capability to predict unseen data accurately.

To delve deeper into the model's performance, we utilised scatter plots, comparing actual to predicted prices from the random forest regressor. A diagonal dashed line served as our perfect prediction benchmark. For clarity, we segmented our analysis into training and test data, with the test data scatter illustrating the model's predictive precision (Figure 7.4).

Another intriguing aspect of random forest is its feature ranking capability. We extracted these importance scores and represented them in a descending bar chart (Figure 7.8). This visualisation, complemented by annotated percentages, provided a lucid snapshot of each feature's significance in the prediction process.

7.4.6 K-Nearest Neighbours Regressor

Within the broad spectrum of regression techniques, K-nearest neighbours (KNN) stands out as an instance-based learning approach. This method hinges on the simple premise that data points with proximate attributes tend to share similar outcomes. Unlike models that rely on a predetermined equation for predictions, KNN evaluates the proximity of an input to its neighbours in the dataset to make informed inferences.

As we navigated this analytical landscape, we incorporated the "KNeighborsRegressor" from the "sklearn.neighbors" module. In pursuit of optimisation, we undertook a meticulous cross-validation procedure to discern the most conducive number of neighbours, culminating in the selection of optimal value of k. With this parameter in place, we trained the model on our chosen training data. Predictions were subsequently elicited from the trained model, spanning both training and testing sets. To gauge the model's efficacy, we harnessed several metrics, namely R^2, Adjusted R^2, MAE, MSE, and RMSE for the training data. This evaluative approach was consistently applied to the test data, furnishing a holistic view of the model's aptitude in handling fresh datasets.

7.4.7 Neural Network Regressor: MLP

The multilayer perceptron (MLP), a class of feedforward artificial neural network, invokes a network of artificial neurons arranged in sequential layers [20]. This meticulously crafted structure allows it to adapt and process intricate relationships within data through an orchestrated flow of computations. An MLP is emblematic of its distinct architecture, consisting of at least three layers: an input layer, one or more hidden layers, and an output layer. The nonlinear activation functions within the hidden layers permitting the network to capture complex nonlinear patterns. This adaptability not only offers versatility in modelling diverse challenges but also makes the MLP adept at regression tasks, moulding it into a potent tool for both classification and continuous predictive analyses.

Before delving into the neural intricacies of the MLP, it is paramount to address its foundational requirement. The MLP thrives on standardised input data, prompting us to apply the "StandardScaler". This normalisation process ensures all input features inhabit a similar scale, enhancing the network's training efficacy and ensuring seamless convergence. Prior to model training, we reserved 20% of the training data for validation, ensuring an unbiased evaluation of the model's fit. This validation set aids in fine-tuning the model's performance before testing.

With our data now harmoniously scaled, we embarked on crafting our MLP using the "keras.Sequential" method. This model's architecture emerges as follows:

- **Input Layer**: There are 256 neurons that are adorned with a ReLU activation function. The inclusion of L2 regularisation (lambda of 0.001) aims to mitigate overfitting, complemented by a 0.3 dropout rate to infuse randomness.

- **Second Layer**: A dense layer with 128 neurons, once more brandishing the ReLU activation, is supported by L2 regularisation and followed by a 0.3 dropout layer.

- **Intermediate Layers**: A 64-neuron dense layer, again with ReLU activations, is coupled with a 0.2 dropout layer, swiftly succeeded by a 32-neuron dense layer with the ReLU signature.

- **Output Layer**: Our ensemble culminates in a single neuron, underscoring our regression task, standing ready to dispense predictions.

Guiding our model's learning phase is the "Adam" optimiser, lauded for its adaptiveness. A calibrated learning rate of 0.0005 ensures steady yet efficient convergence during training.

Once trained, the model flexed its predictive muscles over both training and testing datasets. Metrics such as R^2, Adjusted R^2, MAE, MSE, and RMSE were harnessed to encapsulate its forecasting prowess, shedding light on the model's performance in both familiar and novel scenarios.

7.4.8 Performance Metrics for Model Evaluation

We have used the following metrics for model evaluation.

- **R-squared (R^2)**: The R^2 metric indicates how well our independent factors (features) can explain variations in the dependent factor (house prices). A greater R^2 suggests that our model's predictions align more closely with the actual outcomes. Think of it as a measure of the model's explanatory power.

$$R^2 = 1 - \frac{SS_{Res}}{SS_{Tot}} \tag{7.1}$$

- **Adjusted R-squared**: While the R^2 value tells us about the variance captured by our model, the adjusted version refines this by considering the number of predictors in the model. It is particularly useful when there are many variables in play, ensuring you're not just adding noise.

$$\text{Adjusted } R^2 = 1 - \frac{(1-R^2)(n-1)}{n-k-1} \tag{7.2}$$

- **MAE**: This is a plain and simple way to understand our model's precision. It calculates the mean difference between what our model predicts and the real values. Lower values are preferred, as they signify fewer deviations.

$$\text{MAE} = \frac{1}{n} \sum_{i=1}^{n} \left| y_i - \hat{y_i} \right| \tag{7.3}$$

- **MSE**: A bit different from MAE, this metric squares the differences between predicted and actual values. This means it is especially sensitive to big mistakes. A model with a lower MSE is more reliable.

$$\text{MSE} = \frac{1}{n} \sum_{i=1}^{n} \left(y_i - \hat{y_i} \right)^2 \tag{7.4}$$

- **RMSE**: Think of this as the average error our model might make in its predictions. It is derived from the MSE and provides insights into the spread of residuals or errors the model produces. Again, smaller values here are better.

$$\text{RMSE} = \sqrt{\text{MSE} = \frac{1}{n} \sum_{i=1}^{n} \left(y_i - \hat{y_i} \right)^2} \tag{7.5}$$

7.5 RESULTS AND DISCUSSIONS

In this section, we delve into the performance of a diverse set of regression models and neural network applied to H4M real estate data. By comparing a mixture of traditional and advanced models, we aim to understand which algorithms best capture the nuances of our dataset. Detailed model performance metrics are presented in Table 7.4.

TABLE 7.4 Model Performance Metrics Overview

Method	R^2	Adjusted R^2	MAE	MSE	RMSE
Linear regression	0.3651	0.3632	15235	402302484	20057
XGBoost regressor	0.8770	0.8766	5721	77956264	8829
AdaBoost regressor	0.4647	0.4631	14789	339217236	18418
CatBoost regressor	0.8778	0.8774	5718	77455852	8801
Random forest regressor	0.8937	0.8934	4931	67333749	8206
K-nearest neighbours regressor	0.8066	0.8060	6276	122545585	11070
MLP neural network	0.8380	0.8375	6829	102670766	10133

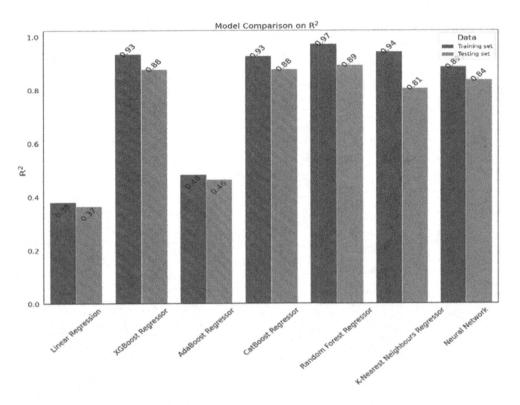

FIGURE 7.2 R^2 performance of all the models.

Figures 7.2 and 7.3 show the R^2 and RMSE performance visualisation of all the models. Model visualisations in terms of predicted vs. actual values and feature importance graphs are shown in Figures 7.4–7.8.

7.5.1 Individual Model Analysis

In this section, we analyse the experimental results of different models.

- **Linear Regression**:

    - **Benchmark Comparison**: Our linear regression model's R^2 (Equation 7.1) of 0.3651 on the test set closely matches the findings from [5], setting a reference point for further comparisons (refer to Table 7.4 and Figure 7.2 for detailed outputs and visualisations, respectively).

    - **Error Insights**: The test set MAE (Equation 7.3), MSE (Equation 7.4), and RMSE (Equation 7.5 and Figure 7.3) values stand at 15,235, 402,302,484, and 20,057 respectively.

    - **Visualisations Interpretation**: As shown in Figure 7.5, the "predicted vs. actual" plot for linear regression reveals significant scatter and deviation from the ideal diagonal line, underlining the challenges faced by this model in accurately predicting the real estate values for our dataset.

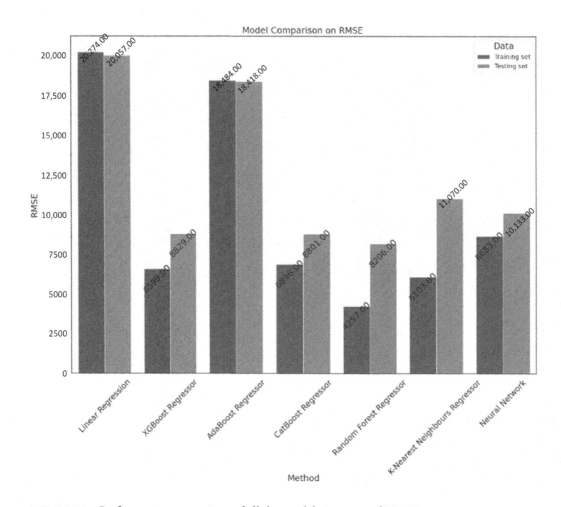

FIGURE 7.3   Performance comparison of all the models in terms of RMSE.

- **XGBoost Regressor**:
  - **Benchmark Comparison**: Our metrics align well with the benchmarks presented by Zhao et al. [5], showcasing XGBoost's consistent ability to handle complex data (refer to Table 7.4 and Figure 7.2 for detailed outputs and visualisations, respectively).

  - **Error Insights**: On the test set, the model produced a commendably low MAE of 5721 and an RMSE of 8829 (Figure 7.3).

  - **Visualisations Interpretation**: As shown in Figure 7.6, the feature importance chart underscores that the count of educational institutions nearby emerges as a prime influencer at 19.17%, reiterating the emphasis on local education facilities. This is followed by the geographical coordinates with latitude registering 14.12% and longitude at 11.72%. Moreover, the count of neighbouring tourist spots at

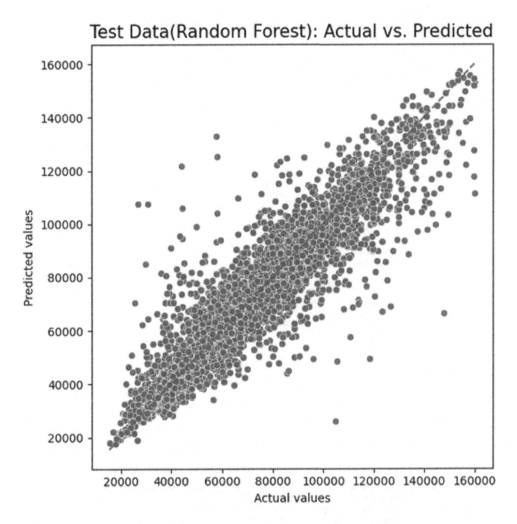

FIGURE 7.4 Predicted vs. actual values for the best performing model for the random forest regressor.

13.13% further accentuates the significance of a property's surrounding attractions. Collectively, these factors highlight the pivotal role of location and adjacent amenities in determining real estate values.

- **AdaBoost Regressor**:

  - **Performance Insights**: With an R^2 of 0.4647 on the test set, AdaBoost demonstrates reasonable predictive capabilities (refer to Table 7.4 and Figure 7.2 for detailed outputs and visualisations, respectively).

  - **Error Insights**: Test set MAE and RMSE values come in at 14,789 and 18,418, respectively.

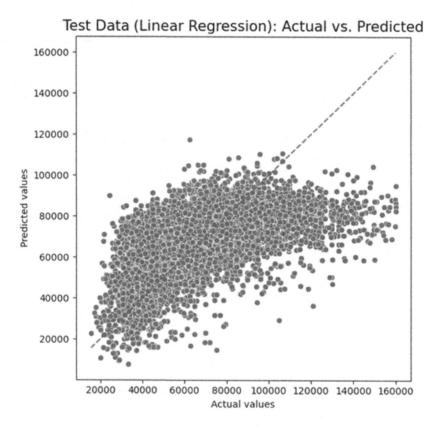

FIGURE 7.5   Predicted vs. actual values for the worst performing model for linear regression.

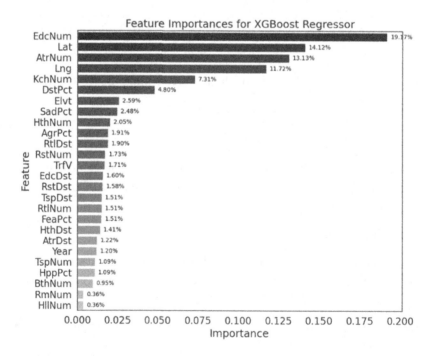

FIGURE 7.6   Feature importance for XGBoost regressor.

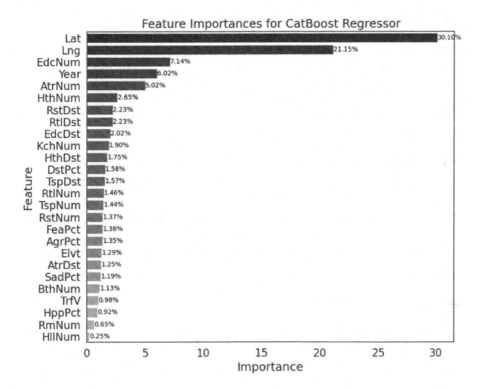

FIGURE 7.7 Feature importance for CatBoost regressor.

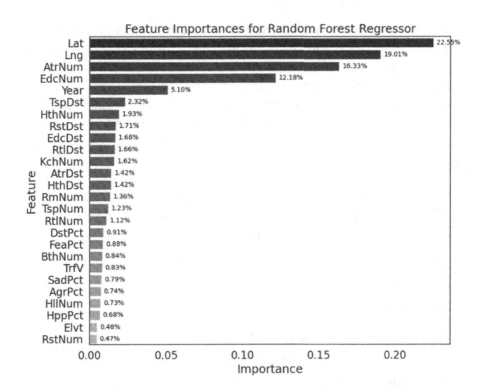

FIGURE 7.8 Feature importance for random forest regressor.

- **CatBoost Regressor**:

  - **Performance Insights**: Boasting an R^2 of 0.8778 on the test set, a marginal yet valuable improvement over the XGBoost benchmark [5] (refer to Table 7.4 and Figure 7.2 for detailed outputs and visualisations, respectively).

  - **Error Insights**: It competes closely with XGBoost, evidenced by the nearly equivalent MAE and RMSE values on the test set.

  - **Visualisations Interpretation**: As shown in Figure 7.7, the feature importance analysis for the CatBoost model reveals that geographical factors are pivotal, with latitude leading at 30.10% and longitude closely following at 21.15%. Additionally, the presence of nearby educational institutions, with an influence score of 7.14%, underlines the consistent emphasis on the importance of local educational facilities. Together, these determinants underscore the central role of a property's location and the educational landscape in shaping real estate valuations.

- **Random Forest Regressor**:

  - **Stellar Performance**: Notably, our random forest model achieved an R^2 of 0.8937 on the test set, marking a clear advancement over benchmarks from Zhao et al. [5] (refer to Table 7.4 and Figure 7.2 for detailed outputs and visualisations, respectively).

  - **Error Insights**: The model boasts the lowest MAE and RMSE values on the test set at 4931 and 8206, respectively.

  - **Visualisations Interpretation**: As shown in Figure 7.4, the "predicted vs. actual" graph for the random forest regressor showcases a nearly perfect diagonal line, reinforcing the model's exceptional performance on this dataset. The feature importance graph in Figure 7.8 highlights that a property's geographical location (latitude at 22.55% and longitude at 19.01%) plays a paramount role in predictions, closely followed by nearby tourist spots (16.33%) and educational institutions (12.8%), emphasising the value of location and local amenities in real estate.

- **KNN**:

  - **Performance Insights**: The KNN model yielded an R^2 of 0.8066 on the test set, reflecting its strength in modelling local patterns (refer to Table 7.4 and Figure 7.2 for detailed outputs and visualisations, respectively).

  - **Error Insights**: MAE and RMSE values on the test set are 6276 and 11,070, respectively.

- **Neural Network Regressor: MLP**:

  - **Performance Insights**: The MLP model achieved an R^2 of 0.8380 on the test set (refer to Table 7.4 and Figure 7.2 for detailed outputs and visualisations, respectively).

  - **Error Insights**: Test set MAE and RMSE values are 6829 and 10,133, respectively.

7.5.2 Model Performance Discussion

Linear regression might fall short due to its linear assumptions, which cannot always model the intricate, nonlinear relationships often present in real estate data. AdaBoost's performance might not be on par with other ensemble methods due to its sensitivity to outliers and noise in the dataset [22]. KNN relies heavily on distance metrics and might be less efficient when dealing with high-dimensional datasets. Feature scaling is essential, and any irrelevant features can heavily influence predictions. The neural network regressor (MLP) may require more meticulous hyperparameter tuning, a different architecture, or a larger dataset to train on to achieve peak performance. The results draw attention to the superiority of ensemble models, especially random forest, CatBoost, and XGBoost, for this dataset. The nature of these models, which combine multiple individual predictions, offers them a unique ability to reduce both variance and bias. We will further delve into the implications of these findings in the conclusion.

7.6 CONCLUSIONS AND FUTURE WORK

Real estate prediction, as our study has demonstrated, remains a multifaceted task where traditional methods, while informative, may sometimes falter against the depth and complexity of modern datasets. Among the many ML methods that have been used on the H4M dataset, ensemble models—especially the random forest, CatBoost, and XGBoost—have proven to be the most effective. These models combine many individual predictions to reduce both variance and bias at the same time. Our research affirms the pivotal role of geographical factors, notably latitude and longitude, in determining property valuations. This assertion is further strengthened by the high scores of latitudes, longitudes, and proximity features such as nearby tourist spots and educational institutions in the feature importance visualisations of our three best performing models: random forest, CatBoost, and XGBoost (refer to Figures 7.8, 7.7, and 7.6 for the visualisations, respectively). This underscores the imperativeness of evaluating a property within its broader context. While advancements in algorithms have enhanced prediction accuracy, it is evident that the rich tapestry of location, amenities, and socioeconomic dynamics plays a crucial role in understanding property valuations in their entirety.

7.6.1 Future Work

The current models have demonstrated commendable performance, yet there is still room for optimisation. Advanced techniques for hyperparameter tuning can be employed to refine these models, pushing the boundaries of predictive accuracy further [22]. Particularly, there is significant potential to enhance the MLP neural network. By adjusting its core design, experimenting with varied activation methods, and exploring new training techniques, it might be possible to improve its prowess in predicting real estate valuations. Additionally, there are numerous factors that influence the multifaceted field of real estate valuation. The incorporation of more varied datasets, such as time-series data reflecting economic growth, historical pricing trends, or in-depth neighbourhood profiles, can offer a richer context. This, in turn, can be pivotal in boosting the model's predictive accuracy.

Continuing on this trajectory the rapid influx of diverse data streams, like live traffic updates, local events, and air quality indices, presents an opportunity for data augmentation. Integrating these dynamic elements into the existing dataset can further sharpen the model's predictive edge [21]. Additionally, while the ensemble methods have been impressive, there is intrigue in the possible synergies between ensemble models and neural networks [22]. Venturing into hybrid architectures may unearth even more profound insights [20]. As data science techniques evolve relentlessly and data sources continue to expand, the realm of real estate analytics remains ripe with opportunities for further exploration and innovative breakthroughs.

REFERENCES

[1] Smith, H., & Frost, G. (2023). "Will house prices fall in 2023?" *Times Money Mentor*. [Online Available]. https://www.thetimes.co.uk/money-mentor/buying-home/will-house-prices-fall-uk

[2] You, Q., Pang, R., Cao, L., & Luo, J. (2017). Image-based appraisal of real estate properties. *IEEE Transactions on Multimedia*, 19(12), 2751–2759.

[3] Poursaeed, O., Matera, T., & Belongie, S. (2018). Vision-based real estate price estimation. *Machine Vision and Applications*, 29(4), 667–676.

[4] McGreal, S., Adair, A., McBurney, D., & Patterson, D., 1998. Neural networks: The prediction of residential values. *Journal of Property Valuation and Investment*, 16, 57–70.

[5] Zhao, Y., Ravi, R., Shi, S., Wang, Z., Lam, E. Y., & Zhao, J. (2022). PATE: Property, amenities, traffic and emotions coming together for real estate price prediction. *2022 IEEE 9th International Conference on Data Science and Advanced Analytics (DSAA)*, pp. 1–10. IEEE.

[6] Fu, Y., Xiong, H., Ge, Y., Yao, Z., Zheng, Y., & Zhou, Z.-H. (2014). Exploiting Geographic Dependencies for Real Estate Appraisal: A Mutual Perspective of Ranking and Clustering. *Proceedings of the 20th ACM SIGKDD International Conference on Knowledge Discovery and Data Mining*, pp. 1047–1056.

[7] Zhou, B., Liu, J., Cui, S., & Zhao, Y. (2022). Largescale traffic congestion prediction based on multimodal fusion and representation mapping. *IEEE International Conference on Data Science and Advanced Analytics*. IEEE.

[8] Fan, R., Zhao, J., Chen, Y., & Xu, K. (2014). Anger is more influential than joy: Sentiment correlation in Weibo. *PLoS One*, 9(10), e110184.

[9] Gill, S. S., Wu, H., Patros, P., Ottaviani, C. et al. (2024). Modern computing: Vision and challenges. *Telematics and Informatics Reports*, 13, 100116.

[10] Wardrip, K. (2011). Public Transit's Impact on Housing Costs: A Review of the Literature. http://www.reconnectingamerica.org/assets/Uploads/TransitImpactonHsgCostsfinal-Aug1020111.pdf

[11] Cortright, J. (2009). *Walking the Walk: How Walkability Raises Home Values in US Cities*. CEOs for Cities.

[12] Hamilton, E., & Dourado, E. (2018). The premium for walkable development under land use regulations. *SSRN Electronic Journal*, 1–22,.

[13] Wang, W., Yang, S., He, Z., Wang, M., Zhang, J., & Zhang, W. (2018). Urban perception of commercial activeness from satellite images and streetscapes. *Companion Proceedings of the Web Conference 2018*, pp. 647–654.

[14] Hristova, D., Aiello, L. M., & Quercia, D. (2018). The new urban success: How culture pays. *Frontiers in Physics*, 6, 27.

[15] De Nadai, M., & Lepri, B. (2018). The economic value of neighbourhoods: Predicting real estate prices from the urban environment. *2018 IEEE 5th International Conference on Data Science and Advanced Analytics (DSAA)*, pp. 323–330. IEEE.

[16] Zhao, Y., Ravi, R., Shi, S., Wang, Z., Lam, E. Y., & Zhao, J. (2022). H4m: Heterogeneous, multi-source, multimodal, multi-view and multi-distributional dataset for socioeconomic analytics in case of Beijing. *IEEE International Conference on Data Science and Advanced Analytics*. IEEE.

[17] Gill, S. S., Xu, M., Ottaviani, C. et al. (2022). AI for next generation computing: Emerging trends and future directions. *Internet of Things*, 19, 100514.

[18] Gill, S. S., & Kaur, R. (2023). ChatGPT: Vision and challenges. *Internet of Things and Cyber-Physical Systems*, 3, 262–271.

[19] Nandhakumar, A. R., Baranwal, A. et al. (2024). Edgeaisim: A toolkit for simulation and modelling of AI models in edge computing environments. *Measurement: Sensors*, 31, 100939.

[20] Dhingra, S., Singh, M., Vaisakh, S.B. et al. (2023). Mind meets machine: Unravelling GPT-4's cognitive psychology. *BenchCouncil Transactions on Benchmarks, Standards and Evaluations*, 3(3), 100139.

[21] Singh, R. & Gill, S. S. (2023). Edge AI: A survey. *Internet of Things and Cyber-Physical Systems*, 3, 71–92.

[22] Walia, G. K., Kumar, M., & Gill, S. S. (2024). AI-empowered fog/edge resource management for IoT applications: A comprehensive review, research challenges and future perspectives. *IEEE Communications Surveys & Tutorials*, 26(1), 619–669.

CHAPTER 8

Stock Market Price Prediction

A Hybrid LSTM and Sequential Self-Attention-Based Approach

Karan Pardeshi, Sukhpal Singh Gill, and Ahmed M. Abdelmoniem

8.1 INTRODUCTION

Utilising historical stock prices within a certain time period is the most crucial step for investors and businesses to forecast future sales and any potential negative earnings. Many researchers and investors who desire to speculate within the stock exchange are lured to that since its fundamentals include high risk and great returns [1]. In the past, the main methods used for determining the value of a developing business were to estimate the profits and incomes and then apply the appropriate cash flow discount rate to those predictions [2]. However, an organisation may use this conventional method for forecasting earnings, provided that it has enough data on performance, positive earnings, or comparable enterprises. We try to solve this issue by giving financial managers and investors the information and algorithms they require to make wise business decisions.

Researchers have tried to anticipate the longer-term condition of the exchange using models that may analyse historical exchange data due to the supply of both past and present securities market data [3]. This historical data typically includes Date, Open, High, Low, Close, Adjusted Close Prices, and Volume as shown in Figure 8.1. Using some statistical analysis approaches, daily data could be examined, and the exchange's future condition might be predicted. The exchange data are additionally naturally noisy and unpredictable because of non-economic variables like natural disasters and political actions. The shortcoming of not accurately capturing the connection between future and past prices is another factor contributing to the unpredictability of the stock data. It would be difficult to forecast the longer-term price of a corporation due to the insufficient information surrounding the stock exchange data, which is often described as noisy features, as explained by the researcher [4, 5]. The necessity for suitable algorithms and techniques to attenuate risks and maximise profits grew along with the fast expansion of commerce and investment.

This chapter tackles these difficulties in predicting stock prices. The target is to attenuate risks for investors within the stock exchange and decision-makers within the financial

DOI: 10.1201/9781003467199-11

	Date	Open	High	Low	Close	Adj Close	Volume
0	2012-05-02	214.600006	216.740005	212.100006	213.945007	191.394974	2968820
1	2012-05-03	213.100006	213.100006	207.660004	208.520004	186.541763	5035860
2	2012-05-04	206.410004	206.945007	198.500000	199.360001	178.347244	5911990
3	2012-05-07	193.600006	203.755005	188.100006	202.615005	181.259155	9728110
4	2012-05-08	204.000000	204.949997	193.000000	195.895004	175.247467	8083050
...	...	...	...	...	...	...	...
2479	2022-05-24	462.000000	466.700012	460.200012	462.350006	455.250031	449676
2480	2022-05-25	461.399994	464.549988	452.149994	454.200012	454.200012	473896
2481	2022-05-26	457.399994	470.000000	452.549988	469.000000	469.000000	916936
2482	2022-05-27	471.950012	474.950012	467.149994	469.000000	469.000000	817811
2483	2022-05-30	473.799988	476.700012	471.200012	474.450012	474.450012	533868

FIGURE 8.1   SBIN stock data snapshot from May 2012 to May 2022.

sector while capturing difficult and constantly changing pricing more promptly. Using the State Bank of India (SBIN) historical stock data [1] as an example, our study compares several statistical forecasting techniques including bidirectional long short-term memory (BiLSTM), convolutional neural network (CNN), Facebook Prophet, LSTM-CNN, and autoregressive integrated moving average (ARIMA) models to exactly predict the longer-term values of the stock [6]. The prediction results of the proposed LSTM-sequential self-attention mechanism (SSAM) model accurately track the daily "adjusted closing" prices of the SBIN stock market index, which dramatically raises the bar for developing effective business plans. And, we use certain significant technical indicators just like the simple moving average (SMA) as supplementary forecasts to extend the robustness of our pro-posed approach.

8.1.1 Motivation

The main motivation for trying to predict stock market prices is the potential return on investment. Even a fraction of a second's knowledge of a stock's price can result in large earnings [2]. Researchers and investors are continually looking for the stock's future price that will provide them with the highest profits. You can add a level of certainty by trying to understand the historical trend of a particular stock that is available on the Internet. To minimise losses and maximise profits, our approach can be very helpful in increasing the accuracy of stock market price predictions [3]. The prediction techniques we outline here are up-to-date and are deemed to be extremely helpful in identifying prospective buying and selling opportunities for the stock of interest. This allows investors to choose when to invest their money to get more returns.

8.1.2 Contributions

Our contributions can be summarised as follows:

- We study and analyse the problem of stock prediction and present the prominent existing methods used for this purpose.

- We propose a hybrid LSTM and self-attention-based approach to tackle this problem, which presents a novel solution to the problem.

- Using common stock datasets, we evaluate the proposed approach and compare them with the existing methods to show its effectiveness.

- Our results show that the proposed approach shows superior performance and can accurately predict future stock prices.

8.2 RELATED WORKS

This section discusses the related work of different types of machine learning models.

8.2.1 Long Short-Term Memory (LSTM)

LSTMs can analyse both individual data points (images) and whole data sequences (videos, time series, etc.). LSTM is a type of recurrent neural network (RNN), which was first introduced recently, and has gained appeal among financial specialists [7]. Similar to conventional RNN frameworks, the LSTM model may learn data over one or more layers [8]. LSTM networks were developed to address the exploding and vanishing gradient problems that can occur when training traditional RNNs, so they are appropriate for making predictions based on time-series data. This is because there may be lags of unknown length between significant events in a time series. In contrast to LSTM, machine learning requires a great deal of time. One of the researchers used the LSTM model to forecast the values of S&P 500 equities from 1992 to 2015 [9]. He used 3 years of data to train the LSTM model and the following year to evaluate it. In his study, the model beat the logistic regression classifier, random forest [9]. On the other hand, a study using the LSTM model was done on the Chinese stock market to anticipate prices [10]. The LSTM model, an algorithmic approach for interpreting time-series data, assumes that the underlying process is unknown. The LSTM model was more accurate in predicting stock price variations than the classification and regression tree (CART) model in the study conducted by [11]. This is because the LSTM model has the capacity to use deep learning to assess sequential input, extract useful information, and discard irrelevant information. When evaluating the LSTM model, the work only considered the basic LSTM model [11].

8.2.2 Bidirectional Long Short-Term Memory (BiLSTM)

Although LSTM is capable of gathering information about long-distance features, it only makes use of data that is accessible before output time. When creating predictions for time series, it is essential to fully take into consideration the forward and backward information law of the data, because this may greatly improve forecast accuracy [12]. The two halves of

BiLSTM are forward and backward LSTM. BiLSTM may utilise the past and future data to draw conclusions that are more extensive and accurate because it considers the changing laws of the data both before and after data transfer, as opposed to the one-way-state transmission in the ordinary LSTM. It has shown exceptional performance and some work used it in applications for water-level prediction [13].

8.2.3 Convolutional Neural Network (CNN)

CNN is used in a variety of applications, including vision, time-series analysis, and the extraction of predictive characteristics from data [13]. The traditional CNN has layers for convolution, activation, and pooling [14]. An effective convolution method is used to abstract the original input while representing data characteristics in a higher-level form. The majority of CNN is made up of both the pooling layer and the convolution layer. Each convolution layer consists of several convolution kernels, which can be calculated as shown in Equation (8.1).

$$l_t = \tanh(x_t * k_t + b_t) \tag{8.1}$$

where:
l_t = output value after convolution
tanh = activation function
x_t = input vector
k_t = weight of the convolution kernel
b_t = bias of the convolution kernel

After the convolution operation of the convolution layer, the features of the data are retrieved; however, the extracted feature dimensions are quite high. To solve this problem and reduce the cost of network training, a pooling layer is added after the convolution layer to reduce the feature dimension.

8.2.4 Autoregressive Integrated Moving Average (ARIMA)

Originally introduced and developed by Box and Jenkins (1976) [15], the general model incorporates the autoregressive (AR), differencing (I), and moving average (MA) components. It involves a variety of stages for finding, developing, and assessing ARIMA models using time-series data [16]. It is sometimes known as the Box-Jenkins technique. One of the approaches for financial forecasting is most frequently used in this model [17–19]. For short-term forecasting, ARIMA models have proven to be helpful [20]. They consistently outperformed complicated structural models in terms of short-term prediction [21]. ARIMA has three main parameters namely *p, d, q*, where:

1. p is a kind of order of AR part for correlation within itself.

2. d is the number of times that raw observations are contrasted; this is considered as "I" – integrated with ARIMA.

3. q is the moving average parameter.

8.2.5 Facebook Prophet Tool

AR models are among the most frequently used to forecast future predictions [22]. Briefly, the output variable is linearly dependent on both its own prior values and a stochastic component in the AR model (an imperfectly predictable term). The Prophet model was recently proposed by Facebook in an effort to create a model that could identify seasonality in time-series data [23]. This model is openly accessible. By using additive regression models, Prophet can track seasonality on a daily, monthly, and annual basis as well as the effects of holidays. For trend forecasting, Prophet uses a piecewise linear model. The mathematical equation for the Prophet model is as follows:

$$y(t) = g(t) + s(t) + h(t) + e(t) \tag{8.2}$$

where:
  $g(t)$ = trend
  $S(t)$ = recurring changes (weekly, monthly, or yearly)
  $H(t)$ = symbol for the impacts of holidays (recall: holidays impact businesses)
  $e(t)$ = error term

Even when dealing with thousands of observations, prophet model fitting procedures are typically faster and do not require any data preprocessing. Missing data and outliers are also addressed [23]. In Facebook Prophet, both linear and nonlinear time functions are supported. In exponential smoothing, a similar method of modelling seasonality as an additive component is applied [24]. This library is so important that it can address problems with seasonality and stationary properties in data. There are a few restrictions with Facebook Prophet, such as the need for input columns with the identifiers "ds" and "y", where "ds" stands for Date and "y" for the target variable. In this scenario, a trend might be rising or falling, positive or negative [21].

8.3 METHODOLOGY

In this section, we discuss the methodology towards our proposed model and approach for stock price prediction.

8.3.1 Dataset

The stock used in this study is in the form of historical data of the SBIN stock data, which includes "open, low, high, close, and adjusted close prices and trading volume". The daily price data used, which spans a period of 10 years and includes 2484 observations, is taken from Yahoo Finance [1]. We consider the "adjusted close" price because the closing price refers to the cost of share at the end of the day, whereas the adjusted closing price accounts for items like dividends, stock splits, and new stock offerings. It might be considered that the adjusted closing price is a more accurate indicator of the stock value as it starts where the closing price ends. To study the general trend of the stock, we have divided the dates into months and by observing the graph shown in

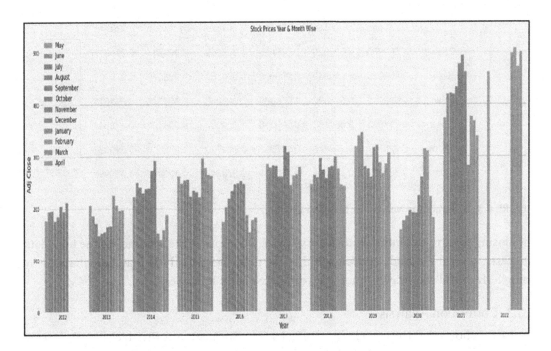

FIGURE 8.2   General trend of SBIN stock market per month and year.

Figure 8.2, we can say that from November until February the stock price of SBIN is high due to festivals and year-end closing.

8.3.2 Feature Engineering
The original data of the stock has the following fields:

- **Date**: Trading date.
- **Open**: The price at which the stock is initially traded.
- **High**: The day's peak trading price.
- **Low**: Lowest price during the trading day.
- **Close**: The final price at which the stock changed hands throughout the trading day.
- **Adjusted Close**: The price changes in response to corporate activities on the closing price.
- **Volume**: The total number of shares that were traded throughout the day.

For our model, we concentrate on "date" and "adjusted close" prices. An adjustment to the computation is made to the closing price of a stock, resulting in the adjusted closing price. Compared with the closing price, it is more detailed and precise. Because external circumstances might have caused changes in the genuine price, the adjustment made to

	Open	High	Low	Close	Adj Close	Volume
Open	1.000000	0.999025	0.999015	0.997905	0.996717	-0.386017
High	0.999025	1.000000	0.998690	0.999163	0.998049	-0.370782
Low	0.999015	0.998690	1.000000	0.999030	0.997647	-0.392613
Close	0.997905	0.999163	0.999030	1.000000	0.998720	-0.378548
Adj Close	0.996717	0.998049	0.997647	0.998720	1.000000	-0.390092
Volume	-0.386017	-0.370782	-0.392613	-0.378548	-0.390092	1.000000

FIGURE 8.3 Correlation values for SBIN stock data.

the closing price represents the stock's true price. To improve the accuracy of the final data forecasts, several methods and algorithms are used. Data analysis may be enhanced by using SMAs, and root-mean squared error (RMSE) and R^2 scores.

8.3.3 Correlation Analysis

Figure 8.3 shows that the correlation coefficients between several variables is called a correlation matrix. The correlation between any two variables is displayed in each column of the table as shown in Figure 8.3. The values indicate how each column relates to the other column. The table demonstrates the strong correlation between practically all the fields in the dataset, except for the volume.

8.3.4 Simple Moving Average (SMA)

SMA calculates the average value of the previous n data points. It is a useful tool that may help determine if a stock price trend will continue or reverse. Equation (8.3) shows how SMA is calculated:

$$\frac{(A_1 + A_2 + \cdots + A_n)}{n} \tag{8.3}$$

where:
$(A_1, A_2, ..., A_n)$ = prices
n = number of total periods

The number of periods in that range is used to calculate the percentage of an elected assortment of prices, or routinely closing prices. A SMA lowers volatility and makes it easier to identify a stock's price trend. A rising SMA indicates that the stock price is also rising. If it is heading downward, the price of the stock is falling, which can be viewed in Figure 8.4. The smoother the SMA, the longer the time period for the moving average.

8.3.5 Root-Mean Square Error (RMSE)

RMSE is used in this instance to determine the most appropriate moving average for the data. A low RMSE value represents low error. In climatology, forecasting, and regression

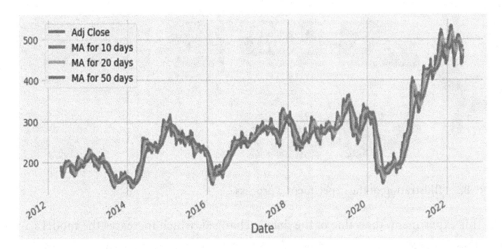

FIGURE 8.4   Calculating moving average for 10, 20, and 50 days.

analysis, root means the square error is frequently used to validate experimental results. Equation (8.4) for RMSE is obtained as follows:

$$\text{RMSE} = \sqrt{\frac{1}{n} \sum_{i=1}^{n} \left(f_i - o_i \right)^2} \tag{8.4}$$

where:
   $\sum$ = summation of all values
   f = predicted value
   i = observed or actual value
   $(f_i - o_i)^2$ = difference between predicted and observed values and squared
   n = total sample size

8.4 ANALYSIS

This section discusses experimental design with other configurations and proposed algorithm.

8.4.1 Experimental Design

The study is divided into six sections: data collection, data preprocessing, model training, model saving, model testing, and prediction findings. Figure 8.5 displays the conceptual flowchart for the method analysis and design. Because the original Yahoo Finance dataset cannot be used directly for model training and testing, data preprocessing is necessary. The issue of inconsistent data magnitude is then addressed by using data normalisation. Finally, a useful dataset for the experiment may be created. Data normalisation entails transforming the data into a specified interval and scaling the data to a particular scale.

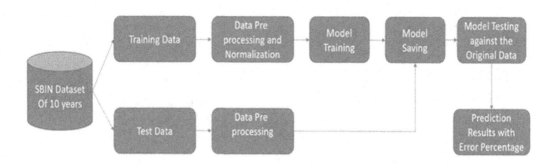

FIGURE 8.5   Illustration of the experimental process.

In this experiment, the value of the data is changed, which increases the model's accuracy and convergence speed. Equation (8.5) of the transformation function is as follows:

$$x^* = \frac{x - min}{max - min} \tag{8.5}$$

where:

max and *min* = sample data's maximum and minimum values, respectively

8.4.2 Experimenting with Other Algorithms and Configurations

The algorithms used for time series are LSTM, BiLSTM, CNN, Facebook (FB) Prophet, ARIMA, and hybrid algorithms [25]. Our study finds that LSTM is very effective and it can more accurately forecast future values and capture previous trend patterns successfully. The configurations of the algorithms are listed in Table 8.1.

8.4.3 The Proposed Algorithm – LSTM with Sequential Self-Attention Mechanism (LSTM-SSAM)

In the following, we will discuss the key components of the proposed LSTM-SSAM approach.

- **Long Short-Term Memory**: Using Google's open-source Tensor Flow software, the LSTM model was developed in Python using Keras, a high-level neural network Application Programming Interface (API) [26]. It uses the aforementioned dataset, which consists of SBIN data points for the time periods 2 May 2012 through 31 May

TABLE 8.1   Configuration of Other Algorithms

Algorithms	Configuration
LSTM (Unit 1)	The number of hidden units 1
LSTM (Unit 50)	The number of hidden units 50
CNN + BiLSTM	Conv1d + MaxPooling +BiLSTM units 50 + Dropout + dense
LSTM + CNN	LSTM unit 50 + Conv1d + MaxPooling + Flatten + Dense *2
Facebook Prophet	Trends of Seasonality
ARIMA	p,d,q(0,1,0)

2022, and splits it into training and test data in proportions of 90% and 10%, respectively. The output (Y) is a forecast of the "Adj Closing" price for the upcoming day using the selected feature(s) of the present and previous number of days (equal to the time step) as input (X). Our model is built using a sequential model with one LSTM layer and one dense layer. We have set LSTM return sequences to be true value, and the LSTM utilises 50 units (dimensionality of the output space). When the return sequences argument is set to True, all of the time steps' hidden states are output [27]. The array's content consists of all the hidden states for each LSTM layer time step. For the purposes of this study, different parameter settings have been developed by trial and error. As a result, many parameter choices were attempted and tested by repeatedly running the model, and values for the hyperparameters that balance the trade-offs between time efficiency and performance are chosen.

In the selection process, several settings that reduced the difference between high and low values were tested. A value of **10** was the best batch size, both in terms of performance and efficiency, after various batch sizes were tested (i.e., the number of samples per gradient update). A value of **50** was chosen as the number of times to loop through the whole dataset because epoch sizes above 50 showed little to no improvements. The mean squared error (MSE) is applied to the loss function. Adam optimiser was chosen among the different optimisers available as Adam gave us the best results. Adam optimiser, which iteratively changes network weights in training data, performed better than Stochastic Gradient Decent (SGD). On the other hand, SGD keeps a constant learning rate during all weight changes. Adam was used because empirical data showed that it is effective in practice and even compares favourably to other stochastic optimisation techniques. The architecture of the LSTM is shown in Figure 8.6. A gradient may transfer from one hidden layer to the next without decreasing due to the memory of LSTM units, which also tackles the problem of vanishing gradients. The cells are a representation of the transport line that runs through each cell (the top line in Figure 8.6), connecting data from previous modules and the current module. It has been established that LSTMs are more powerful than standard RNNs. The LSTM layer is made up of four neural network layers that interact in a certain way.

A typical LSTM device consists of three distinct parts: *a cell, an escape door,* and *a forgotten door.* Cells' main responsibilities are to categorise values over a range of arbitrary periods and to keep track of the data flow in and out of them. To regulate the state of each cell, each LSTM needs three different kinds of doors: between 0 and 1, Forget Gate generates a number, with 1 denoting "to keep that completely" and 0 denoting "to ignore it altogether". Memory Gate selects the most recent data that needs to be processed in the cell. The values that are modified are then determined by a sigmoid layer called the "input layer". After that, a "tanh" layer generates a new candidate value vector that might be added to the state. Each cell's output is determined by the gate output.

An LSTM will have three separate dependencies depending on the data it receives:

1. The prior condition of the cell (specifically, the data that remained in the memory following the previous time step).

2. The previous hidden state (this is the same as what the previous cell's output was, for example).

3. The input for the current time step (i.e., the most recent data being input at that moment).

These dependencies may be explained as follows in relation to the field of financial asset price prediction:

- **The Previous Cell State**: The stock's trend of the previous day.

- **The Previous Hidden State**: The stock's price of the previous day.

- **The Input at the Current Time Step**: Other elements that may have an impact on price. These can be daily investment news alerts that are released publicly.

The horizontal line c_t in the diagram shown in Figure 8.6 stands for the cell state, which symbolises the LSTM's memory. This is consistent with the stock's previous day's pattern, as we immediately noted in (1). These data will be processed by the cell, which will also handle any other data that comes in. In our stock prediction scenario, the data from earlier time steps, in particular, the stock price from the previous day, will be present in the line denoted by c_{t-1}, which is the Hidden State stated in (2).

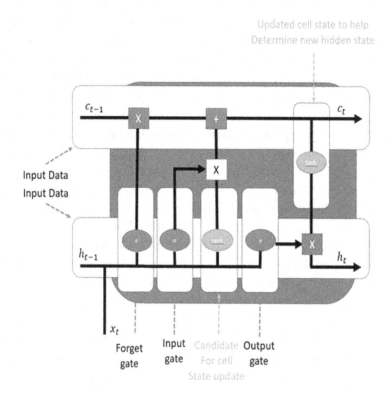

FIGURE 8.6   Architecture of long short-term memory.

The horizontal line shown by h_{t-1} represents the input during this time, which is the stock price at the present moment as stated in (3). The LSTM will provide a result based on information from prior stock prices (Hidden State), the current price in combination with the trend from the previous day (Cell State), and so on.

- **Self-Attention Mechanism:** The self-attention model allows inputs to interact with one another (i.e., calculate the attention of all other inputs with regard to one input) as illustrated in Figure 8.7. While producing output, the attention mechanism enables output to concentrate attention on input. The first phase involves multiplying each of the encoder input vectors by each of the three weight matrices (*W(Q), W(K), and W(V)*) that we trained throughout the training process [19, 26]. For each of the input vectors, this matrix multiplication will produce three vectors: *the key vector, the query vector,* and *the value vector*.

  The second phase of calculating self-attention is the Query vector from the current input, which is multiplied by the key vectors from other inputs. The third phase involves multiplying the score by the square root of the dimensions of the key vector (d_k). This is done because when we use the softmax function in the future, certain self-attention scores end up being extremely low. In the fourth phase all of the self-attention scores will be subjected to the softmax function. In the fifth phase, the value vector is multiplied by the determined vector from the previous step. In the last phase, the weighted value vectors obtained in the stage before are added to provide the self-attention output.

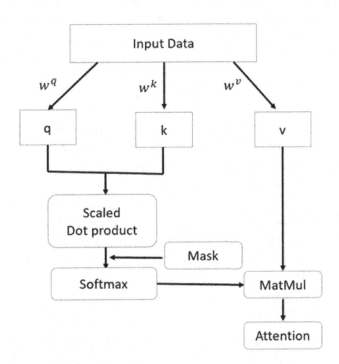

FIGURE 8.7   Self-attention mechanism architecture.

All input sequences are subjected to the aforementioned method [18]. The self-attention matrix for the input matrices *(Q, K, and V)* is determined mathematically by Equation (8.6):

$$\text{Attention}(Q,K,V) = \text{softmax}\left(\frac{QK^T}{\sqrt{d_k}}\right)V \tag{8.6}$$

where the vectors for the query, key, and value are combined together as *Q, K,* and *V.*

- **Q = Query**: Queries are a collection of vectors that you obtain by merging the input vector with the query weights (*Wq*), and you wish to calculate attention for these vectors.

- **K = Key**: keys are a collection of vectors that are produced when you combine the input vector with the key weights; these are the vectors that you will use to measure attention.

- **V = Value**: When you combine an input vector with value weights, you obtain a collection of vectors called values. These vectors are then multiplied by the softmax attention probabilities. Value vectors enable the selection of pertinent terms.

Rectified linear unit (ReLU) function is the best activation function to utilise for forecasting individual stock returns because it is most frequently used in the literature and empirical investigations [28]. ReLU allows nonlinear properties in the data, giving us more alternatives with our dataset. The ReLU function is described as follows in Equation (8.7):

$$\text{ReLU}(x) = \begin{cases} 0 & \text{if } x < 0 \\ x & \text{otherwise} \end{cases} \tag{8.7}$$

As a result, the ReLU activation function only requires the total weight inputs from each layer. In the absence of adequate data, it outputs zero; in the presence of sufficient data, it receives an *x* value. For the specific issue we are dealing with, we use this as the last layer because the linear activation function is always defined as the last layer output for regression issues. After building the network structure and the relative activation functions [29], it is essential to provide a measure to assess the model's performance to increase prediction accuracy. There are a number of hyperparameters that must be determined, including the number of flattened and dense neurons in each layer, as shown in Table 8.2.

8.5 EXPERIMENTAL RESULTS

To verify the effectiveness of the proposed model, different models including LSTM (Unit 1), LSTM (Unit 50), CNN-BiLSTM, and LSTM-CNN are compared on the SBIN stock dataset collected for this work. The predicted results are shown in Figure 8.8, which presents on

TABLE 8.2   Parameters Setting of the Proposed Method

Layer	Output Shape	Parameters
LSTM (Unit 50)	(None, 10, 50)	10400
Seq_self_attention	(None, 10, 50)	3265
Flatten	(None, 500)	0
Dense	(none, 1)	501

the x-axis the "Date" and on the y-axis the "Adj Closed" price. As shown in Figure 8.8, the dark line is the test data of the "Adj Close" price of the stock which is the actual value, and the other lines are the predicted values of the "Adj Closed" price.

The prediction errors of different models on the SBIN stock dataset are listed in Table 8.3. As shown in this Table 8.3, LSTM (Unit 50) has a higher predictive power than the others.

We can take LSTM (Unit 50) and augment it with the self-attention mechanism to enhance the performance of the LSTM mode [30]. We present the results in Table 8.4 which verify the effectiveness of the LSTM-SSAM model. It can achieve superior performance compared with the LSTM model over all the metrics (i.e., RMSE, time, and R^2 score). And, the values of actual data and predicted data are in the same range and the error difference is lower compared with other algorithms. Figure 8.9 shows the red line in the same range of Test_data (actual price from June 2021 to May 2022).

Table 8.5 gives the values for the forecast error between the actual price and the predicted price and its error percentage. The results show that the error is significantly low and its percentage is less than ~3%. The forecast error is calculated by subtracting the actual values and the predicted values as shown in Equation (8.8):

$$\text{Forecast Error} = \left[\text{Actual Price}\right] - \left[\text{Predicted Price}\right] \tag{8.8}$$

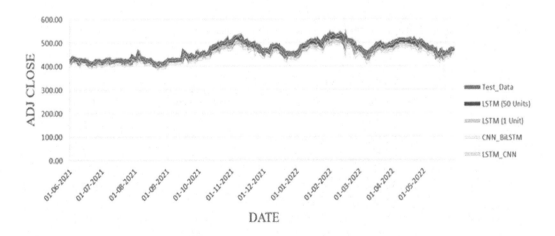

FIGURE 8.8   SBIN graphical representation of other algorithms.

TABLE 8.3   Comparison of Algorithms on SBIN

Algorithm	RMSE	Time (Sec)	R² Score
LSTM (Unit 1)	14.37	144.0	0.83
LSTM (Unit 50)	10.80	144.1	0.905
CNN+BiLSTM	21.32	144.0	0.63
LSTM+CNN	19.78	144.2	0.67
FB_Prophet	88.64	7.4	−0.08
ARIMA	49.82	–	−0.09

TABLE 8.4   Comparison of LSTM (Unit 50) and Proposed Model

Algorithm	RMSE	Time (Sec)	R² Score
LSTM (Unit 50)	10.80	144.1	0.905
Proposed model	8.17	108.2	0.946

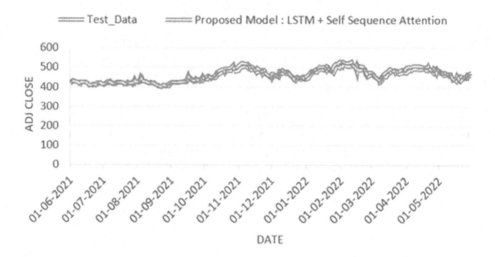

FIGURE 8.9   Graph of proposed model predicting the values of SBIN test dataset from June 2021 to May 2022.

TABLE 8.5   Proposed Model Predictions from June 2021 to May 2022

Date	Test_Data	Predicted	Forecast Error	Error Percentage
01-06-2021	422.060	414.115	7.945	1.882
02-06-2021	426.548	421.643	4.904	1.150
03-06-2021	432.899	425.945	6.953	1.606
04-06-2021	426.942	432.451	−5.510	1.291
07-06-2021	425.760	427.028	−1.268	0.298
08-06-2021	420.591	426.185	−5.595	1.330
09-06-2021	414.978	421.085	−6.107	1.472
23-05-2022	453.872	454.919	−1.047	0.231

(Continued)

TABLE 8.5 (*Continued*)   Proposed Model Predictions from June 2021 to May 2022

Date	Test_Data	Predicted	Forecast Error	Error Percentage
24-05-2022	455.250	452.759	2.491	0.547
25-05-2022	454.200	454.959	−0.759	0.167
26-05-2022	469.000	453.817	15.183	3.237
27-05-2022	469.000	468.350	0.650	0.139
30-05-2022	474.450	467.755	6.695	1.411

Similarly, the forecast percentage is calculated by dividing forecast error and actual price multiplied by 100 as in Equation (8.9):

$$Forecast\ Error\ (\%) = Abs\left(\frac{[Forecast\ Error]}{[Actual]}\right) \times 100 \tag{8.9}$$

where:

Abs = absolute value of the number

We have also compared the same algorithms with two different stock data, namely HDFC BANK and BANKBARODA datasets. Table 8.6 shows the results of testing the various study models and we observe that the proposed model outperforms the other models and has the best accuracy. Here also we can observe that LSTM (Unit 50) has greater accuracy than other algorithms, and our proposed model LSTM-SSAM model outperforms the LSTM mode with accuracies of 90.74% for HDFCBANK and 96.08% for BANKBARODA.

Finally, the graph in Figures 8.10 and 8.11 compares the Test_Data and the proposed model predicted price. It shows that the proposed model has the least error and demonstrates its effectiveness in the future price of these two stocks.

In summary, the experimental results show that the proposed hybrid LSTM and attention model (i.e., LSTM-SSAM) achieves the best accuracy and robustness with the least error over the various benchmarks and datasets.

TABLE 8.6   Results for (HDFCBANK and BANKBARODA) Stocks

Algorithm	HDFC RMSE	R² Score	BANK BARODA RMSE	R² Score
LSTM(Unit 1)	28.07	87.90	3.51	91.50
LSTM(Unit 50)	27.65	88.26	3.13	93.25
CNN+BiLSTM	39.51	76.04	2.67	95.08
LSTM+CNN	44.26	69.99	2.70	94.95
FB_Prophet	524.80	−6.39	126.41	−0.99
ARIMA	124.53	−0.90	17.71	−0.001
Proposed Model	24.55	90.74	2.38	96.08

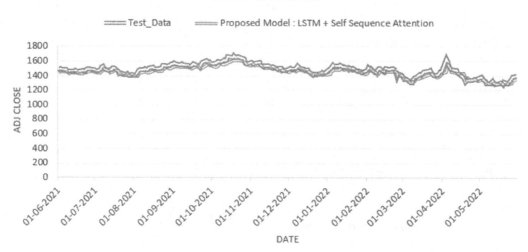

FIGURE 8.10   Graph of proposed model predicting the values of HDFC test dataset from June 2021 to May 2022.

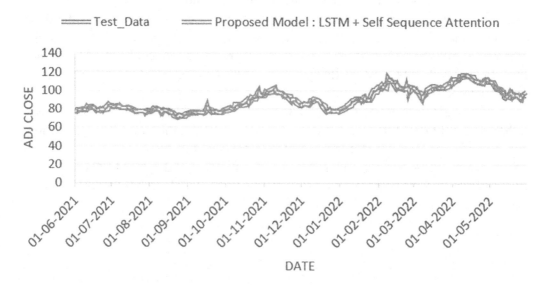

FIGURE 8.11   Graph of proposed model predicting the values of BANKBARODA test dataset from June 2021 to May 2022.

8.6 CONCLUSIONS AND FUTURE WORK

For the stock market, learning the future price is very important for making investment decisions. This chapter establishes a forecasting framework to predict the "Adj Close" prices of stock. Compared with other approaches, we offer a novel stock market time-series forecasting model called LSTM-SSAM, in which the self-attention model can more precisely analyse the sequential stock attributes. The experimental findings demonstrate that our proposed model has a lower RMSE and improved accuracy of prediction outcomes when compared with the widely used time-series models. The fact that historical data alone cannot be used to reduce stock market volatility is still an open question for our future study in several directions, but other aspects of the current environment, such as the most recent news in politics and the economy, also need to be examined. In this chapter, we have only focused on stocks related to the banking sector. Therefore, we can add data predictions related to stock news and Twitter sentiment analysis to enhance the stability and accuracy of the model in the case of a major event [31]. We also envision that the proposed approach could be made more practical by deploying it in a distributed fashion using recent machine learning paradigms such as distributed machine learning or federated learning approaches [20] to provide for more dynamic and adaptive stock price prediction systems.

REFERENCES

[1] The State Bank of India (SBIN) dataset stock data. Available at: https://finance.yahoo.com/quote/SBIN.NS/history?p=SBIN.NS

[2] Vo, T. V., & Gill, S. S. (2022). GRAPES: Semi-automatic approach for forecasting models to predict GameStop prices using cloud computing and machine learning. *International Journal of Grid and Utility Computing*, 13(5), 538–550.

[3] Dhingra, S., Singh, M., Vaisakh, S.B. et al. (2023). Mind meets machine: Unravelling GPT-4's cognitive psychology. *BenchCouncil Transactions on Benchmarks, Standards and Evaluations*, 3(3), 100139.

[4] Xing, T., Sun, Y., Wang, Q., & Yu, G. (2013). The analysis and prediction of stock price. *IEEE International Conference on Granular Computing (GrC)*, pp. 368–373.

[5] Deboeck, G. J. (Ed.). (1994). *Trading on the Edge: Neural, Genetic, and Fuzzy Systems for Chaotic Financial Markets*. Wiley.

[6] Muñoz, E. (2020). *Attention Is All You Need: Discovering the Transformer Paper*. Published in Towards Data Science.

[7] Abu-Mostafa, Y. S., & Atiya, A. F. (1996). Introduction to financial forecasting. *Applied Intelligence*, 996(6), 205–213.

[8] Hargreaves, C., & Chen, L. (2020). Stock prediction using deep learning with long-short-term-memory networks. *International Journal of Electronic Engineering and Computer Science*, 5(3), 22–32. http://www.aiscience.org/journal/ijeecs

[9] Hochreiter, S., & Schmidhuber, J. (2006). Long short-term memory. *The MIT Press Journals*, 9, 1735–1780. https://doiorg.libproxy1.nus.edu.sg/10.1162/neco.1997.9.8.1735

[10] Lui, Y. (2019). Novel volatility forecasting using deep learning long-short-term-memory recurrent neural networks. *Expert Systems with Applications*, 132, 99–109.

[11] Fischer, T., & Krauss, C. (2018). Deep learning with long-short term-memory networks for financial market predictions. *European Journal of Operational Research*, 270, 654–669.

[12] Gill, S. S. et al. (2024). Modern computing: Vision and challenges. *Telematics and Informatics Reports*, 13, 100116.

[13] Chen, K., Zhou, Y., & Dai, F. (2015). An LSTM-based method for stock returns prediction: A case study of China stock market. *IEEE International Conference on Big Data (Big Data)*, pp. 2823–2824.

[14] Nie, Q., Wan, D., & Wang, R. (2021). CNN-BiLSTM water level prediction method with attention mechanism. *Journal of Physics: Conference Series*, IOP Publishing, 2078, pp. 1–8

[15] Hipel, K. W., McLeod, A. I., & Lennox, W. C. (1977). Advances in Box-Jenkins modeling: 1. Model construction. *Water Resources Research*, 13(3), 567–575.

[16] Garlapati, A., Krishna, D. R., Garlapati, K., Srikara Yaswanth, N., Rahul, U., & Narayanan, G. (2021). Stock price prediction using Facebook prophet and Arima models. *2021 6th International Conference for Convergence in Technology (I2CT)*, Maharashtra, India.

[17] Meyler, A., Kenny, G., & Quinn, T. (1998). *Forecasting Irish Inflation Using ARIMA Models.* Central Bank of Ireland Research Department, *Technical Paper*, 3/RT

[18] Tabachnick, B. G., & Fidell, L. S. (2001). *Using Multivariate Statistics* (4th ed.). Pearson Education Company.

[19] Rangan, N., & Titida, N. (2006). ARIMA Model for Forecasting Oil Palm Price. *Proceedings of the 2nd IMT-GT Regional Conference on Mathematics, Statistics and Applications*, University Sains Malaysia.

[20] Singh, R. & Gill, S. S. (2023). Edge AI: A survey. *Internet of Things and Cyber-Physical Systems*, 3, 71–92.

[21] Li, M., Ning, D. J., & Guo, J. C. (2019). CNN-LSTM model based on attention mechanism and its application. *Computer Engineering and Applications*, 55(13), 20–27.

[22] Walia, G. K. Kumar, M., & Gill, S. S.. (2024). AI-empowered fog/edge resource management for IoT applications: A comprehensive review, research challenges and future perspectives. *IEEE Communications Surveys & Tutorials*, 26(1), pp. 619–669

[23] Lee, W., Kim, K., Park, J. et al. (2018). Forecasting solar power using long-short term memory and convolutional neural networks. *IEEE Access*, 6, 73068–73080.

[24] Loukas, S. (2020). Time-Series Forecasting: Predicting Stock Prices Using Facebook's Prophet Model. Available at:https://towardsdatascience.com/time-series-forecasting-predicting-stock-prices-using-facebooks-prophet-model-9ee1657132b5

[25] Gill, S. S., Xu, M., Ottaviani, C. et al. (2022). AI for next generation computing: Emerging trends and future directions. *Internet of Things*, 19, 100514.

[26] Merh, N., Saxena, V. P., & Pardasani, K. R. (2010). A comparison between hybrid approaches of ANN and ARIMA for Indian stock trend forecasting. *Journal of Business Intelligence*, 3(2), 23–43.

[27] Vaswani, A., Shazeer, N., Parmar, N., Uszkoreit, J., Jones, L., Gomez, A. N., Kaiser, L., & Polosukhin, I. (2017). "Attention Is All You Need." arXiv:1706.03762.

[28] Bergström, C., & Hjelm, O. (2019). Impact of time steps on stock market prediction with LSTM (Dissertation). Retrieved from http://urn.kb.se/resolve?urn=urn:nbn:se:kth:diva-262221

[29] Hansen, C. (2019). Activation Functions Explained - GELU, SELU, ELU, ReLU and more. Available at: https://mlfromscratch.com/activation-functions-explained/

[30] Self -attention in NLP. (2020). Available at: https://www.geeksforgeeks.org/self-attention-in-nlp/

[31] Gill, S. S., & Kaur, R. (2023). ChatGPT: Vision and challenges. *Internet of Things and Cyber-Physical Systems*, 3, 262–271.

CHAPTER 9

Federated Learning for the Predicting Household Financial Expenditure

Ho Kuen Lai, Ahmed M. Abdelmoniem, and Sukhpal Singh Gill

9.1 INTRODUCTION

Financial management is crucial to our welfare [1]. Although young adults in this generation have increased their awareness of budget management, they have less experience practicing basic financial skills, for example, budgeting and saving plans in the long term [2]. Most young adults purchase items based on their desires instead of their needs [3]. These financial behaviours among young adults will lay the foundation for future household financial habits. As young adults are in transition from financial dependence to independence, their financial habits inevitably influence household expenditure [4]. Given the influential role of households as key decision-makers in financial markets, their expenditure patterns significantly impact economies. Accurate prediction of household financial expenditure is, therefore, essential not only for personal empowerment but also for stakeholders like banks, financial institutions, and governments. Such predictions guide policy decisions, optimise resource allocations, and foresee potential financial risks [5].

Traditional machine learning (TML) has already been widely used in multiple fields for a decade, such as psychology, information technology, statistics, etc. [6]. However, predicting household financial expenditures while maintaining privacy poses a significant challenge. The TML approach often requires centralising sensitive financial data in one place. In 2014, JPMorgan Chase suffered data leakage, which exposed more than 75 million households' personal details [7, 8]. Another incident is the 2013 breach of Target Corporation's network, resulting in significant financial losses [9, 10]. In our increasingly digital era, more data need to be handled, which implies a higher chance of sensitive information being leaked [10]. These incidents and emerging concerns underscore the pressing need to explore alternative methodologies that prioritise data privacy without compromising on prediction accuracy.

Federated learning (FL), on the other hand, is an alternative approach for predicting while addressing data privacy concerns [11]. FL shifts from training models on a server to

DOI: 10.1201/9781003467199-12

individual client devices [12]. This decentralisation ensures that sensitive data like financial data will remain on clients' devices, addressing privacy concerns associated with centralised data storage [13].

Given this context, the core objective of this research is to compare the performance of FL in predicting household financial data with the TML approach using the same model [14]. Our primary focus is determining whether FL, while inherently offering enhanced data privacy, can achieve similar or superior accuracy levels to the TML approach. Through this comparative analysis, we aim to shed light on the potential of FL as a robust alternative in financial predictions, providing a balance between accuracy and privacy.

9.2 RELATED WORK

In this section, we discuss the existing related work in different categories.

9.2.1 TML in Financial Prediction and Its Importance

Many researchers have focused on financial prediction as it is an important area of finance, economics, and government policy. This surrounds areas like the stock market, budget forecasting, economic growth, and expenditure predictions. Predictions not only support financial decision-making but also steer strategic governmental policies. Several studies have used the same TML approach with different models to predict finance. Yadav et al. [15] used the long short-term memory (LSTM) model for time-series prediction in the Indian stock market. Their emphasis on the utility of these predictions for increasing profits underscores the relevance of accurate forecasting in financial data. Emsia and Coskuner [16] also conducted a study by exploring the economic growth within Turkey's gross domestic product (GDP). They found that the estimated accuracy of using a genetic algorithm-support vector regression (SVR) model with more than 0.91 as R^2 and lower than 0.025 as the root-mean squared error (RMSE). This indicates that using the TML model obtains effective results in budget planning. Also, Zheng et al. [17] conducted research on forecasting health expenditures in China by using historical data from 1978 to 2017 by harnessing the autoregressive integrated moving average (ARIMA) model. Their findings pointed towards rapidly escalating healthcare costs, emphasising the need for accurate forecasting for optimal resource allocation in healthcare. Muremyi et al. [18] also found that the TreeNet model has the highest accuracy with 87% compared with the multivariate adaptive regression splines (MARS) model with 50.16%, decision tree model with 74%, random forest model with 83%, and gradient boosting with 81%, all of which are based on RMSE. They concluded and suggested the government increase expenditures on public health. These studies gave us insights into the prevalent use of the TML approach in diverse financial forecasting areas.

9.2.2 Importance of Household Expenditure

Households, as the foundation economic units, play a crucial role in shaping the financial landscapes of economies. Their spending patterns, influenced by various socioeconomic and behavioural factors, are vital indicators of economic health and consumer behaviour. Predicting household expenditure has tangible implications for policymaking [19]. Accurate predictions can provide insights into consumer behaviours, thereby influencing the direction and effectiveness of financial and economic policies. Ahmad and Fatima [19] emphasised the importance of understanding these patterns for policy creation, using a classification-based neural network approach. While they addressed the classification aspect, there lies a gap in predicting precise household expenditure figures, signalling a more detailed exploration need.

9.2.3 The Rising Data Privacy Concerns, TML and FL

The digital age has brought forth an augmented awareness of data privacy, especially in areas involving sensitive information. Chua et al. [20] conducted a survey and found out finance has the second highest mean rank, 4.30 out of 5.00. This implies that finance has a high privacy concern, which indicated the importance of protecting sensitive financial data. Moreover, the introduction of initiatives like General Data Protection Regulation (GDPR) [21] shows there is an evident global move towards protecting personal data. Based on past studies, financial prediction has predominantly leveraged TML models. Models such as SVR, MARS, and TreeNet have found applications in predicting household and government health expenditures, as well as a country's GDP growth. Conversely, time-series data, particularly in the stock market, has often employed models like ARIMA and LSTM. However, the innate process of TML, which involves direct data transmission to a central server for model training, poses a significant challenge [22]. This centralisation especially becomes problematic when handling inherently sensitive data like financial, healthcare, or home application information [23].

Given the privacy constraints of TML, FL is a promising alternative. The core difference lies in the data handling approach. Whereas TML centralises data, sending it directly to a server for training and aggregation, FL does the opposite by decentralising the data. In FL, ML models are trained locally on client nodes or devices. Once the training is completed, only the model updates will be sent to the central server for aggregation, not the raw data. A global model will be formed by aggregating from each client's updated models. The process will be iterated as many times as desired [23]. Because only updated models were sent to the server, the raw data of clients will remain on their devices, which makes FL a more privacy-friendly method than TML [24]. Thus, the decentralised approach showed that FL is a better substitution for TML when handling sensitive information [25].

9.2.4 Existing Studies on FL and Its Advantage

Research has commented and performed FL on medical health industry. Rieke et al. [26] concluded that FL can obtain accurate and unbiased models on the digital healthcare industry and also think FL is beneficial for sensitive data. Dayan et al. [27] conducted a study by collecting 20 organisations around the world to train on an FL model, which is used to predict future the oxygen requirement of symptomatic patients who suffer from COVID-19. The result from the ANOVA test of the FL model had a high prediction score. These findings suggested that FL can be a new approach for predicting sensitive data. Pourroostaei Ardakani et al. [28] used FL to predict stock market trends. They found the best model for the MSE score for FL is random forest, the second is linear regression, and the last is support vector machine (SVM) [29]. In the centralised MSE score result, linear regression performed better than random forest. While these findings stem from stock market predictions, household financial expenditure predictions, though within the financial area, present different challenges [30]. Given linear regression's efficacy in centralised environments, it would be insightful to test its applicability to household expenditure predictions. To ensure whether FL's performance can meet match the results, we need a strong baseline TML model with which to compare the results.

9.2.5 Current Research

The existing research has offered insights into the effectiveness of various modelling techniques in financial predictions, with a prominent emphasis on TML. However, due to the rising privacy concerns, simply relying on traditional methods may no longer be sustainable, especially in areas involving sensitive household financial data [31]. There exists an important need to incorporate methodologies that ensure not only predictive accuracy but also to prioritise data privacy.

FL presents itself as a novel alternative that promises the preservation of data privacy by allowing model training locally, without sharing raw data. There is limited knowledge on the practical effectiveness of FL in the domain of household financial predictions.

Hence, the present study aims to bridge this gap by comparing the performance of FL in the area of household expenditure predictions with the TML approach using the same linear regression model. This comparison will shed light on whether FL, while inherently providing data privacy, can match or even exceed the prediction capabilities of the TML method.

9.3 METHODOLOGY

In this section, we discuss the methodology used in this research work.

9.3.1 Research Design

The primary objective of this study is to test whether the performance of the FL approach matches TML's performance. To conduct a fair comparison analysis for both methods, we need to apply the same model; in this case the linear regression model will be used. The "Region" column in the dataset is used for partitioning data within the FL approach. However, to maintain consistency across both approaches, this column is exempted from the correlation-based feature selection.

Performance evaluations between FL and TML are assessed using MSE and R^2. Both approaches operate on identical feature variables and target variables to ensure a fair comparison. It should be noted that while the "Region" column is used as partitioning in the FL setup, a normalisation technique was not included because it mimics the real-world scenario. While normalisation scales data might reduce the impact of outliers, it can also inadvertently skew the representation of different social classes in the dataset. This skewness could introduce bias and potentially affect the model's generalisation.

9.3.2 Data Collection

We found a dataset from Kaggle called the "Filipino Family Income and Expenditure" [32]. This dataset contains anonymised household financial data from 41,544 households in the Philippines. The dataset is collected from the Family Income and Expenditure Survey

	Total Household Income	Region	Total Food Expenditure	Main Source of Income	Agricultural Household indicator	Bread and Cereals Expenditure	Total Rice Expenditure	Meat Expenditure	Total Fish and marine products Expenditure	Fruit Expenditure	...	Number of Refrigerator/Freezer	Number of Washing Machine	Number of Airconditioner	Number of Car, Jeep, Van	Number of Landline/wireless telephones	Number of Cellular phone	Number of Personal Computer	Number of Stove with Oven/Gas Range	Number of Motorized Banca	Number of Motorcycle/Tricycle
0	480332	CAR	117848	Wage/Salaries	0	42140	38300	24676	16806	3325	...	1	1	0	0	0	2	1	0	0	1
1	198235	CAR	67766	Wage/Salaries	0	17329	13008	17434	11073	2035	...	0	1	0	0	0	3	1	0	0	2
2	82785	CAR	61609	Wage/Salaries	1	34182	32001	7783	2590	1730	...	0	0	0	0	0	0	0	0	0	0
3	107589	CAR	78189	Wage/Salaries	0	34030	28659	10914	10812	690	...	0	0	0	0	0	1	0	0	0	0
4	189322	CAR	94625	Wage/Salaries	0	34820	30167	18391	11309	1395	...	1	0	0	0	0	3	0	0	0	1

5 rows × 60 columns

FIGURE 9.1 Sample Kaggle dataset.

across the entire 17 regions across the country. The dataset contains 60 columns of variables that related to a family's demographics, expenses, and their house conditions, for example, type of building, number of owned items, other relevant financial indicators, etc. Figure 9.1 is a sample of the dataset.

9.3.3 Data Cleaning and Preprocessing

To ensure data quality and integrity, we removed two columns with null values, "Household Head Occupation" and "Household Head Class of Worker". Given the absence of an explicit target variable for total expenditure, we synthesised the column named "Total Household Expenditure" by aggregating 20 expenditure categories, as illustrated in Figure 9.2. Subsequently, to eliminate redundancy, columns used in this aggregation were removed. Moreover, due to the presence of categorical data, one-hot encoding was applied, transforming these "object" datatype into numerical values suitable for prediction tasks. Notably, the "Region" column was not subjected to this encoding.

```
# Compute the total expenditure
expenditure_columns = ['Total Food Expenditure',
                       'Bread and Cereals Expenditure',
                       'Total Rice Expenditure',
                       'Meat Expenditure',
                       'Total Fish and  marine products Expenditure',
                       'Fruit Expenditure',
                       'Vegetables Expenditure',
                       'Restaurant and hotels Expenditure',
                       'Alcoholic Beverages Expenditure',
                       'Tobacco Expenditure',
                       'Clothing, Footwear and Other Wear Expenditure',
                       'Housing and water Expenditure',
                       'Imputed House Rental Value',
                       'Medical Care Expenditure',
                       'Transportation Expenditure',
                       'Communication Expenditure',
                       'Education Expenditure',
                       'Miscellaneous Goods and Services Expenditure',
                       'Special Occasions Expenditure',
                       'Crop Farming and Gardening expenses']
df['Total Household Expenditure'] = df[expenditure_columns].sum(axis=1)
df = df.drop(expenditure_columns, axis=1)
```

FIGURE 9.2 Code for computing total household expenditure.

9.3.4 Feature Selection

Post one-hot encoding, the result consists 134 columns that pose a threat to overfitting. To mitigate this, a correlation matrix was calculated, guiding us to select the top 20 features that exhibited the highest correlation with "Total Household Expenditure". A heatmap matrix and the final dataset sample is presented in Figures 9.3 and 9.4.

9.3.5 Multivariate Linear Regression (MLR)

Multivariate linear regression (MLR) predicts a dependent variable based on multiple independent variables. It encapsulates the linear relationship between these variables as a weight sum, as presented in the equation:

$$y = b_0 + (b_1 \times x_1) + \cdots + (b_n \times x_n)$$

where:

y = dependent variable

x_1 to x_n = denote the independent variables

b_0 = intercept

b_1 to b_n = coefficients

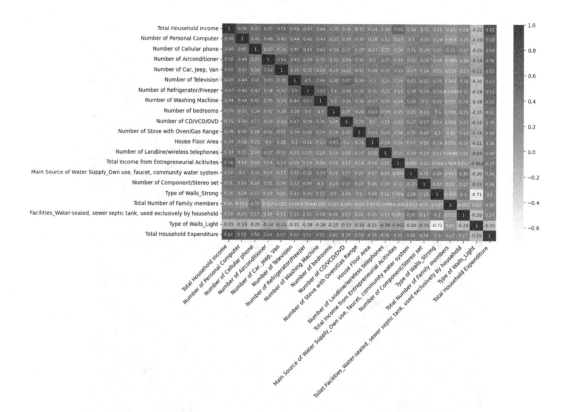

FIGURE 9.3 Top 20 features that correlated with "Total Household Expenditure".

	Total Household Income	Number of Personal Computer	Number of Cellular phone	Number of Airconditioner	Number of Car, Jeep, Van	Number of Television	Number of Refrigerator/Freezer	Number of Washing Machine	Number of bedrooms	Number of CD/VCD/DVD	...	Number of Landline/wireless telephones	Total Income from Entrepreneurial Acitivites	Main Source of Water Supply_Own use, faucet, community water system	Number of Component/Stereo set	Type of Walls_Strong	Total Number of Family members	Toilet Facilities_Water-sealed, sewer septic tank, used exclusively by household	Type of Walls_Light	Total Household Expenditure	Region
0	480332	1	2	0	0	1	1	1	3	1	...	0	44370	1.0	0	1.0	4	1.0	0.0	465737	CAR
1	198235	1	3	0	0	1	0	1	2	1	...	0	0	1.0	1	1.0	3	1.0	0.0	200600	CAR
2	82785	0	0	0	0	0	0	0	1	0	...	0	0	0.0	0	0.0	6	0.0	1.0	185494	CAR
3	107589	0	1	0	0	1	0	0	1	0	...	0	15580	1.0	0	0.0	3	0.0	1.0	230271	CAR
4	189322	0	3	0	0	1	1	0	3	0	...	0	75687	1.0	0	0.0	4	1.0	0.0	299544	CAR

5 rows × 22 columns

FIGURE 9.4 Final dataset sample.

MLR was selected as the predictive modelling technique for this study, with "Total Household Expenditure" serving as the target variable, whereas the other 20 variables, which bear the most correlation with the target, act as predictors. Given linear regression's efficacy in centralised and FL environment [28], MLR is used for both FL and TML in predicting "Total Household Expenditure".

9.3.6 Performance Evaluation

To measure the performance of our MLR model, we rely on two statistical metrics, R^2 and MSE. R^2 measures how well the variations in the predictor variables explain the variations in the dependent variable, which in our case is the "Total Household Expenditure". A higher R^2 value indicates that the model explains a significant portion of the variability in the dependent variable based on the independent variable. MSE calculates the average of squares of the errors or deviations between the predicted and the actual values. Essentially, it captures the average squared difference between what our model predicts as the expenditure and what is actually observed. Low MSE value is desirable as it indicates smaller errors between predicted and observed values, denoting a more accurate model.

9.3.7 TML Settings

For the TML approach, we employed the MLR model using Python's scikit-learn library. After cleaning the dataset, we denoted the feature set as "X", which comprises all columns except the "Total Household Expenditure". The target set, "y", represents the "Total Household Expenditure" column.

We partitioned the dataset into training and test subsets by using an 80-20 split, where 80% of the data was used for training and the remaining 20% for testing purposes. This splitting was accomplished using the "train_test_split" function from the scikit-learn library, setting the "random_state" parameter to 42 to ensure consistent splitting across multiple runs. Then, the MLR model was initialised and trained on the "X_train" and "y_train" dataset. The ".fit()" method was applied to optimise the model's parameters using the training data. After training, the model's predictive accuracy was assessed on the test set. Predicted values for "Total Household Expenditure" were obtained using the ".predict()" method.

9.3.8 FL Settings

For the FL approach, the primary dataset was segregated into 17 distinct partitions based on the "Region" column. This approach was adopted to mimic the real-world scenario in which data from different regions is stored locally and not centrally. Figure 9.5 visually represents these 17 partitions.

For each regional partition, we allocated data into training and testing sets using an 80:20 ratio, using a consistent random seed for reproducibility. Both training and testing datasets, along with their corresponding target values for each partition, were transformed into PyTorch tensors. These tensors were then loaded into DataLoader objects to facilitate batch processing during model training and evaluation. Our predictive model MLR, defined as "MultiLinearRegressionModel" class, originates from the "nn.module" of PyTorch. It consists two layers, input and output. The input layer is designed to accept tensors matching the dimensions of the selected 20 features. The output layer computes a single continuous value representing our target variable, "Total Household Expenditure".

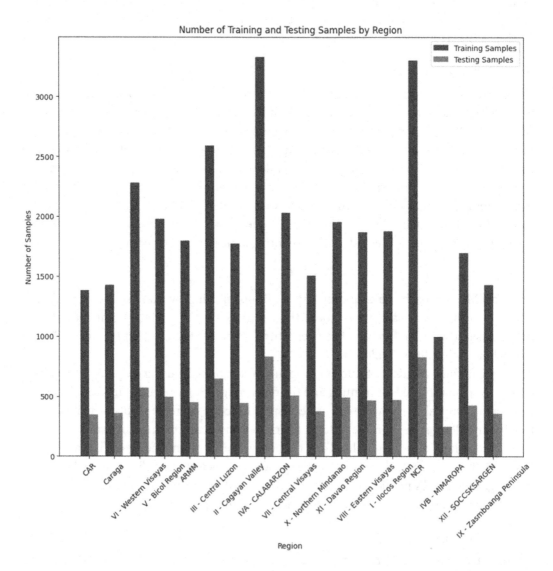

FIGURE 9.5 Training and testing distribution for 17 regions into which clients were partitioned.

We use Flower simulation framework to implement the FL paradigm. Flower is an FL framework that offers both simulated research and real-world applications, streamlining the process of conducting FL with minimal effort [33]. Flower helps in arranging the FL process between clients and the central server, ensuring smooth and efficient model aggregation and distribution. For the Client design, each of the 17 regional data partitions acted as a distinct client. To ensure uniformity and ease of management across all these regional partitions, we devised a custom-designed "FlowerClient" class. This class will perform three tasks, local model training, evaluation, and sharing. After training their local MLR models, each client evaluated the performance using regional testing data. At the end of each round, clients forwarded their model updates to the central server. For our server setup, we employed the built-in federal averaging (FedAvg) strategy by using "fl.server. strategy.FedAvg". Following each training round, the server averaged the received model weights from all clients to produce an updated global model, representing insights from all regions.

To evaluate the predictive capability of the FL approach, we conducted a series of training sessions spread over 30 rounds. During each of these rounds, all 17 regional clients actively participated, with both "fraction_fit" and "fraction_evalute" parameters set to the full value of 1.0. This method was designed with the intention of capitalising the wealth of insights that each region's data offer. As the rounds progressed, model updates from all clients were combined using the FedAvg strategy. This iterative process continually refined our global model. After each round, this enhanced model was then sent back to all participating clients, setting the stage for the subsequent round of training. Upon completing the training rounds, the model was independently tested against each region's dataset and the resulting performance metrics were then aggregated. These aggregated metrics offer a better understanding of the global model's predictive capability across various regional datasets.

9.4 RESULTS

In this section, we discuss the result outcomes of this research work.

9.4.1 Traditional Machine Learning Approach

Using the MLR model, we aimed to predict the "Total Household Expenditure" based on multiple features in the dataset. Our evaluation focused on two essential metrics, MSE and R^2. The MSE, a measure of average squared differences between the predicted and actual values, was found to be 10,317,380,458.57. While an ideal MSE would be zero, indicating perfect prediction, our value suggests that there are notable differences between the predicted and actual expenditures. Such a high value for the MSE implies that there are substantial deviations in some predictions, although it is difficult to interpret the magnitude without contextual benchmarks or comparisons. Our R^2 value stood at 0.7862, which can be interpreted as approximately 78.6% of the variability in the "Total Household Expenditure", which is explained by our model's independent variables. An R^2 value of 1 would denote a perfect fit, so our model's value suggests a reasonably strong relationship between features and the target variable, demonstrating a good model fit. Both MSE and

TABLE 9.1   Traditional Machine Learning Results

Evaluation Metrics	Results
R^2	10,317,380,458.57 (1.03×10^{10})
MSE	0.786 (78.6%)

R^2 observations are supported by Table 9.1. An analysis of the scatterplot (Figure 9.6) offers more insight into the model's performance. The concentration of points in the lower left indicates the model's high accuracy in predicting lower expenditure values. However, as the true expenditure value increases, our model's predictions become less precise, indicating potential challenges in modelling higher expenditure households.

9.4.2 Federated Learning

Using the FL paradigm, the MLR model was trained in a decentralised manner to predict the "Total Household Expenditure" across different nodes. These nodes periodically synchronised with a central sever, which aggregated the models into a global model. The performance metrics used for evaluation were MSE and R^2. Over 30 rounds of FL cycles, the MSE demonstrated a declining pattern. It started at approximately 1.59×10^{10} and eventually stabilised around 2.005×10^8 by the 30th round. In terms of R^2, the model began with a value in the negative domain at around –3.721. However, as training progressed,

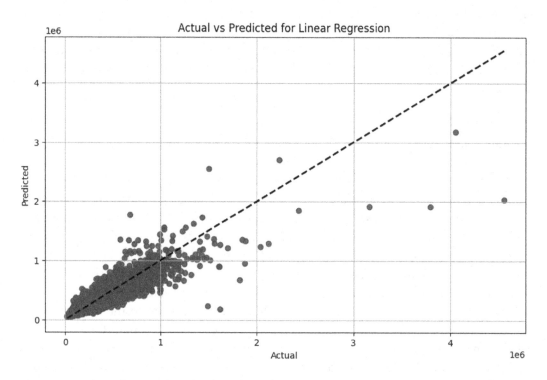

FIGURE 9.6   Actual vs. predicted value of total household expenditure scatterplot in traditional machine learning.

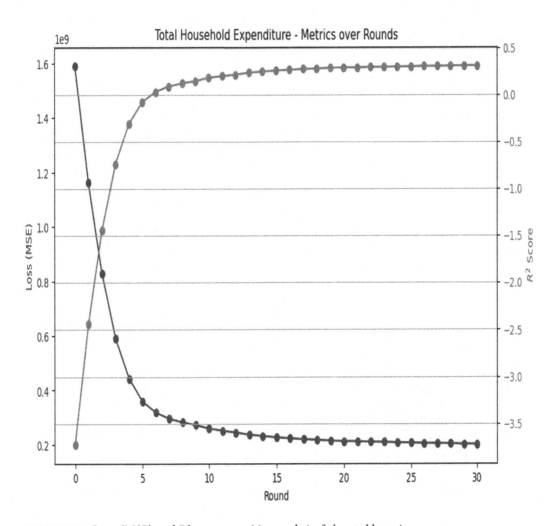

FIGURE 9.7   Loss (MSE) and R^2 score over 30 rounds in federated learning.

this metric showed significant improvement. By the 30th round, an R^2 value of around 0.307 was achieved, suggesting that about 50.7% of the variance in the "Total Household Expenditure" was explained by the model's features. Both metrics for each round are shown in Figure 9.7.

The scatterplot (Figure 9.8) for the global model, which compares actual against predicted expenditure, showed a similar pattern observed in TML approach. Notably, however, there were certain data points in the plot that were distanced from the main concentration compared with TML scatterplot.

9.4.3 Comparing Both Approach Performance

Based on the results, comparing both approaches, TML shows higher R^2 than FL in the 30th round at 0.786 > 0.307. This indicated that TML accounted for a greater percentage of the variance in the "Total Household Expenditure", suggesting a stronger linear relationship

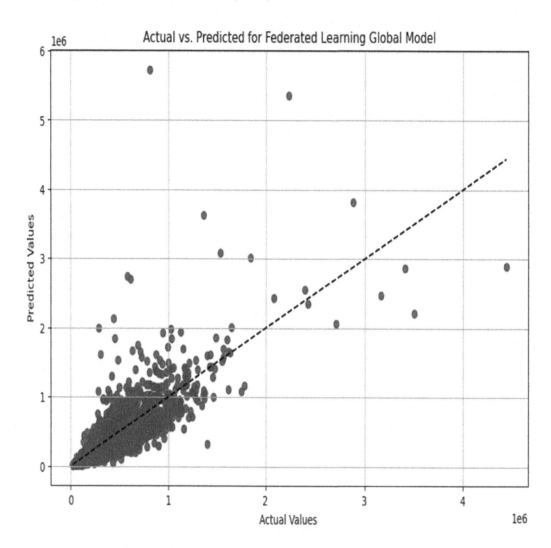

FIGURE 9.8 Actual vs. predicted value of total household expenditure scatterplot in federating learning global model.

with the data. However, TML has a higher MSE score compared with FL at $1.03 \times 10^{10} > 1.86 \times 10^{8}$; FL's MSE score is significantly lower than TML's MSE score. This means that FL's prediction is closer to the actual values despite its lower R^2. Both comparative results are shown in Table 9.2. The implication of these results and potential applications will be further explored in the following section.

TABLE 9.2 Comparative Result for Both Approach

Evaluation Metrics	TML Results	FL Results on 30th round
R^2	0.786 (78.6%)	0.307 (30.7%)
MSE	10,317,380,458.57	20053807.318889
	1.03×10^{10}	1.86×10^{8}

9.5 DISCUSSION

Our study was designed to assess the comparative performance of FL against the TML approach in forecasting household expenditures. We encountered several noteworthy observations and challenges. Upon evaluation, the TML approach exhibited a stronger predictive capability, accounting for approximately 78.6% of variations in expenditures. This indicates that the TML effectively utilises the dataset's features for forecasting. Conversely, despite 30 iterations, FL's predictive accuracy was only achieved at about 30.7%. While TML demonstrated a high ability to capture variations, it also had significant prediction errors. In contrast, FL, despite its lower overall accuracy, was more precise in its expenditure prediction. This highlights the importance of not solely relying on one metric but considering both the overall accuracy and precision of predictions. Although the results showed that FL using the MLR model does not match or outperform all the metrics in the TML approach, it shed light on the potential challenges and limitations for further improvement in future work.

A significant observation was our reliance on the MLR model. Given FL's iterative nature, it may benefit from a more flexible modelling approach. Recent studies, like Pourroostaei Ardakani et al. [28], have identified that alternative models such as SVR and decision trees might offer superior performance in FL settings, especially in stock market prediction. Furthermore, based on Figures 9.6 and 9.8, data points in both approaches concentrated in the lower left, which indicates the model's accuracy in predicting lower expenditure values but not across other expenditure levels. This observation can be attributed to a higher number of households with lower income levels, leading to a non-uniform distribution across the dataset.

In addition, our FL approach was premised on 17 regions, a small number that could limit the comprehensive simulation of FL performance. This also suggested that acquiring more data points is essential. Moreover, based on Figure 9.5, we can see that the data distribution across 17 regions is not identical, which introduces a non-identical and independent data distribution (non-IID) challenge. Zhao et al. [34], highlighted that FL's performance decreased by over 50%. This suggests that the non-IID regional subsets could be impacting our outcomes. While FL inherently addresses data privacy concerns through localising training and testing, data remain on the clients' devices. However, Hao et al. [35] stated that malicious hackers can violate personal data when the parameters are shared. For example, attackers can access patients' healthcare data through wearable devices. A small amount of sensitive information exchange from model to server can lead to malicious attacks stealing raw data, hence invading privacy [36]. Because one of the special features of FL is data privacy, in our FL setup we did not include any privacy-preserving techniques. This could produce a serious privacy concern if it happens in a real-world situation. Both FL and TML offer their own strengths and challenges; the quest for an optimised predictive model for household expenditures requires further exploration in the future.

9.6 FUTURE WORK

To address the modelling section, a comparative analysis should be conducted in the future work. Only exploring the MLR model as the baseline model for comparison is not enough.

By applying a more complex model might suit better in the complex nature of the dataset in household financial prediction. For example, based on the research results of Pourroostaei Ardakani et al. [28], applying random forest might increase our understanding of using only one model for comparison on both approaches in the context of predicting household financial expenditure. Also, because of the nature of the FL process, using a more advanced model like a neural network might obtain a better performance and understanding. Therefore, in future work, we should include a variety of models to continue testing the performance of both approaches. Also, integrating more regions could provide a robust evaluation framework, effectively simulating FL's capabilities. Because the Philippines only has 17 regions in total, perhaps looking into the household datasets of other countries, such as the USA, might provide a greater amount of partitioning. Also, a non-IID challenge is essential to impacting the performance in the FL approach, as exploration of a solution is required. Given the privacy concerns raised, employing methods like differential privacy in future studies can help strengthen the data protection in an FL setting. The differential privacy technique protects an individual client's privacy by adding noise to the data, which ensures a decrease in the chance of an attack on an individual's personalised data [37]. Also, including other metrics, like RMSE, MAE, etc., in the study can provide a more compressive evaluation.

9.7 CONCLUSIONS

To conclude, our study compared the FL approach in predicting household financial expenditure with the TML approach. Results show that FL did not match or outperform in all the metrics when compared with the TML approach, using the MLR model. TML demonstrated better predictive capability capturing a higher variance in expenditures, whereas FL, despite its decentralised nature, showcased better precision. Challenges such as non-IID data distribution in FL and the need for diverse model selections were evident. Privacy concerns in FL highlighted the importance of robust protection mechanisms like differential privacy [38].

REFERENCES

[1] Prihartono, M. R. D., & Asandimitra, N. (2018). Analysis factors influencing financial management behaviour. *International Journal of Academic Research in Business and Social Sciences*, 8(8), 308–326.

[2] Mien, N. T. N., & Thao, T. P. (2015, July). Factors affecting personal financial management behaviors: Evidence from Vietnam. *In Proceedings of the Second Asia-Pacific Conference on Global Business, Economics, Finance and Social Sciences (AP15Vietnam Conference)*, Vol. 10, No. 5, pp. 1–16.

[3] Jennifer, J., & Widoatmodjo, S. (2023). The influence of financial knowledge, financial literacy, and financial technology on financial management behavior among young adults. *International Journal of Application on Economics and Business*, 1(1), 344–353.

[4] Shim, S., Xiao, J. J., Barber, B. L., & Lyons, A. C. (2009). Pathways to life success: A conceptual model of financial well-being for young adults. *Journal of Applied Developmental Psychology*, 30(6), 708–723.

[5] Gomes, F., Haliassos, M., & Ramadorai, T. (2021). Household finance. *Journal of Economic Literature*, 59(3), 919–1000.

[6] Nasteski, V. (2017). An overview of the supervised machine learning methods. *Horizons. b*, 4, 51–62.

[7] Silver-Greenberg, J., Goldstein, M., & Perlroth, N. (2014). JPMorgan Chase Hacking Affects 76 Million Households. *New York Times*, 2.

[8] Tripathi, M., & Mukhopadhyay, A. (2020). Financial loss due to a data privacy breach: An empirical analysis. *Journal of Organizational Computing and Electronic Commerce*, 30(4), 381–400.

[9] Weiss, N. E., & Miller, R. S. (2015, February). The target and other financial data breaches: Frequently asked questions. *Congressional Research Service, Prepared for Members and Committees of Congress February*, Vol. 4, p. 2015.

[10] Cheng, L., Liu, F., & Yao, D. (2017). Enterprise Data breach: Causes, challenges, prevention, and future directions. *Wiley Interdisciplinary Reviews: Data Mining and Knowledge Discovery*, 7(5), e1211.

[11] Zhang, C., Xie, Y., Bai, H., Yu, B., Li, W., & Gao, Y. (2021). A survey on federated learning. *Knowledge-Based Systems*, 216, 106775.

[12] Gill, S. S. Wu, H., Patros, P., Ottaviani, C. et al. (2024). Modern computing: Vision and challenges. *Telematics and Informatics Reports*, 13, 100116.

[13] Li, L., Fan, Y., Tse, M., & Lin, K. Y. (2020). A review of applications in federated learning. *Computers & Industrial Engineering*, 149, 106854.

[14] Gill, S. S., Xu, M., Ottaviani, C. et al. (2022). AI for next generation computing: Emerging trends and future directions. *Internet of Things*, 19, 100514.

[15] Yadav, A., Jha, C. K., & Sharan, A. (2020). Optimizing LSTM for time series prediction in Indian stock market. *Procedia Computer Science*, 167, 2091–2100.

[16] Emsia, E., & Coskuner, C. (2016). Economic growth prediction using optimized support vector machines. *Computational Economics*, 48(3), 453–462.

[17] Zheng, A., Fang, Q., Zhu, Y., Jiang, C., Jin, F., & Wang, X. (2020). An application of ARIMA model for predicting total health expenditure in China from 1978–2022. *Journal of Global Health*, 10(1), 1–8.

[18] Muremyi, R., Haughton, D., Kabano, I., & Niragire, F. (2020). Prediction of out-of-pocket health expenditures in Rwanda using machine learning techniques. *Pan African Medical Journal*, 37(1), 1–14.

[19] Ahmad, Z., & Fatima, A. (2011). Prediction of household expenditure on the basis of household characteristics. *Islamic Countries Society of Statistical Sciences*, 21, 351–367.

[20] Chua, H. N., Ooi, J. S., & Herbland, A. (2021). The effects of different personal data categories on information privacy concern and disclosure. *Computers & Security*, 110, 102453.

[21] Truong, N., Sun, K., Wang, S., Guitton, F., & Guo, Y. (2021). Privacy preservation in federated learning: An insightful survey from the GDPR perspective. *Computers & Security*, 110, 102402.

[22] Dhingra, S., Singh, M., Vaisakh, S.B. et al. (2023). Mind meets machine: Unravelling GPT-4's cognitive psychology. *BenchCouncil Transactions on Benchmarks, Standards and Evaluations*, 3(3), 100139.

[23] Mammen, P. M. (2021). Federated Learning: Opportunities and Challenges. *arXiv preprint* arXiv:2101.05428.

[24] Blanco-Justicia, A., Domingo-Ferrer, J., Martínez, S., Sánchez, D., Flanagan, A., & Tan, K. E. (2021). Achieving security and privacy in federated learning systems: Survey, research challenges and future directions. *Engineering Applications of Artificial Intelligence*, 106, 104468.

[25] Altexsoft. (2020). Federated Learning: The Shift from Centralized to Distributed On-Device Model Training. [Image]. Available at: https://www.altexsoft.com/blog/federated-learning/ [Accessed 23 Aug. 2023].

[26] Rieke, N., Hancox, J., Li, W., Milletari, F., Roth, H. R., Albarqouni, S., Bakas, S., Galtier, M. N., Landman, B. A., Maier-Hein, K., & Ourselin, S. (2020). The future of digital health with federated learning. *NPJ Digital Medicine*, 3(1), 119.

[27] Dayan, I., Roth, H. R., Zhong, A., Harouni, A., Gentili, A., Abidin, A. Z., Liu, A., Costa, A. B., Wood, B. J., Tsai, C. S., & Wang, C. H. (2021). Federated learning for predicting clinical outcomes in patients with COVID-19. *Nature Medicine*, 27(10), 1735–1743.

[28] Pourroostaei Ardakani, S., Du, N., Lin, C., Yang, J. C., Bi, Z., & Chen, L. (2023). A federated learning-enabled predictive analysis to forecast stock market trends. *Journal of Ambient Intelligence and Humanized Computing*, 14(4), 4529–4535.

[29] Walia, G. K., Kumar, M., & Gill, S. S. (2024). AI-empowered fog/edge resource management for IoT applications: A comprehensive review, research challenges and future perspectives. *IEEE Communications Surveys & Tutorials*, 26(1), 619–669.

[30] Singh, R & Gill, S. S. (2023). Edge AI: A survey. *Internet of Things and Cyber-Physical Systems*, 3, 71–92.

[31] Gill, S. S., & Kaur, R. (2023). ChatGPT: Vision and challenges. *Internet of Things and Cyber-Physical Systems*, 3, 262–271.

[32] Flores, F. P. (2017). Filipino Family Income and Expenditure. [Online]. Available at: https://www.kaggle.com/datasets/grosvenpaul/family-income-and-expenditure [Accessed Date 27 May. 2023].

[33] Beutel, D. J., Topal, T., Mathur, A., Qiu, X., Fernandez-Marques, J., Gao, Y., Sani, L., Li, K. H., Parcollet, T., de Gusmão, P. P. B., & Lane, N. D. (2020). Flower: A Friendly Federated Learning Research Framework. *arXiv preprint* arXiv:2007.1439.

[34] Zhao, Y., Li, M., Lai, L., Suda, N., Civin, D., & Chandra, V. (2018). Federated Learning with Non-IID Data. *arXiv preprint* arXiv:1806.00582.

[35] Hao, M., Li, H., Luo, X., Xu, G., Yang, H., & Liu, S. (2019). Efficient and privacy-enhanced federated learning for industrial artificial intelligence. *IEEE Transactions on Industrial Informatics*, 16(10), 6532–6542.

[36] Lyu, L., Yu, H., Ma, X., Chen, C., Sun, L., Zhao, J., Yang, Q., & Philip, S. Y. (2022). Privacy and robustness in federated learning: Attacks and defenses. *IEEE Transactions on Neural Networks and Learning Systems*, 1–21. DOI: https://doi.org/10.1109/TNNLS.2022.3216981

[37] El Ouadrhiri, A., & Abdelhadi, A. (2022). Differential privacy for deep and federated learning: A survey. *IEEE Access*, 10, 22359–22380.

[38] Golec, M., Ozturac, R., Pooranian, Z. et al. (2021). iFaaSBus: A security-and privacy-based lightweight framework for serverless computing using IoT and machine learning. *IEEE Transactions on Industrial Informatics*, 18(5), 3522–3529.

IV

Computing and Business

CHAPTER 10

Deep Neural Network-Based Prediction of Breast Cancer Using Cloud Computing

Sindhu Muthumanickam and Sukhpal Singh Gill

10.1 INTRODUCTION

Breast cancer is the most commonly diagnosed cancer among women globally, with millions of new cases reported each year [1]. While the majority of cases occur in women, men can also develop breast cancer, albeit at lower rates. Its far-reaching impact extends beyond the individual, touching families, communities, and healthcare systems. The journey through diagnosis, treatment, and recovery presents not only medical challenges but also emotional and psychological hurdles that demand a comprehensive and empathetic approach. In the fight against this complex and multifaceted disease, deep learning, a subset of artificial intelligence (AI), has emerged as a potent tool capable of unlocking new dimensions of understanding, detection, and treatment. This chapter delves into the convergence of deep learning and breast cancer research, exploring how advanced computational techniques are reshaping the landscape of medical science and transforming our approach to addressing this formidable challenge.

Breast cancer is an extremely varied disease with many different molecular subgroups and clinical manifestations. It develops when breast tissue cells grow out of control and form a tumour [2]. For a successful intervention and better patient outcomes, early detection and correct diagnosis are essential. However, the complexity of breast cancer's appearance makes using conventional diagnostic techniques difficult. Let us introduce deep learning, a ground-breaking technology that has the power to transform the industry. AI has recently made unheard of advances in healthcare thanks to the accessibility of enormous and varied datasets as well as exponential advances in processing capacity. Deep learning, which is characterised by neural networks that can decipher complex patterns from data, has demonstrated astounding proficiency in a variety of fields, including image identification and natural language processing. Deep learning's capacity to draw conclusions from complicated and high-dimensional datasets offers a special chance to understand the complexity of the disease in the context of breast cancer.

DOI: 10.1201/9781003467199-14

10.1.1 Motivation and Contributions

A major driving force for the research was having experienced the struggles, victories, and emotions of a breast cancer survivor. Being an integral part of the patient right from the diagnosis, treatment, and ultimately winning the disease prompted an in-depth research on breast cancer and to find ways to detect the disease early. Early detection saves patient's lives and reduces the toll of the disease on the patients both physically and emotionally. As per Cancer Research UK statistics [2], it is predicted that one in seven UK females will be diagnosed with breast cancer in their lifetime and around three in four (75.9%) women diagnosed with breast cancer in England survive their disease for 10 years or more. With early diagnosis, the survival rate of the cancer patients can be increased further. The *main contributions* of this research article are as follows:

- Exploring and understanding the Wisconsin Breast Cancer dataset (WBCD) (readily available in sklearn.datasets package of Python),

- Extracting and selecting the most important features using principal component analysis (PCA),

- Building various classification models and a deep neural network (DNN) to predict breast cancer, and

- Building a user-friendly interface to predict breast cancer using DNN built.

10.2 RELATED WORKS

This section will highlight some similar work that has been done in the past employing a dataset on breast cancer using various machine learning techniques. Ten recent research papers have been evaluated in this article to examine machine learning and computational approaches. Research by Yue et al. [3] examined the use of Machine Learning (ML) in the analysis and prediction of breast cancer. The WBCD was employed, and the researcher concentrated on different machine learning models, including K-nearest neighbours (KNNs), decision trees (DTs), artificial neural networks (ANNs), and support vector machines (SVMs). These ML models significantly increased prediction and classification accuracy. The content in the paper is quite understandable and straightforward, and it is presented in a table format with supporting details like classification accuracy, algorithms, and example techniques. Researchers claim that even though many algorithms deliver excellent results with great accuracy, further testing is still required to make algorithms better. To develop an intelligent Friedreich's ataxia (FRDA) healthcare system, the researchers planned to conduct further ML analysis of the FRDA dataset.

To predict breast cancer, Banu & Thirumalaikolundusubramanian [4] employed a different classifier algorithm. The researcher concentrated on Bayes classifiers, such as boosted augmented naïve Bayes (BAN), Bayesian belief network (BBN), and tree augmented naïve Bayes (TAN), and claimed that these might be utilised to obtain enhanced classification and accuracy. This study employed the 569 occurrences and 32 characteristics of WBCD. Here, all classifiers were blended using the gradient boosting (GB) model to increase classification accuracy. Comparing the combined GB results to the other three models' nearly identical accuracy of 90%, the combined GB results were improved. The performance of the classifier was assessed based on its sensitivity, specificity, and accuracy of prediction. The obtained results demonstrated that employing TAN was unquestionably advantageous in classifying breast cancer because it improved the outcome. Chaurasia et al. [5] also used the WBCD collection to develop cancer prediction algorithms that can forecast whether breast cancer will be malignant or benign. The research was assessed by Waikato Environment for Knowledge Analysis (WEKA). To create their cancer prediction models, the researchers used three well-known data mining methods, namely the radial basis function (RBF) network, J48, and naïve Bayes (NB). The researchers employed ten-fold cross-validation techniques to calculate the unbiased estimate of the three constructed prediction models for performance comparison reasons. The method's accuracy and efficacy were used to determine the model's performance assessment. All three models performed well in this experiment, with the RBF network and J48 achieving accuracy levels of 96.77% and 93.41%, respectively. However, the NB model outperformed the others, achieving a classification accuracy of 97.36%. The researchers also performed a specificity and sensitivity analysis to better understand the relative contributions of the independent variables to the prediction of breast cancer survival. The prognosis factor "Class" played the most significant predictor, according to the sensitivity result. A hybrid breast cancer prediction model was developed by Chidambaranathan [6] utilising the extreme learning machine (ELM) and k_means algorithms. Using features extracted from the data, the k_means algorithm precisely clusters tumours. Each cluster denotes a distinct tumour pattern. Single-layer feedforward neural networks (SLFNs) are an expanded form of ELM that detects cancer more quickly and accurately. After SVM classifies an image, the extracted columns are fed into a hybrid technique that combines k_means and ELM. This technique figures out things like sensitivity, specificity, accuracy, and the Jaccard distance. The proposed hybrid system functioned more accurately than the others, according to the results.

Oskouei et al. [7] conducted a thorough analysis of 45 articles that used machine learning and data mining approaches in the detection, treatment, and prognosis of breast cancer. Based on their research topic, the researcher categorised the publications into four groups. According to this study, 21 articles looked into the classification accuracy of the models, 12 articles looked into breast cancer detection, and 1 article looked into and used a regression model to diagnose breast cancer in its earliest stages. Eleven articles were devoted to developing prediction models for early breast cancer detection. The findings of the study demonstrated that no tool exists that can automatically identify breast cancer and recommend an effective course of treatment for the patient. As a result, the researchers saw a necessity for creating a cutting-edge tool that can automate the diagnosis process and suggest essential therapies. Akinsola et al.'s [8] breast cancer prediction app was created to assist physicians in determining whether a patient's tumour is malignant or benign based on their medical records. The Lagos Federal Government Hospital provided the dataset. The researchers classified the dataset using three supervised learning algorithms from the WEKA toolkit: multilayer perceptron (MLP), C4.5, and NB. The performance of the researchers was assessed based on forecast accuracy and building time. The C4.5 model outperformed the other models in terms of speed and efficiency. It took 0.28 seconds and had a 93.9% accuracy rate. It was proposed that more features should be added in the future to improve the patient's usability.

To create the cancer prediction system, Majal et al. [9] used classification and association techniques on the Wisconsin dataset. There are nine characteristics and 699 data points in this particular dataset. The frequent pattern growth algorithm (FP) was used in conjunction with the rule mining methodology to discover the frequent patterns of cancer. A DT-based algorithm was also utilised to predict outcomes based on a few predictor factors, including gender, age, and the severity of the symptoms. The researchers discovered that the model they used had a high accuracy that was reasonable and suitable for use by doctors. In their study, Laghmati et al. [10] presented the various ML algorithms benchmarked to distinguish between sick and healthy breast cancer patients. After evaluating and comparing the results using various parameters, they found that the ANN is a more successful model in determining the severity of breast cancer when compared with SVM, KNN, or DT. Their results yielded an accuracy of 84%. Based on data gathered from hospitals in the Gaza Strip by authors in [11], a model was presented to assist in resolving the challenge of establishing the level of illness risk and to obtain best practices, lifespan, and effect purposes of advanced wellness. The model's application of classification algorithms like SVM, ANN, and KNN to the acquired breast cancer data determines the severity of breast cancer. The accuracy of the model utilising the aforementioned classification strategies on the breast cancer dataset was 77% after evaluation and testing.

However, to predict breast cancer, researchers in [12] used eight different data mining algorithms. Wisconsin Prognostic Breast Cancer Data (WPBC) served as the study's dataset, and experiments were conducted using the four classification algorithms SVM, DT C5.0, Bayes network (BN), and KNN, as well as the four clustering techniques such as Expectation-Maximization (EM), K-means, partitioning around medoids (PAM), and fuzzy c-means. Using the R programming language, the experiment was carried out. The results revealed that classifying algorithms perform better than clustering algorithms, with SVM and DT (C5.0) having the best accuracy of 81% and fuzzy c-means having the lowest accuracy of 37% among the tested algorithms. In contrast, the researchers in [13] described how they used three data mining techniques to categorise breast cancer as either malignant or benign. The following methods were used on the WDBC breast cancer dataset: logistic regression (LR), NB, and DT. According to their data, their classification accuracy is 97.90%, which is higher than the classification accuracy provided by our study, which has a higher prediction accuracy, and the other two tested classifiers. Table 10.1 shows the comparison of proposed work with existing studies for predicting breast cancer.

TABLE 10.1   Comparison of Proposed Work with Existing Studies for Predicting Breast Cancer

Study	Machine Learning Models	Feature Selection	Feature through PCA	DNN Built
[3]	SVM, KNN, ANN	X	X	X
[4]	TAN, BAN, BBN	X	X	X
[5]	Naïve Bayes	X	X	X
[6]	K-means, ELM	X	X	X
This work	SVM, Random Forest Classifiers (RFC), Gradient boosting classifier (GBC)	✓	✓	✓

10.3 PROPOSED TECHNIQUE

The proposed technique contributes to better model performance, reduced overfitting, faster computation, interpretability, and a deeper understanding of the data, ultimately leading to more effective and efficient machine learning models [14]. The selected features are used in basic classification models and a DNN model, and the accuracy of the models is compared [15]. The model with the highest accuracy is chosen and deployed to a website to be used for prediction.

10.3.1 Model Building Process

The following steps have been followed for model building process:

- Detailed exploratory data analysis (EDA),

- Feature selection using PCA, and

- Selected features are used in random classifier, support vector classifier, gradient boosting classifier (GBC), and DNN.

DNNs are a type of ANN with numerous layers of interconnected nodes, or neurons [16]. To learn hierarchical features, each layer of neurons examines the input data and sends it through a series of nonlinear modifications. The DNN architecture contains the following components:

- **Input Layer:** This is the network's first layer; it is where input data is fed into the network. The number of neurons in this layer is proportional to the size of the input data.

- **Hidden Layers:** These are the layers between the input and output layers; this is where most of the computation and feature extraction take place. Each hidden layer consists of multiple neurons, and the number of hidden layers can vary based on the complexity of the problem and the architecture design. Each neuron in a hidden layer takes inputs from the previous layer, performs a weighted sum of inputs, applies an activation function, and passes the result to the next layer.

- **Activation Function:** Every neuron in the hidden layers has an activation function. Rectified linear unit (ReLU), sigmoid, and tanh are examples of common activation functions. These functions give the model nonlinearity, allowing it to discover complicated relationships within the data.

- **Weights and Biases:** These define the connections between neurons. Each link is assigned a weight, which affects the strength of the connection. During the training process, the network learns the ideal weights and biases to minimise the error between expected and actual outputs.

- **Output Layer:** The network's final layer generates output based on the information learned from the preceding layers. The number of neurons in the output layer is determined by the job for which the network is created. For example, in binary

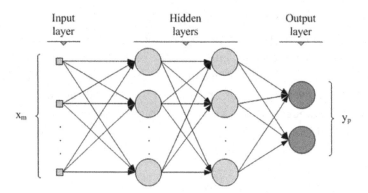

FIGURE 10.1   General DNN architecture.

classification, one neuron may have a sigmoid activation function, whereas in multi-class classification, numerous neurons may have softmax activation.

- **Loss Function:** This computes the difference between the predicted and actual output values. It measures how well the network performs and is used to update the weights and biases during the training phase.

- **Optimisation Algorithm:** The optimisation algorithm (e.g., gradient descent) is used to iteratively update the network's weights and biases during training to minimise the loss function.

- **Backpropagation:** This is the process of propagating errors from the output layer backward through the network to change weights and biases. It allows the network to learn from its mistakes and adjust its parameters as needed.

Figure 10.1 shows the pictorial representation of a DNN architecture.

To solve the problems in this study, a feedforward neural network with three linear layers and ReLU activation functions is built [17]. This is then followed by a sigmoid activation function.

10.3.2 Application and Deployment

A web application is developed in the ASP.NET framework that utilises the model with the highest accuracy to predict breast cancer. We have used the Google Cloud Platform (GCP) to implement the machine learning models in this research work for better performance [16].

10.4 PERFORMANCE EVALUATION

This section discusses the dataset, model implementation, graphical user interface (GUI), and experimental results.

10.4.1 Dataset

The dataset used is the well-known WBCD, which was originally obtained from medical image analysis of breast cancer biopsies. It includes features extracted from digitised

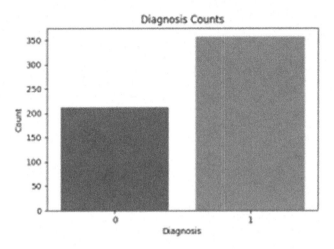

FIGURE 10.2   Data distribution graph.

images of fine-needle aspirates (FNAs) of breast masses. The dataset contains a total of 30 features, which are computed from the cell nucleus characteristics present in the images [18]. These features include measures such as radius, texture, smoothness, compactness, concavity, symmetry, and fractal dimension. The primary objective of the dataset is to classify tumours as either benign (non-cancerous) or malignant (cancerous).

10.4.2 Detailed Exploratory Data Analysis

As the first step of EDA, a data overview is carried out by viewing the dataset, comprehending the data's data type, reviewing its summary statistics, and examining any missing values [19]. Data visualisation is carried out as the second phase in EDA using the distribution of the data, histograms of features grouped by target, box plots of features grouped by target, and correlation heatmaps. The distribution of given data grouped by target is visualised through bar graphs (Figure 10.2).

As per the graph (Figure 10.2), it is evident that the data are not a balanced dataset. Through all these EDAs, we can conclude that we have more benign (non-cancerous) samples compared with malignant (cancerous) samples. We can also note that there are not many outliers that impact the prediction. Also, out of the 30 parameters, not all are correlated and impact the decision-making process.

10.4.3 Feature Selection Using Principal Component Analysis (PCA)

PCA is a method used for selecting a smaller collection of features from the original dataset by using the components produced by PCA. By using this method, the most significant details are retained while removing the less significant ones. A PCA elbow graph is a visualisation tool that aids in choosing the right number of primary components to keep when using PCA to reduce the number of dimensions. The number of major components can be chosen by looking at the "elbow", which is the region in which the explained variance begins to level out. Figure 10.3 shows the generated elbow graph. Based on the graph

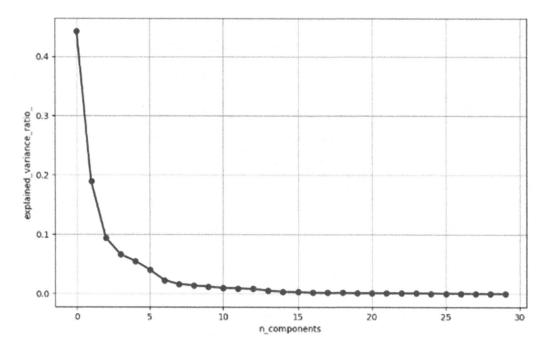

FIGURE 10.3   Elbow graph.

(Figure 10.3), the n_components are selected as 2. Visualising the 2 principal components through a scatterplot is shown in Figure 10.4. When distinct clusters of data points are seen in the scatterplot, it is possible that the number of major components selected is effectively encapsulating significant data structures. According to the scatterplot (Figure 10.3), clusters of data are visible with very little to no overlapping of the data points, hence the n_components selected as 2 is correct.

10.4.4 Model Building and Comparison of Accuracy

The following machine learning models were created using the chosen features.

- Random forest classifier

- Support vector classifier

- GBC

Because the models' best accuracy was 98%, a DNN with three hidden layers is built to increase accuracy even more. An accuracy of 100% is anticipated because the model's goal is to forecast cancer, one of the deadliest diseases. The DNN model that is built is one designed for classification tasks, in which input data are converted via several layers to create a probability score for each class. The DNN model built here consists of three hidden layers, each followed by a ReLU activation function. The final output is obtained by passing the processed data through a sigmoid activation function. The hyperparameters like the

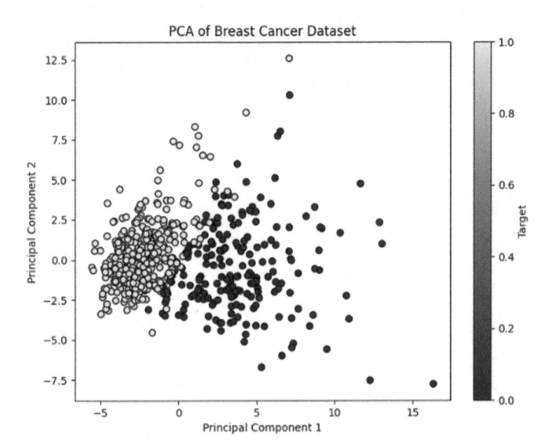

FIGURE 10.4   Scatterplot to view n_components.

optimiser and learning rate are tuned to increase the accuracy of the model. This DNN model is specifically built for binary classification tasks, which is the target of this work. The neural network model's accuracy is 99.12%. Table 10.2 shows the accuracy comparison of the models.

10.4.5 Justification to Use a Deep Neural Network

Though all the models perform fairly well in the prediction, which is evident from the test accuracy, the DNN has the highest accuracy. The models must be able to handle enormous amounts of data when they are used in practical applications. Machine learning algorithms will take longer to predict when dealing with massive amounts of data, delaying the

TABLE 10.2   Accuracy Comparison of Models

Model	Accuracy (%)
Random forest classifier	98.25
Support vector classifier	96.49
Gradient boosting classifier	98.25
Deep neural network	99.12

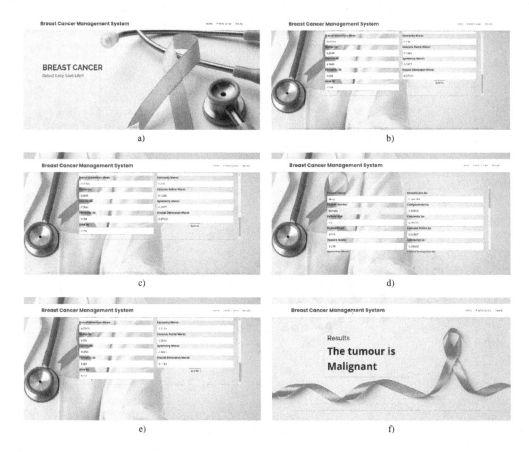

FIGURE 10.5 Implementing using GUI. (a) Landing page of the website; (b) Entering the details of Tumour of the patient for prediction; (c) Submitting the details of patient; (d) Entering the details of Tumour of the patient for prediction; (e) Submitting the details of patient; and (f) Results page.

diagnosis [20]. DNNs can effectively manage vast amounts of data and will solve the time delay issue [21]. Also, neural networks do not need to undergo extensive re-engineering to adapt to and learn from fresh inputs [22]. They are therefore appropriate for applications involving dynamic or developing datasets.

10.4.6 Implementing Using GUI

A website is developed using ASP.NET technology, using CSS, HTML, and C#. When the values are entered, the website uses the DNN to predict whether a tumour is benign or malignant. Screenshots of the website are shown in Figure 10.5.

10.5 CONCLUSION AND FUTURE WORK

Finally, the creation of a deep learning model to predict breast cancer using cloud computing shows enormous promise for improving early diagnosis and treatment outcomes for this common disease. Significant advances in producing accurate and timely forecasts have been made through the use of large-scale datasets and the processing capacity provided by cloud platforms. The model's performance, as indicated by its high sensitivity and specificity rates, highlights its potential as a significant tool in the medical profession. More balanced data for training the model can be used in further work. Also, incorporating multiple types of medical imaging data, such as mammograms, ultrasounds, and magnetic resonance images (MRIs), in the future will produce a more comprehensive and accurate prediction model. Information fusion from many modalities has the potential to increase diagnosis accuracy. Although the built application has a good visual aesthetic, its usability might be enhanced to make it more interactive [21]. The web application can be expanded with other features, such as the ability to gather more information about the patient, their cancer, and their treatment, as well as to display the statistics through graphs that can serve as a foundation for future research [22].

REFERENCES

[1] Siegel, R. L., Miller, K. D., Wagle, N.S. et al. (2023). Cancer statistics, 2023. *CA: A Cancer Journal for Clinicians*, 73(1), 17–48.

[2] Zhou, L., Zhang, Z., Chen, Y. C. et al. (2019). A deep learning-based radionics model for differentiating benign and malignant renal tumours. *Translational Oncology*, 12, 292–300.

[3] Yue, W., Wang, Z., Chen, H., Payne, A., & Liu, X. (2018). Machine learning with applications in breast cancer diagnosis and prognosis. *Designs*, 2(2), 13.

[4] Banu, B., & Thirumalaikolundusubramanian, P. (2018). Comparison of bayes classifiers for breast cancer classification. *Asian Pacific Journal of Cancer Prevention (APJCP)*, 19(10), 2917–2920.

[5] Chaurasia, V., Pal, S., & Tiwari, B. B. (2018). Prediction of benign and malignant breast cancer using data mining techniques. *Journal of Algorithms & Computational Technology*, 12(2), 119–126.

[6] Chidambaranathan, S. (2016). Breast cancer diagnosis based on feature extraction by hybrid of k-means and extreme learning machine algorithms. *ARPN Journal of Engineering and Applied Sciences*, 11(7), 4581–4586.

[7] Oskouei, R. J., Kor, N. M., & Maleki, S. A. (2017). Data mining and medical world: Breast cancers diagnosis, treatment, prognosis and challenges. *American Journal of Cancer Research*, 7(3), 610–627.

[8] Akinsola, A. F., Sokunbi, M. A., & Onadokun, I. O. (2017). Data mining for breast cancer classification. *International Journal of Engineering and Computer Science*, 6(8), 22250–22258.

[9] Majali, J., Niranjan, R., Phatak, V., & Tadakhe, O. (2015). Data mining techniques for diagnosis and prognosis of cancer. *International Journal of Advanced Research in Computer and Communication Engineering*, 4(3), 613–616.

[10] Laghmati, S., Tmiri, A., & Cherradi, B. (2019). Machine learning based system for prediction of breast cancer severity. *In 2019 International Conference on Wireless Networks and Mobile Communications (WINCOM)* (pp. 1–5). Fez, Morocco.

[11] Ahmad, L. G., Eshlaghy, A. T., Poorebrahimi, A., Ebrahimi, M., & Razavi, A. R. (2013). Using three machine learning techniques for predicting breast cancer recurrence. *Journal of Health & Medical Informatics*, 4, 124.

[12] Tafish, M. H., & El-Halees, A. M. (2018). Breast cancer severity degree predication using data mining techniques in the Gaza strip. *2018 International Conference on Promising Electronic Technologies (ICPET)*, Deir El-Balah, pp. 124–128.

[13] Gill, S. S., Wu, H., Patros, P. et al. (2024). Modern computing: Vision and challenges. *Telematics and Informatics Reports*, 13, 100116.

[14] Gill, S. S., Xu, M., Ottaviani, C., Patros, P., Bahsoon, R., Shaghaghi, A. et al. (2022). AI for next generation computing: Emerging trends and future directions. *Internet of Things*, 19, 100514.

[15] Dhillon, A., Singh, A., Vohra, H. et al. (2022). IoTPulse: Machine learning-based enterprise health information system to predict alcohol addiction in Punjab (India) using IoT and fog computing. *Enterprise Information Systems*, 16(7), 1820583.

[16] Moqurrab, S. A., Tariq, N., Anjum, A. et al. (2022). A deep learning-based privacy-preserving model for smart healthcare in internet of medical things using fog computing. *Wireless Personal Communications*, 126(3), 2379–2401.

[17] Iftikhar, S., Golec, M., Chowdhury, D. et al. (2022). FogDLearner: A deep learning-based cardiac health diagnosis framework using fog computing. *Proceedings of the 2022 Australasian Computer Science Week*, pp. 136–144.

[18] Desai, F., Chowdhury, D., Kaur, R. et al. (2022). HealthCloud: A system for monitoring health status of heart patients using machine learning and cloud computing. *Internet of Things*, 17, 100485.

[19] Ojha, U., & Goel, S., (2017). A study on prediction of breast cancer recurrence using data mining techniques. *2017 7th Int. Conf. on Cloud Computing, Data Science & Engineering—Confluence* (pp. 527–530). IEEE.

[20] Singh, R. & Gill, S. S. (2023). Edge AI: A survey. *Internet of Things and Cyber-Physical Systems*, 3, 71–92.

[21] Gill, S. S., & Kaur, R. (2023). ChatGPT: Vision and challenges. *Internet of Things and Cyber-Physical Systems*, 3, 262–271.

[22] Ginanjar, S., Wibowo, A., & Sarwoko, E. A. (2020). The best architecture selection with deep neural network (DNN) method for breast cancer classification using MicroRNA data. *Journal of Physics: Conference Series*, 1524(1), 012106.

CHAPTER 11

Performance Analysis of Machine Learning Models for Data Visualisation in SME

Google Cloud vs. AWS Cloud

Jisma Choudhury and Sukhpal Singh Gill

11.1 INTRODUCTION

It is 2023, yet machine learning (ML) techniques are not being used in small- to medium-sized enterprises (SMEs) within the United Kingdom, although using advanced ML techniques has potential revenue growth [1]. ML is a vital element in decision-making that can add valuable visualisation quickly into an enormous data set by converting raw data into meaningful material that makes businesses profitable and supports their ability to compete in the trade. The traditional tools and techniques are obsolete for decision support in vast data analysis used to predict data within retail or travel enterprises, whereas ML techniques can be used for pattern recognition as they have key components to recognise the correct object type, such as fish, flowers, etc. [2]. There is much research to provide information on the cloud for SMEs [3]; therefore, the use of the cloud within small businesses is increasing due to publicity. Although small- to medium-sized businesses are using cloud computing, they are not familiar with ML techniques due to less publicity on ML techniques for SMEs. To increase publicity, this chapter is focused on advanced ML techniques. Constructing an efficient ML structure is costly and usually takes several years to implement a project for an organisation. Along with this, the abundance of algorithms also creates complications in selecting a suitable one for creating the solution to a specific business problem.

In this chapter, we propose to build a cost-effective ML model in a cloud computing environment to solve the restraints in the current design approaches. The flexibility of the cloud architecture or services resolves the hardware limitation for the business. This chapter is dedicated to researching and experimenting with advanced ML techniques. The secondary research and experiments prepared for this work ensure outcomes through realistic investigation within a short time frame. The ML model can be reused in various

DOI: 10.1201/9781003467199-15

distinct sections at various phases for efficiency, cost, and time [4]. An effective combination of several methods using appropriate algorithms such as fragmentation, image classifications, linear regression, etc. can be created. To use these ML methods, this work is going to use several cloud platforms, such as Google Cloud Platform (GCP), Amazon Web Services (AWS), Jupyter Notebook, and Colab Notebook, for cloud services [5]. This work has produced a lively, scalable, and convenient architecture for SMEs to encourage them to use ML techniques in their businesses.

11.1.1 Motivation and Our Contributions

The motivation of hybrid ML techniques applied to the business sector's retail parameter is infinite. First, the SME does not have adequate resources to build the business solution due to cost; hence, deploying cost-effective ML techniques is the best way to gain experience with them. This surges advantages and boosts revenues [4]. Secondly, SMEs have little opportunity, as the research that is available is mostly for larger businesses and the dataset is larger in quantity, as a result of SMEs' failure to distinguish the data. Hence, this chapter uses a combination of small- and medium-sized datasets to get the most from hybrid ML to obtain familiarity from the data, permitting SMEs and myself to develop insights into the ML framework to run businesses more efficiently [3]. Also, an advanced ML model can support SMEs in meeting their individual needs as much as it can guide SMEs to perform much better in using a planned decision.

Here, we have shown that it is achievable to involve SMEs such as retail, a seafood company, or a travel agency in the ML framework within the cloud or cloud-related services for their business. To achieve success, we have provided an experiment that includes tools and services from cloud providers, such as appropriate cloud instances from AWS and GCP, and GCP-provided cloud notebooks such as Google Colab [6]. In this way, we have provided a theoretical and practical experiment to visualise how to use ML techniques for their business. For instance, seafood retailers can classify the type of fish, and travel retailers can predict customer information [7]. Therefore, we have explored and found the solution for fish image classification using the advanced algorithm "MobileNet-v-3Large", which is the latest ML technique for Graphics Processing Unit (GPU)-based image classification and the best function of prediction to achieve 100% accuracy [8]. On the other hand, we have used AutoML to perceive the evaluation metrics from GCP and AWS to create an easy experiment for SMEs, and we have submitted an AWS and GCP's AutoML file to Kaggle to determine the better accuracy prediction of AWS and GCP. To obtain the accuracy, we have written code that opens the prediction files given by GCP and AWS and converts them to the correct format to upload to Kaggle. We have provided all ipynb files and shared links in the appendices. This work has provided cost and time analysis while exploring AWS and GCP. Hence, it inspires SMEs to apply ML techniques in their business. We have also achieved classification performance (100% accuracy) using MobileNet-v-3Large in fish classification categories. Finally, we have deployed an application-enabled classification model using deep learning for flower and grass prediction. This achievement also contributes to educating florist business owners about ML techniques for flower classification. Later this work will discuss the ML advanced techniques individually and traditional computing techniques in data classification and prediction and the features, such as storage, instances, etc., of cloud services that are related to this field. In general, this chapter is thoroughly related to the six objective types as follows:

1. Investigate the advantages of ML classification methods on the cloud and compare them with traditional computer vision techniques.

2. Experiment with the features of two different cloud platforms and evaluate their features.

3. Be able to get live predictions from the dataset on the cloud.

4. Train a model on a GPU-based cloud notebook platform to improve accuracy.

5. Deploy a trained model using deep learning techniques.

6. Compare the performance of different cloud providers and their services in terms of cost and time.

11.2 PROBLEM STATEMENT

According to Jain et al. [9], SMEs are the key factor for a country's economic growth and to create jobs in developing countries. The literature demonstrated that only a small quantity of SME is successful with excellent performance and maintainable growth. Hence, it is essential to define the socioeconomic issues that delay their growth.

SMEs like seafood retail spoil fish due to a lack of categorisation and classification of the fish [10]. Considering the quality of fish in retail, categorisation and classification must be carried out thoroughly to avoid spoilage that produces severe human health issues and economic loss [11]. Hence, the illnesses and decline in seafood offerings, with individual symptoms in different species, mainly required the categorisation of species. In this area, the current lengthy and slow traditional methods can be replaced with classifications based on ML and image methods that exhibit fast and precise outcomes [12]. Thus, it is required to design practical and appropriate datasets. Nonetheless, most of the publicly offered datasets do not fit the revealed aim. These types of datasets mostly contain images from underwater species that are usually not consumed. In this chapter, a realistic dataset covering nine individual fish was collected from the Aegean Region of Turkey [13]. Furthermore, complete experiments based on different classification approaches are performed to analyse the usability of this collected dataset [14]. To investigate several methods, various data have been used, such as Titanic data to predict survivors, which will create a concept for data prediction for a travel agency. To support florist enterprises, a flower classification model has been selected to predict accuracy [15]. These experimental consequences demonstrate promising outcomes. Hence, these trained data will be available for further examinations to inspire retail business.

11.3 RELATED WORK

SMEs ensure economic growth in Europe. An estimated 88.8 million people worked for SMEs in the European Union (EU) generating € 3.666 trillion in revenue [16]. The most recent financial crisis and the subsequent economic recession in the EU28 had a significant negative impact on SMEs, making it challenging for them to remain in good standing in the economy [17]. The aim of this previously mentioned research has already been discussed; therefore, this literature review would be related to the research objectives.

ML is the study of computer algorithms that can improve themselves through experience and data use. Data classification is part of the ML technique for predicting the classification of the data; for example, classification predictions are tricky, including a discrete class label output. The classification algorithm is a supervised learning method that can detect a class of new clarifications based on data training [18]. A classification algorithm is a function that evaluates the features of an input so it can separate one class into positive values of an output and negative values for others.

A review of the literature was discussed in the introduction, then were expanded in different sections to categorise modern approaches to ML classification. Three extensive methodologies were explained, including those in which advanced ML algorithms were applied to compete in the retail business domain. For example, mobile apps could use the first training method, the MobileNet algorithm, to tell the difference between the pattern and the seafood-based category [19]. The second experiment used small data to train a classification model called the binary classification set on pre-trained AutoML of the GCP, which gives access to phenomenon cloud tools like Table, Vertex AI, and more on a small dataset to obtain better results. In the third approach, using AWS SageMaker, Autopilot used the same Titanic data as GCP [20]. Therefore, it can define the cloud tools to compare with both AutoML. The next approach is distributing a large dataset, which was pulled from the direct Kaggle website to the S3 bucket. Although, due to instance capacity unavailability and rigidity, the AWS SageMaker distribution was curved, exploring AWS SageMaker delivers an understanding of cloud computing. The fourth approach was a fish classifier using MobiletNet; the prediction accuracy was 100% and the data loss was less than 0.004502 [21]. Finally, the most inspired experiment was deploying a GPU-optimised FastAI library using cnn_learner to predict classifications of dandelion and grass images [22]. The reason for combining several approaches is to experiment with and understand different approaches, as this chapter not only focused on seafood retail but also on florists and travel agencies; hence, these businesses have potential revenue.

11.4 PROPOSED MODEL

In this section, we discuss the proposed model and its components.

- *FastAI* is an advanced deep learning library, founded in 2016, that focuses on deep learning and artificial intelligence [23]. It provides a high level of competence and the outcome of the state of the art in the deep learning domain. It builds new approaches without considerable negotiation in terms of ease of use, performance, and flexibility. It is a new category of transmit system for Python, along with tensors that GPU-optimise new computer visions as an extension of pure Python [24].

- *cnn_learner* helps to get a pre-trained model with a specified architecture through a custom head that suits the data best.

- *XGBoost* uses a gradient boosting framework, which is a decision tree-based cooperative ML algorithm involving prediction problems for unstructured data such as images, text, etc. [25].

- *GCP AutoML* tables take the user's dataset to train their data for various model architectures simultaneously. Hence, this approach allows the AutoML technique to establish the best model architecture for the developer's data quickly without taking consecutive iterations across several achievable model architectures. It helps to clean data, provides missing information, predicts accuracy, and helps to distribute the data. The model architecture's AutoML Table analyses include linear, deep neural networks, gradient-boosted decision trees, etc. [26].

- AWS AutoML with SageMaker Autopilot supports building binary classification models to maximise data accuracy. First it inspects the data using a single Application Programming Interface (API) call, then runs several candidates to understand the optimal combination of data preprocessing steps and ML algorithms [27].

- *Google Colab* is best for many things, from refining Python coding abilities to creating effectiveness with deep learning libraries such as PyTorch, TensorFlow, and Keras. There are many advanced ML algorithms that can provide solutions to prediction problems. MobileNet-v-3Large is one of them. It is the third version of the architecture and has capabilities for image analysis for mobile applications. This architecture can be incorporated with frameworks such as TensorFlow Lite [26].

11.5 PERFORMANCE EVALUATION

This section discusses the dataset and implementation details, along with the experimental results.

11.5.1 Dataset Information

Table 11.1 shows the dataset information.

11.5.2 Implementation

To implement an ML distributed system, first a large dataset must be selected from Kaggle and directly uploaded to the AWS S3 bucket. However, due to instance capacity unavailability, this method has been changed.

TABLE 11.1   Dataset Information

Dataset Name	Source	Size
Gravitational-wave-detection	https://www.kaggle.com/c/g2net-gravitational-wave-detection/overview	73 GB
Fish dataset	https://www.kaggle.com/crowww/a-large-scale-fish-dataset	3 GB
Greenran_image_Classifier	https://www.kaggle.com/code/btphan/greenr-an-image-classifier-in-fastai	205 KB
Titanic	https://www.kaggle.com/c/titanic	165 KB

GCP AutoML: This strategy from GCP's Table provides tools to help ML workflow training, evaluating, and deploying models to make predictions [28]. This function manages the dataset, such as images, tabular text, and video data, and creates a custom model with minimal effort. To deploy the train data, it requires importing data from storage. Thus, this work has imported a dataset from cloud storage [29]. Training the data requires a target column for the model to predict, and the data need to be categorised for AutoML to build a classification model. After running AutoML, the model needs to be exported to evaluate and test the data. Figure 11.1 shows the accuracy of the binary classification model after the train model.

The next step in this implementation is to evaluate the model data. Thus, this GCP tool delivers a test dataset to BigQuery. This section of the implementation includes confusion metrics. Confusion metrics review the success of classification predictions for a model. The ground truth labels are the matrix rows, and the columns are the model's label predictions. It scans each row to resolve the misclassifications that occur; the blue cell specifies

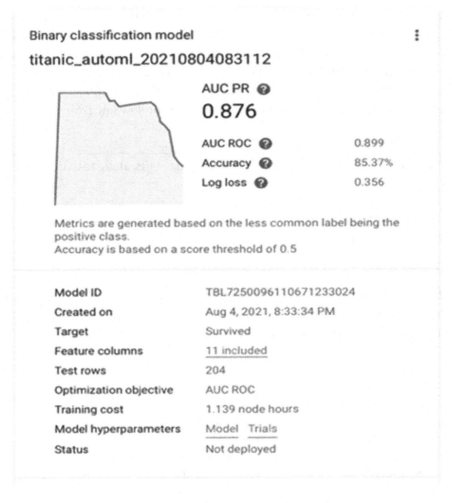

FIGURE 11.1   The accuracy of binary classification.

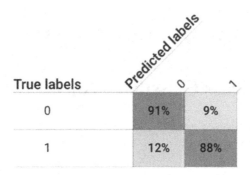

FIGURE 11.2   GCP AutoML Predicted labels.

accurate predictions for the label (true positives or negatives), whereas the grey cells signify the errors (false positives or negatives). Figure 11.2 shows the GCP AutoML-predicted labels.

The evaluation section holds the prediction of targeted data "survived", and the accuracy is shown in Figure 11.3.

The next step is to use online prediction. The model has been deployed to the cloud using deploy to endpoint from the instances to the cloud using AutoML-enabled prebuild API to send Representational State Transfer (REST) requests. Thus, the result shows the prediction. The figure has been used in the test and analysis sections.

- **AWS SageMaker Autopilot**: To train data on AutoML, Autopilot is user-friendly; you just need to create an instance and upload data from the S3 bucket, then run Autopilot. It automatically trains the data.

- **Deep learning deployment**: Python's development on FastAI enables this implementation. This deployment allows users to select and upload an image to predict their classification, as shown in Figure 11.4.

After uploading the result, it shows 72.7% accuracy in Figure 11.5.

This implementation allows users to see the prediction directly on the websites, as shown in Figure 11.6.

11.5.3 Test and Results

Autopilot focused on detailing coding and provided pdfs in the Jupyter Notebook instances [30]. It shows the date created and information about the data. It does not provide specific

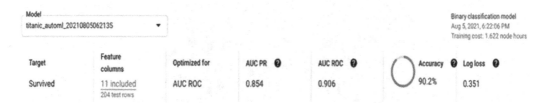

FIGURE 11.3   Binary classification accuracy results.

Jisma Choudhury, Student ID: 200769013

Dandelio and Grass Classifier Project

Is your picture of a dandelion or grass?

Select picture to upload:

1. Choose File   grass 1

2. Upload

Submit picture URL

1. https://images.unsplash.com/photo-1533460004989-cef01064af7e?ixid=Mnwxl

2. Upload

FIGURE 11.4   Select and upload image.

Prediction: **dandelion**

Confidence: [('dandelion', '72.7%'), ('grass', '27.3%')]

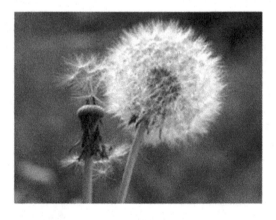

FIGURE 11.5   Outcome of the prediction.

Prediction: **grass**
Confidence: **[('grass', '73.1%'), [('dandelion', '26.9%')]**

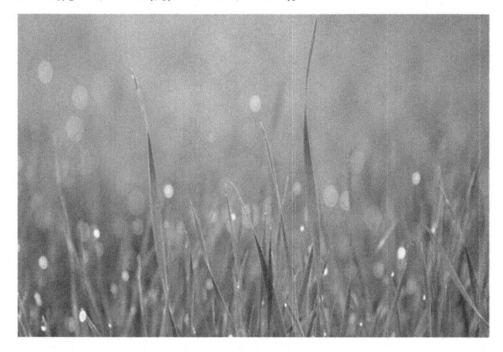

FIGURE 11.6   Predicting images using weblink.

prediction outcomes such as F1, data loss, or accuracy, so it does not meet expectations. GCP AutoML provided live prediction and met expectations by providing specific prediction outcomes such as F1, data loss, and accuracy. Google Colab-trained data testing provided a Colab accuracy of 1.00, which meets the expectations of the proposed solutions as shown in Figure 11.7.

- **Colab**: Data loss is 0.00405 as shown in Figure 11.8. Results of model evaluation are shown in Figure 11.9.

- **Kaggle submission**: Submitting on Kaggle shows the score of AWS and GCP AutoML in Figure 11.10. It makes it easy to compare both services.

11.5.4 Comparison of Cloud Services

GCP plays a crucial role in these experimental results. Firstly, it inspires users to explore the platform provided with a £300 credit. Although AWS offers free-tier services, they are not suitable for ML instances. Here, this chapter critically compares GCP and AWS to guide SMEs in their understanding of cloud-based ML services. Therefore, this chapter looks at their tools and services to compare them. AutoML played a key role in creating a fast initial model. It has been used as a baseline or proof of concept that is useful for manufacturing models. AutoML enables a high-quality custom ML model with a slight effort.

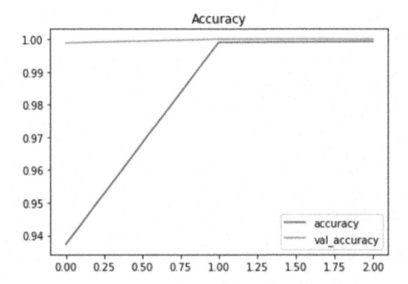

FIGURE 11.7   Colab accuracy.

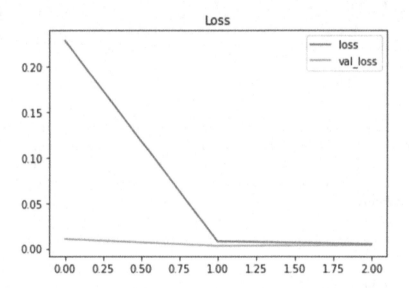

FIGURE 11.8   Data loss.

```
results = model.evaluate(test_images)

print(f"Test Loss: {results[0]:.5f}")
print(f"Test Accuracy: {results[1]:.4f}")

29/29 [==============================] – 485s 17s/step – loss: 0.0041 – accuracy: 1.0000
Test Loss: 0.00405
Test Accuracy: 1.0000
```

FIGURE 11.9   Result of model evaluation.

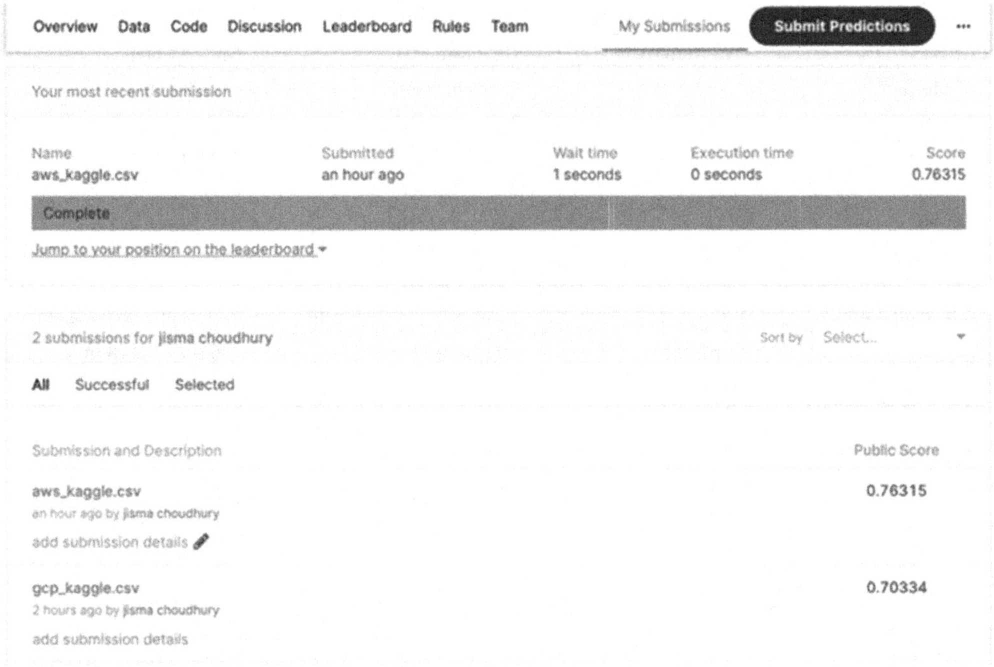

FIGURE 11.10 Kaggle score.

It allows users to define their own selected categories from the list. The online prediction of this method delivers an API to approach the model that is being created to apply in generating predictions. It can be compared with AWS SageMaker Autopilot (AutoML), and GCP. AutoML has better features; it provides details of data, the classification model, predicted accuracy, and details of implementation such as time, cost, etc. On the other hand, AWS SageMaker autopilot does not provide enough instances for on-demand services. Therefore, within the GPU limitation, SageMaker failed to provide details on predicted accuracy, confused metrics, etc. However, elasticity-wise, GCP has greater flexibility to accessibility with no strict limitation on use, while to use AWS instances for SageMaker requires asking the service centre to increase instances. In terms of time, GCP is a much faster way to implement ML models, whereas AWS is not suitable for short-term projects if the project uses on-demand services. In every section of the ML model there are instance limitations for on-demand. To get back the request reply from the AWS service centre it can take up to 72 hours to prove it, thus consuming time for a project. To compare cost, GCP was a great deal; it provides first-time users with £300 in credits, thus allowing this work to explore and experiment with GCP smoothly without cost concerns. In contrast, AWS is costly. To analyse data, this project used FSx at first, and it was four times higher than an ordinary AWS instance, costing £1.80/hr. As this work is experiment-based and it took time to understand the data analysis result using FSx, the total cost was £72. GCP provides Google Colab, which also played a crucial role. It predicted medium-sized data within 9 minutes with no cost and performed well to predict data. Table 11.2 compares AWS AutoML, GCP AutoML, and Google Colab customised ML.

TABLE 11.2   Comparison of AWS AutoML, GCP AutoML, and Colab Cloud Notebook

Criteria	AWS AutoML	GCP AutoML	Google Colab
ML Model	Classification	Classification	Classification
F1 score	0.857	Not specified	N/A
Accuracy	90.2	92.6	1.0000
Precision	83.3	Not specified	N/A
Data loss	0.341	Not specified	0.00405
Confusion metrics	Not specified	True/predicted table 0: 91/1:88	N/A
Code availability	Not specified	Provide code with pdf	Fully self-customised
Time	60 minutes	60 minutes	485 seconds (8 minutes) 17 s/step
Cost	1.139 node hour	0.20 per hour	None
Kaggle rated score	0.70334	0.76315	N/A
Size capacity	124 KB	124 KB	3 GB

11.6 CONCLUSIONS

This chapter is motivated by ML techniques that allow SMEs to be stimulated in their trade to increase business revenue. Hence, it determines cost analysis, prediction performance, and time efficiency using different ML techniques on the GCP, AWS, and Google Colab platforms. Through these cloud service platforms, techniques such as AutoML, customised ML-trained models, GPU-based ML algorithms, and MobileNet3 have helped to improve prediction accuracy. In contrast, this work has deployed a deep learning classifier model. Thus, this work delivers the concept of using cloud-based ML techniques practically. Hence, an analysis has been made on the inspiration of classification performance and several cloud platform tools to visualise the most applicable technique to be used in a cost-effective project.

REFERENCES

[1] Gill, S. S., Xu, M., Ottaviani, C. et al. (2022). AI for next generation computing: Emerging trends and future directions. *Internet of Things*, 19, 100514.

[2] Casturi, N. V. (2019). Enterprise Data Mining & Machine Learning Framework on Cloud Computing for Investment Platforms. Computer Business.

[3] Singh, A., & Gill, S. S. (2020). Measuring the maturity of Indian small and medium enterprises for unofficial readiness for capability maturity model integration-based software process improvement. *Journal of Software: Evolution and Process*, 32(9), e2261.

[4] Gill, S. S. Wu, H., Patros, P. et al. (2024). Modern computing: Vision and challenges. *Telematics and Informatics Reports*, 13, 100116.

[5] Walia, G. K. Kumar, M., & Gill, S. S. (2024). AI-empowered fog/edge resource management for IoT applications: A comprehensive review, research challenges and future perspectives. *IEEE Communications Surveys & Tutorials*, 26(1), 619–669.

[6] Kingsley, M. S. (2023). Comparing AWS, Azure, and GCP. *In Cloud Technologies and Services: Theoretical Concepts and Practical Applications* (pp. 381–393). Springer International Publishing.

[7] Hu, D., Li, Q., Duan, Y., Han, G., Chen, X., & Si, J. (2012). Fish species classification by color texture and multi-class support vector machine using computer vision. *Computers and Electronics in Agriculture*, 88, 133–140.

[8] Nijhawan, R. et al. (2019). A Hybrid Deep Learning Approach for Automatic Fish Classification. *In Proceedings of ICETIT 2019, Emerging Trends in Information Technology* (pp. 427–436). IEEE

[9] Jain, N., Tomar, A., & Jana, P. K. (2018). Novel framework for performance prediction of small and medium scale enterprises: A machine learning approach. *2018 International Conference on Advances in Computing, Communications and Informatics (ICACCI)*, pp. 42–47. https://doi.org/10.1109/ICACCI.2018.8554747

[10] Hasija, M. J., Buragohain, S., & Indu, S. (2017). Fish species classification using graph embedding discriminant analysis. *International Conference on Machine Vision and Information Technology (CMVIT)*. 81–86

[11] Spampinato, D., Giordano, R. D., Salvo, Y.-H. J., Chen-Burger, R. B., Fisher, G., & Nadarajan, G. (2010). Automatic fish classification for underwater species behavior understanding. *Proceedings of the first ACM International Workshop on Analysis and Retrieval of Tracked Events and Motion in Imagery Streams.*

[12] Gill, S. S. (2024). Quantum and blockchain based serverless edge computing: A vision, model, new trends and future directions. *Internet Technology Letters*, 7(1), e275.

[13] Pornpanomchai, B., Lurstwut, P., Leerasakultham, W., & Kitiyanan, W. (2013). Shape and texture based fish image recognition system. *Kasetsart Journal - Natural Science*, 47(4), 624–634.

[14] Ogunlana, O., Olabode, O., Oluwadare, S. A. A., & Iwasokun, G. B. (2015). Fish classification using support vector machine. *African Journal of Computing & ICT*, 8(2), 75–82.

[15] Larsen, R., Olafsdottir, H., & Ersboll, B. K. (2009). Shape and texture-based classification of fish species. *Scandinavian Conference on Image Analysis*, 5575, 745–749

[16] Molnár, I., & Belyó, P. (2015). 17. Improving SME Performance Globally: The Hungarian Case. In Ghauri, P.N., and Kirpalani, V.H., M. eds. *Handbook of Research on International Entrepreneurship Strategy: Improving SME Performance Globally* (pp. 351–383). Edgar Elgar Publishing Limited.

[17] Assante, D., Castro, M., Hamburg, I., & Martin, S. (2016). The use of cloud computing in SMEs. *Procedia Computer Science*, 83, 1207–1212.

[18] Gill, S. S., & Kaur, R. (2023). ChatGPT: Vision and challenges. *Internet of Things and Cyber-Physical Systems*, 3, 262–271.

[19] Pan, H., Pang, Z., Wang, Y., Wang, Y., & Chen, L. (2020). A new image recognition and classification method combining transfer learning algorithm and mobile net model for welding defects. *IEEE Access*, 8, 119951–119960.

[20] Nandhakumar, A. R., Baranwal, A. et al. (2024). Edgeaisim: A toolkit for simulation and modelling of ai models in edge computing environments. *Measurement: Sensors*, 31, 100939.

[21] Olalekan Elesin (2020) Automate the end-to-end AutoML lifecycle with Amazon SageMaker Autopilot and Amazon Step Functions — CD4AutoML. Online Available: Olalekan.medium.com/automate-the-end-to-end-automl-lifecycle-with-amazon-sagemaker-autopilot-and-amazon-step-functions-d5589a569853

[22] Singh, R. et al. (2023). Edge AI: A survey. *Internet of Things and Cyber-Physical Systems*, 3, 71–92.

[23] Rothman, D. (2020). *Artificial Intelligence By Example: Acquire Advanced AI, Machine Learning, and Deep Learning Design Skills*. Packt Publishing Ltd.

[24] Howard, J., & Gugger, S. (2020). Fastai: A layered API for deep learning. *Information*, 11(2), 108.

[25] Li, J., An, X., Li, Q.,Wang, C., Yu, H., Zhou, X., & Geng, Y. A. (2022). Application of XGBoost algorithm in the optimization of pollutant concentration. *Atmospheric Research*, 276, 106238.

[26] Sabharwal, N., & Agrawal, A. (2021). *Up and Running Google AutoML and AI Platform: Building Machine Learning and NLP Models Using AutoML and AI Platform for Production Environment (English Edition)*. BPB Publications.

[27] Das, P., Ivkin, N., Bansal, T., Rouesnel, L., Gautier, P., Karnin, Z., ... & Venkateswar, K. (2020, June). Amazon SageMaker autopilot: A white box AutoML solution at scale. *Proceedings of the Fourth International Workshop on Data Management for End-to-End Machine Learning*, pp. 1–7.

[28] Singh, S., Chana, I., & Singh, M. (2017). The journey of QoS-aware autonomic cloud computing. *IT Professional*, 19(2), 42–49.

[29] Gill, S. S., Chana, I., Singh, M., & Buyya, R. (2019). RADAR: Self-configuring and self-healing in resource management for enhancing quality of cloud services. *Concurrency and Computation: Practice and Experience*, 31(1), e4834.

[30] Boom, B. J., Huang, P. X., He, J., & Fisher, R. B. (2012). Supporting ground-truth annotation of image datasets using clustering. *Proceedings of International Conference on Pattern Recognition*, 1542–1545

V

Security and Edge/Cloud Computing

CHAPTER 12

Enhancing Data Security for Cloud Service Providers Using AI

Muhammed Golec, Sai Siddharth Ponugoti, and Sukhpal Singh Gill

12.1 INTRODUCTION

With the widespread use of Internet technologies, increasing processing power and storage needs have brought with them many technological developments. Digital technology innovation, especially in the Information Technology (IT) sector, has introduced products and services that will perform tasks in a more organised and efficient manner. One of these services is cloud computing [1]. Cloud computing is a computing service in which services such as storage, networking, and processing are offered to users via the Internet [2]. Many companies, including those in the commercial and government sectors, are moving sensitive information to the cloud using cloud service providers (CSPs) such as Microsoft, Google, and Amazon due to the numerous advantages it provides, such as adaptability, extensibility, centralisation, etc. [3]. Many commercial CSPs offer users advantages such as a convenient economic model, dynamic scalability, and low operational complexity with the various delivery models they offer. However, in addition to these advantages, problems such as security, privacy, and cold start are the biggest obstacles to the adoption of cloud computing by everyone [4].

Ensuring security in cloud computing is critical for the universal adoption of this technology. As a result, many researchers have experimented with various methods, including using blockchain and secure communication protocols [5–7]. Another method to increase data security in cloud computing is to combine digital forensics and artificial intelligence (AI) [8]. Digital forensics involves analysing digital data, such as log data, to determine the impact of security problems such as data leakage that may occur in cloud environments [9]. If combined with AI techniques [10], such as *advanced analysis speed*, the size of the digital data collected can reach huge sizes. AI models can process large volumes of data quickly. Combined with *pattern recognition*, with advanced algorithms, AI models can easily detect patterns that digital forensics experts may miss and thus detect potential threats more accurately.

DOI: 10.1201/9781003467199-17

12.1.1 Motivation and Contributions

Although cloud computing offers advantages such as high processing power and storage, it still brings problems such as security and privacy. In applications where sensitive data, such as biometric data, is used [11], the use of the cloud is still a major concern. Therefore, this problem must be solved for the cloud to be adopted by all segments. This chapter presents a digital forensic-based approach to increasing data security in CSPs. This research focuses on the deployment of private cloud infrastructures as well as how services ensure digital security because moving data to the cloud exposes consumers who use their preferred cloud service to special attacks from hackers. Part of this initiative focuses on how to keep data stored in clouds secure. Thus, it is aimed at providing a basis for future studies combining AI and forensic techniques [12]. This article [12] examines how well a cloud user can constantly monitor the CPS's data protection through monitoring and, in the event of a breach of the signed agreement, how the supplier can follow up using forensic techniques. To achieve this, we create technical solutions that will consistently provide users of cloud services with adequate information security while attempting to implement regular audits against the service-level agreements (SLAs) provided by cloud providers at the beginning of the contract. We also use forensic tools to track data security breaches on the CSP's side when such incidents occur. The main contributions of this chapter include

- Using a digital forensics toolkit to enhance data security in cloud computing,

- Laying the foundation for future studies combining AI and digital forensics,

- Monitoring security threats to the cloud architecture by performing cloud auditing on the client side, and

- Using virtual machine (VM) technology to test the proposed approach.

12.2 BACKGROUND

In this section, some basics of cloud computing are explained to the reader.

12.2.1 Cloud Computing's Inception

In 1961, John McCarthy, an Massachusetts Institute of Technology (MIT) professor, proposed the idea of computers as a utility analogous to electricity. Then, in 1969, J. C. R. Licklider, who eventually went on to establish the Advanced Research Projects Agency Network (ARPANET)'s foundation, proposed an "Interplanetary computer network" at ARPA, and Bolt, Beranek, and Newman agreed (BBN). The convergence of McCarthy's utilities computing notion and Licklider's large network laid the groundwork for the further growth of cloud computing [13]. In 2002, Amazon Web Services (AWS) was launched, and it offered a spectrum of cloud-based services ranging from computing to storage. They subsequently introduced the Elastic Compute Cloud (EC2) [14] in 2006, which is a business online service that allows users to rent machines by the hour. "Amazon EC2/S3 was the first globally available cloud computing architecture provider", according to Jeremy Allaire, Chairman of the Board of Brightcove [15]. Google and others began to provide browser-based corporate applications, such as Google Apps, in 2009, which marked a key milestone in cloud computing. The advancement of virtualisation technologies has been a significant factor in the development of cloud computing. High-bandwidth access is another option. The exponential upsurge of smart mobile phones and e-book gadgets is a key part of the mystery that has brought everything together and is signalling a new virtualization paradigm [16].

Beyond these, there are even more sensing or other modern devices implanted in a wide range of physical objects, such as automobiles, utilities, hospital instruments, camera systems, highways, waterways, medicines, and animals. These are connecting the world's largest online and offline infrastructure, resulting in a plethora of new, apps [10]. These are critical characteristics in IT systems as traditional infrastructure is not designed to scale-up or scale-down in response to variations in demand. As a result, the common answer is to over allocate resources, resulting in underutilisation of overall resources. As a result, elasticity is a critical function in cloud services, allowing for automated scaling-up and scaling-down without further work.

12.2.2 On-Demand Self-Service

This is a cloud computing feature that allows a user to set up and utilise a cloud service without interacting with a human and obtain access to the processing power and storage they demand. This avoids the hassles associated with the traditional IT approach, in which each demand for extra capacity necessitates going through the regular bureaucracy of budgeting, obtaining equipment, deploying, and training, among other things. Obtaining this infrastructure, on the other hand, is as straightforward as purchasing a present online using self-service [17].

12.2.3 Pervasive Accessibility (Apps and Beyond)

Another quality the cloud inherits from its online ancestors is ubiquitous access. All entities' capabilities are open and available to anyone using any compatible device or service, according to the idea of seamless access (application). Within and beyond the company, cloud computing is a driving factor for service ubiquity [18].

12.2.4 Comprehensive Virtualisation

The early age of mass acceptance of IT utilising the cloud was marred by a lack of mature technologies and qualified staff, resulting in "VM sprawl". The lack of apparent transparency of connectivity components – to behave as one from the perspective of software engineers and organisational groups – was a missing element in this era. Regardless of a cloud's degree of scale, the ease of dealing with it remains the same, i.e., it remains as simple to manage and develop platforms as if it were a single server. This is the definition of total virtualisation [19].

12.2.4.1 Private Clouds

Inner clouds, usually referred to as private clouds, are IT assets and applications that are possessed, managed, and presumed to be limited to a single enterprise. Generally, the cloud infrastructure is operated within the borders of the owning company [20]. Although the term "private cloud" may appear to be a euphemism in the notion that clouds are designed to be shared, some scenarios do occur where an organisation may want to develop and maintain their own cloud. Therefore, corporations must acquire, create, and operate these clouds, missing out on the cost benefits as well as the less practical experience that public clouds provide. The private cloud, on the other hand, is devoted to a single company; thus, risk monitoring and day-to-day operations of hosts are managed by the company, and defined security standards, rules, and compliance with regulations may be imposed.

12.2.4.2 Public Cloud

A public cloud is a cloud computing installation plan that is available to the masses and is hosted, administered, and maintained by a third cloud computing provider. Individual users or companies are referred to as the general public. With public clouds, the third-party cloud services vendor handles day-to-day administration and performance, leaving the client with very little influence over the cloud's logical and physical safety. Public clouds are a cost-effective choice for businesses because they deliver instant cost reductions [21]. This is because cloud deployments relieve the corporation of the burden of managing IT infrastructures and enable access to cutting-edge capabilities without debilitating capital investment costs. The clouds that were offered were largely public clouds like Amazon, Google, and Salesforce, and they tended to specialise in delivering services on certain tiers. Amazon, for example, concentrates on connectivity services, whereas Google and Salesforce concentrate on software solutions.

12.3 RELATED WORK

This section's main goal is to examine the body of prior writing on the topic with respect to this work. To identify areas of variance from those of the project, it evaluates previously linked technological schemes and approaches involved in keeping data safe in a world where losing sensitive or secret information exposes one to the danger of fraud or copyright violations, as well as the potential for immediate damage to an organisation's brand. In comparison to the outdated method of storing data utilising magnetic tapes (such as those found in floppy drives), hard drives, and mainframes, Judith Hurwitz's [22] presentation offers superior storage in terms of capacity and security to some extent. This article explores the advantages of cloud services, including scalability through dynamic, or "on-demand", purveying of resources on a fine-grained basis, where customers serve themselves in close proximity to real time without the users having to plan ahead for peak loads, performance, maintenance, and scalability, among others. Due to the aforementioned facts, additional cloud computing research work examines how to secure cloud services, and from the user's perspective, we embrace this service based on trust. But this work goes a step further by examining how to make sure that from the user's perspective we do not just adopt these services based on trust, hoping that our data are kept secured in the cloud and that these data are not compromised in terms of security, but also making sure that we can audit and also carry out forensic investigations in places that matter and when it is necessary, especially in cases where there is a breach of security measure(s) in the cloud [23].

12.3.1 Market for Cloud Computing

After defining cloud computing, we will now examine the many vendors who provide cloud computing services and what they have to offer.

12.3.1.1 Amazon Web Services (AWS)

One of the first businesses to make cloud computing services available to the general public is Amazon, which offers the most comprehensive cloud service. Amazon has made significant investments in data centres that it previously solely utilised for its own operations before deciding to offer these computer capabilities to the general public. Consequently, the public will be able to benefit from Amazon's computer infrastructure [14, 21]. Amazon provides a variety of cloud services, such as the following:

EC2 is a web service that enables scalable application deployment by offering an interface through which a user can build VMs and additional central processing unit (CPU) cycles to load any necessary software. The customer then pays by the hour for active servers and receives scalable application deployment [14]. You may store and retrieve anything up to 5 GB in size using Amazon's virtual storage service using the *Simple Storage Service (S3)* web services interface. *Simple Queue Service (SQS)* is a distributed queue messaging service that uses a message passing API to enable communication between several computers over the Internet [24]. A content delivery network called Cloud Front uses a worldwide network of edge points to provide content [25].

12.3.1.2 Microsoft Azure Services Platform

The public cloud implementation, called the Windows Azure platform, is part of Microsoft's cloud service and is run on Microsoft's global data centres. An operating system called Windows Azure is used to run apps and services that end users employ for hosting, administration, and development of IT infrastructure. The end user uses the offered libraries in conjunction with programmes like Visual Studio to create the needed Azure-based apps [21, 26].

12.3.1.3 Google Cloud Platform (GCP)

With the help of Google App Engine, developers may create web applications that run on Google's network. Python and Java are the programming languages that are currently supported. Google App Engine makes it simple to deploy web apps by supplying computer resources as needed [26]. Utilising Bigtable and other parts of Google's scalable architecture through the Google App Engine makes it simpler to adjust to changes [27].

12.4 SECURITY ISSUES AND METHODOLOGY

As we saw in the last section, cloud computing has many amazing advantages, including cost savings and simple access to cutting-edge resources. However, security issues are a major obstacle when thinking about deploying key applications and sensitive data to a public cloud environment. The cloud services provider must now handle these security issues by creating security measures that are on par with or better than those that the business would employ in their own private enterprise. We explore these security issues in this chapter and offer a method that would allow a user of a cloud service to be sure that the service provider upholds this service level [28].

12.4.1 Cloud Computing Risks

In the article "Seven Cloud Computing Risks", published by Gartner[1], it is stated that certain concerns regarding the security of the cloud service should be brought up with the seller.

The following are some cloud computing risks:

- **User access:** Due to insider threats, access control is a major consideration when discussing cloud computing services. The employment practices and logical and physical network access at the service provider's end are out of the user's control when using a cloud service. As a result, the user is vulnerable to compromise by others who are also responsible for providing the service [29].

- **Regulatory compliance:** Despite the fact that the service provider stores the cloud user's data, it is still the user's responsibility to ensure its security and integrity. Customers must check that these services can comply with regulatory obligations as a result, or they face legal action.

- **Location of data:** While utilising cloud services, a consumer runs the risk of having their data stored abroad. Additionally, the criteria and limitations that must be applied to data access vary for each country. For instance, whereas other nations might not even have any restrictions, the European Economic Area (EEA) has the Data Protection Act. The cloud user therefore runs the danger of falling short of the legal requirements for compliance [21].

- **Data separation:** Users who utilise cloud services incur the risk of having their data kept in a shared environment with data from other users. Data are encrypted both during transit and at rest; however, encryption may or may not be offered. Despite the effectiveness of encryption, its availability is weakened [10].

- **Recovery:** When using cloud services, disaster recovery is crucial. Users may not be aware of the actual location of their data, but it is there and it is exposed to hazards like fire, water, and other natural catastrophes. Customers are thus quite concerned because they have no idea what may happen to their data.

- **Support for investigations:** In the event of a security breach, accessing logs and data is typically challenging because multiple customers are frequently co-located and because the information about the customer may be dispersed across various servers and data centres, making it challenging to conduct an investigation.

12.4.2 Top Threats to Cloud Computing

The biggest dangers to cloud computing, according to the Cloud Security Alliance, are as follows:

- **Threat 1: Cloud computing abuse and nefarious usage:** Because service providers have little control over who uses their services, criminals may use the vast resources to carry out evil deeds like hosting Trojans and botnets [10].

- **Threat 2: Unsecure APIs and interfaces:** A consumer may be exposed to security risks as a result of using the software interface and APIs offered by service providers, which might jeopardise the confidentiality, integrity, and accessibility of their data.

- **Threat 3: Negative insiders**: Customers may be exposed to potential harmful insiders who may have access to their sensitive information because the providers do not have stringent recruiting policies or access control structures.

- **Threat 4: Shared technology issues**: Cloud providers make use of virtualisation technology to make their services scalable, therefore exposing the customer to flaws from the hypervisor and insufficient isolation.

- **Threat 5: Hijacking an account or service**: Attackers who are able to get client security credentials can damage data integrity and steer users away from the genuine site and towards a malicious one.

- **Threat 6: Risk profile unknown**: Giving over management of its infrastructure to a cloud provider exposes a company to the possibility of security safeguards failing [23].

12.4.3 Investigation of Cloud Services

With the use of computer forensic evidence, computer crime offenders may be prosecuted. Computer forensics is the use of scientific techniques and computing tools to verify the presence or non-occurrence of a suspected event. Analysing storage media like CDs or hard drives is a step in the acquisition of forensic evidence.

The following steps are included in forensic analysis:

1. Confirming that an occurrence has indeed occurred.

2. Collecting evidence and making sure that the chain of custody of the evidence is upheld using methods designed particularly to preserve the integrity of the evidence.

3. Examining and analysing the data.

4. Results reporting.

5. Computer forensics must be conducted in a way that preserves the standards of evidence that may be used as acceptable evidence in a court of law [23].

12.4.4 Challenges of Digital Forensics in the Cloud Ecosystem

Although proponents of cloud computing highlight its scalability and cost-effectiveness as reasons to utilise cloud services, forensic scientists consider this a forensic issue due to the scale and variety. The following are the difficulties in performing a forensic investigation in a cloud environment:

- Determining the computing and storage capabilities necessary for the research,

- Distinguishing consumer data sources when gathering evidence,

- Cloud-based forensic analytic methodologies adaptation,

- Developing live analytic methods,

- Developing better methods for log production and analysis, and

- Gaining a thorough grasp of processes, their interdependencies, and how they are distributed throughout various cloud ecosystem systems.

Figure 12.1 shows the solution's architecture in detail. Three VMs running on a VMware Workstation must be used to achieve this solution. Two of the VMs are configured to operate in a client-server configuration and are running Windows 10 and Ubuntu operating systems. The FortiGate security gateway virtual appliance, which is set up to guarantee the security of the cloud deployment, is the third VM. The forensic toolbox was put in place to analyse server-side digital evidence on the client side. By adding AI models to the framework we propose in the next stages, server-side digital evidence can be analysed and prediction results with higher accuracy can be produced.

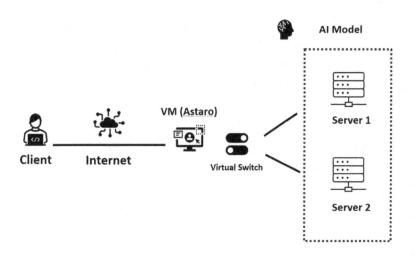

FIGURE 12.1   The main architecture.

12.4.5 Software Components

The following are the main software components considered in this work:

- **VMware Server Workstation:** Virtualisation software such as VMware Workstation is used to help in the rapid installation of several VMs on a real server. Figure 12.2 shows the design overview of the VM. Hardware and programs supported by VMware Server include:

  - Any standard x86-compatible or x86-64-compatible personal computer

  - Windows, Linux, Solaris, and other guest operating systems (both 32-bit and 64-bit)

  - Two-way Virtual Symmetric Multi-Processing (SMP)

  - Intel Virtualisation Technology (Intel VT)

  - AMD-Virtualisation (AMT-V)

- **FortiGate Security Gateway:** A virtual appliance called FortiGate Security Gateway is made to function in VMware settings. It was the first unified threat management software with VMware compatibility. It enables quick and simple implementation of a comprehensive security solution. Industry-leading security features including an intrusion prevention system (IPS), web filtering, secure sockets layer (SSL) inspection, and automated threat protection are combined by FortiGate next-generation firewalls (NGFWs) to provide security-driven networking [28].

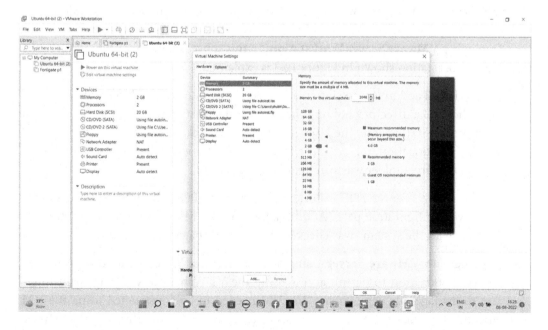

FIGURE 12.2 Design overview.

- **Forensic Toolkit (FTK):** This is a computer forensics programme that offers top-notch password cracking, decryption, and computer forensic analysis. It is an enterprise-class scalability, speed, and analytics-driven digital investigative platform that has received judicial validation [22].

12.5 IMPLEMENTATION

We outline the procedures followed in this chapter to accomplish the previously mentioned goals. Forensic analysis of the cloud deployment also entails setting up the virtual environment, configuring the security components, and deploying the FTK. The goal of this solution is to offer a safe cloud infrastructure that enables client-side forensic investigation of the server. The client-server arrangement of this work is a good representation of the cloud infrastructure. After the installation, the setup follows involving various design elements, including the FortiGate Security Gateway, the FTK, the Windows 10 and Ubuntu VMs, and the VMware Server Workstation.

12.5.1 Solution Design

The aim of this chapter is to present a new study that increases security in the cloud for AI forensics, which is still in its infancy. The client-server arrangement of this work is a good representation of the cloud infrastructure. Then, we set up the various design elements, including the FortiGate Security Gateway, FTK, Windows XP and Ubuntu VMs, VMware Workstation, and VMs for those two operating systems [30].

12.5.1.1 Setup and Configuration

The main steps to setting up configurations for performance evaluation are as follows:

- **Deploying VMware Server Workstation:** In this subsection, the configuration of the server workstation shown in Figure 12.3 is explained.

   1. The initial action was to sign in as the Administrator on the Microsoft Windows 11 host. The directory holding the downloaded installation file was then chosen from the Start menu. The User Account Control dialogue box was then used to give authorisation to launch the installation, after which the license is approved and the target folder was specified for installation.

   2. The FQDN, Server HTTP Port, and Server HTTPS Port were entered on the Server configuration page. Additionally, "Allow VMs to start and stop automatically with the system" was checked on that same page [31].

- **Logging Into VMware Server Using VI Web Access:** We configured the VMware Server Workstation to permit access using the VI Web Access management interface to manage our deployment. The VM needed to be constructed using the VM wizard before the operating system was installed to deploy the VMs on the VMware Workstation.

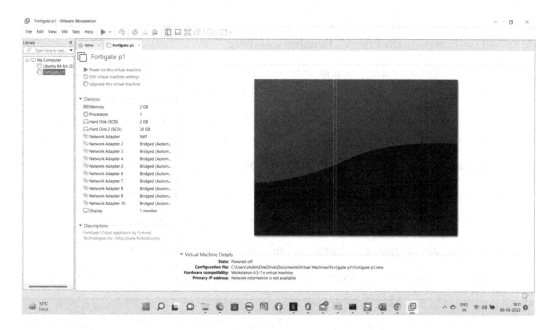

FIGURE 12.3   VMware Server Workstation configuration overview.

- **A New VM Can Be Created:** Figure 12.4 shows the creation of a new VM using the following steps:

  1. Create VM was selected in the host workspace's commands section after logging in to the Web Access management interface.

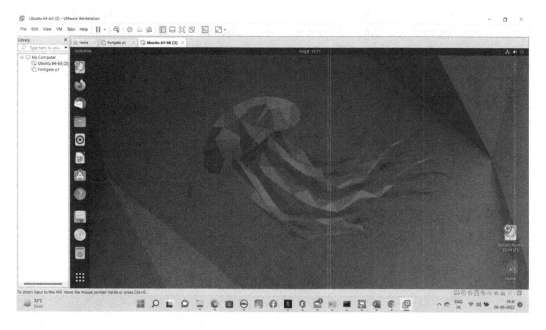

FIGURE 12.4   VM running Ubuntu.

2. A datastore was chosen from a list of available datastores on the Name and Location page after the VM's name was input.

3. The kind of operating system to be installed on the new VM and its version were chosen on the Guest Operating System tab.

4. The hardware version 7 (the default) was chosen under the Product Compatibility header so that the VM could run the newest VMware Workstation.

- **Deploying the Windows 10 and Ubuntu VMs on VMware Workstation**

1. From the already existing datastore, the ISO Image was chosen.

2. The Virtual Device Node section's SCSI or IDE device node was also chosen.

3. The virtual computer was powered once the modifications were stored.

4. The Console tab was selected to finish installing the guest operating system using VMware Remote Console.

5. To complete installation, the procedures applicable to Windows XP and Ubuntu O.S. were followed.

- **Deploying FortiGate on VMware Workstation:** Figure 12.5 shows *FortiGate homepage and* Figure 12.6 shows *Ubuntu IP address.*

1. The Infrastructure Client was launched to log into the VMware Workstation administration interface once the downloaded package was unzipped in the VMachines directory [29].

2. The VMX file for FortiGate was chosen and added to the Inventory from the context menu under the datastore area where the virtual FortiGate is situated.

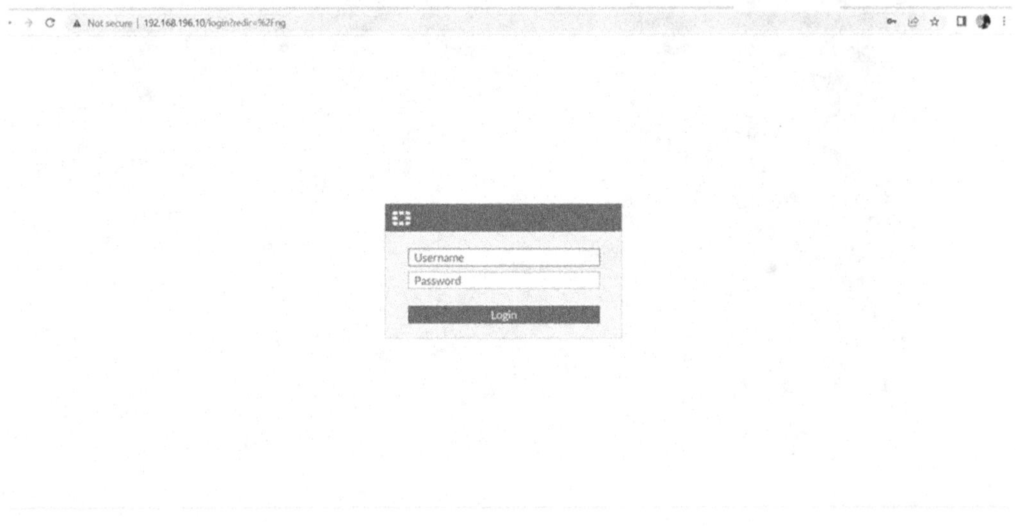

FIGURE 12.5   FortiGate homepage.

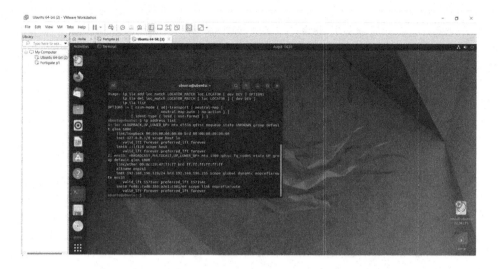

FIGURE 12.6   Ubuntu IP address using ipconfig on terminal.

3. After selecting a name for the FortiGate, the VMware Add to Inventory Wizard launched.

4. The VM's operating system was then defined as the VMware Workstation, and the Add to Inventory Wizard was finished.

5. After that, the required IP address settings were completed.

6. The SSL certificate was approved once the web browser was given the valid URL.

7. A strong password and a legitimate email address were supplied for the administrator account because this was the first time FortiGate's online front end (named WebAdmin) had been launched.

8. The Perform Basic System Setup button was clicked to continue logging in and the admin username and password specified was entered.

9. After logging in, the Dashboard of WebAdmin appeared, providing us with all system status information of the FortiGate Security Gateway unit.

   – Network configuration information

   – Windows 10-VM1 – 192.168.206.1

   – Ubuntu-VM2 – 192.168.196.128/24

   – FortiGate – 192.168.196.10/24

- **HTTP/S:** FortiGate was set up as an HTTP/S caching proxy using the HTTP/S tab. Simple cache services, web filtering, etc. are provided by the HTTP/S of FortiGate.

- **Firewall:** The firewall's packet filter rules were created and managed using the packet filter. Figure 12.7 shows the statistics of FortiGate.

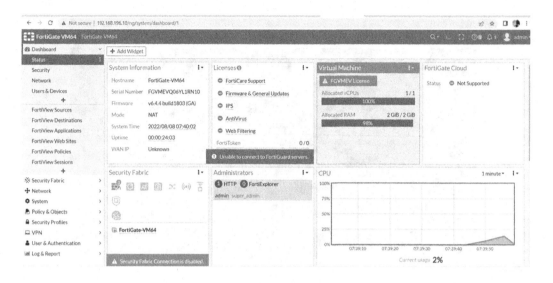

FIGURE 12.7   FortiGate network security statistics.

- **Events:** The firewall's IPS rules were set forth on the Events tab. The IPS is a signature-based IPS that analyses all traffic before automatically thwarting assaults in their attempts to infiltrate the network. Figure 12.8 shows the statistics of the FortiGate event system.

- **VPN Logging:** The Events tab in FortiGate was used to enable VPN logging. All system interactions, including FTP Data connections, Admin messages, IPS warnings, etc. were enabled on the computer. Figure 12.9 shows the FortiGate events system.

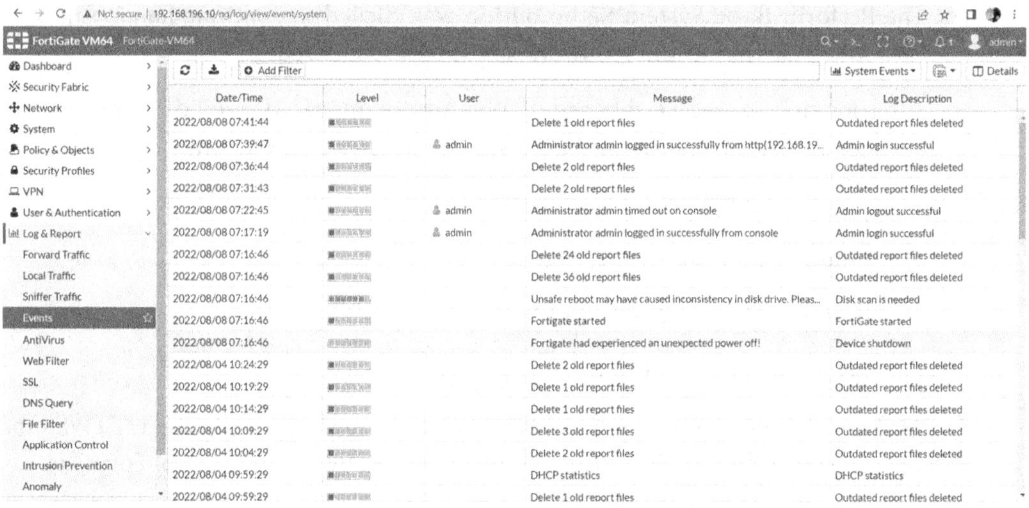

FIGURE 12.8   FortiGate event system statistics.

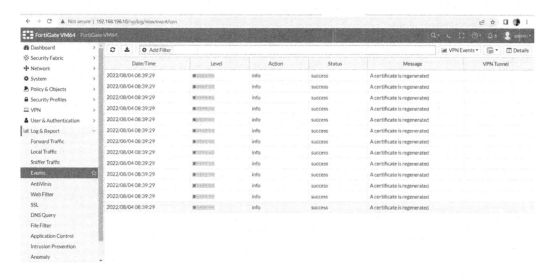

FIGURE 12.9   FortiGate events system.

- **Turning on Audit in Windows 10:** Local auditing and logging in Windows 10 must be enabled to support forensic analysis.

    1. After accessing the control panel and logging in as the administrator, the local security policy was enlarged to show the various policy settings.

    2. The needed type of auditing was then enabled.

- **FTK Deployment:** The goal of FTK is to provide a comprehensive computer forensics solution. It provides a collection of the most popular forensic tools in one location for investigators/cyber security analysts. One of the most important procedures in a digital forensic investigation is forensic imaging. Making an archive or backup copy of the complete hard disk is what it is all about; it is a storage file with all the data required to start the operating system. However, for this imaged disk to function, the hard drive must be used. Disk image files cannot be used to recover a hard drive because they need to be opened and loaded on the drive using an imaging application. Several disk images can be stored on a single hard drive [15]. Flash drives with more storage space can also be used to store disk images. FTK will have you covered whether you are attempting to break a password, examine emails, or search for certain characters in files. And just to sweeten the deal even more, it also has a user-friendly GUI. The following actions were done in order to install and execute FTK:

    - **Configure Access Data FTK Imager:** Access data software installation was completed when the installation wizard was run, the instructions were followed, and all defaults were accepted.

    - **Setup FTK:** FTK was then installed by selecting Autorun once Access data software had been installed. The location for the FTK components was chosen after

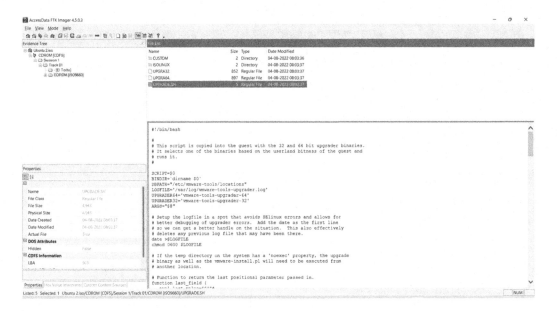

FIGURE 12.10   FTK running forensic analysis on the server logs.

reading and accepting the Access data license agreement. The programme was successfully installed by following the on-screen instructions.

- **Run FTK:** To add the schema to the database, FTK was then executed. Figure 12.10 shows *running forensic analysis logs*.

If there was any security threat or discrepancy in the data, it would have been highlighted in red, which would help us be aware of any potential data breach. Create full-disk forensic pictures and handle a variety of data types from many sources, including network data, Internet storage, data from mobile devices, and data from hard drives. This is a technique for extracting and dumping a volatile content's contents onto a non-volatile storage medium to keep them for later analysis. Only when the acquisition has been carried out correctly without distorting the picture of the volatile memory can a RAM analysis be carried out properly [28]. Because the volatile data will not be around when the system reboots, the investigator must exercise caution when collecting it at this point. All of this is done in a centralised, secure database. Parse Windows system information files and registry files in a tab that is simple to read, interactive, and reportable. Label, bookmark, and export each item separately for each category to make finding, filtering, and reporting simple. Use visualisation technology that presents your data in timelines, cluster graphs, pie charts, geolocations, and other ways to help you understand events better.

12.6 CONCLUSIONS AND FUTURE WORK

Cloud computing is a technological development that has entered our lives in many areas, including military and civilian applications, and has been used in academia and the private sector for many years. Because it still has some security flaws, application developers have not fully adopted it. The main focus of this chapter is to identify the challenges in ensuring security in cloud computing and to present a prototype solution aimed at solving this problem. To do this, we propose an approach that will be the basis for studies combining AI and digital forensic studies, which are still in their infancy. To set up the test environment, we implement a virtual security gateway that offers firewalls, web security, and intrusion detection. Additionally, we modified the forensic toolkit to perform forensic analysis in the cloud to track breaches.

In the future, the proposed approach can be applied to a real-world cloud environment such as Amazon EC2. This will enable real-world testing and evaluation using real data. Digital data can be analysed by adding AI models with high prediction performance to this research [32]. Thus, advantages such as automated analysis, data recovery, and reconstruction provided by digital forensics and AI can be beneficial. By increasing data security for CSPs, more users will be able to be included in the cloud environment.

NOTE

1 https://www.infoworld.com/article/2652198/gartner-seven-cloud-computing-security-risks.html

REFERENCES

[1] Gill, S. S. Wu, H., Patros, P. et al. (2024). Modern computing: Vision and challenges. *Telematics and Informatics Reports*, 13, 100116.

[2] Walia, G. K. Kumar, M., & Gill, S. S. (2024). AI-empowered fog/edge resource management for IoT applications: A comprehensive review, research challenges and future perspectives. *IEEE Communications Surveys & Tutorials*, 26(1), 619–669

[3] Golec, M., Gill, S. S., Parlikad, A. K., & Uhlig, S. (2023). HealthFaaS: AI based smart healthcare system for heart patients using serverless computing. *IEEE Internet of Things Journal*, 10(21), 18469–18476.

[4] Singh, R. & Gill, S. S. (2023). Edge AI: A survey. *Internet of Things and Cyber-Physical Systems*, 3, 71–92.

[5] Doyle, J., Golec, M., & Gill, S. S. (2022). Blockchainbus: A lightweight framework for secure virtual machine migration in cloud federations using blockchain. *Security and Privacy*, 5(2), e197.

[6] Golec, M., Chowdhury, D., Jaglan, S., Gill, S. S., & Uhlig, S. (2022, May). AIBLOCK: Blockchain Based Lightweight Framework for Serverless Computing Using AI. 2022 *22nd IEEE International Symposium on Cluster, Cloud and Internet Computing (CCGrid)* (pp. 886–892). IEEE.

[7] Golec, M., Gill, S. S., Golec, M. et al. (2023). BlockFaaS: Blockchain-enabled serverless computing framework for AI-driven IoT healthcare applications. *Journal of Grid Computing*, 21(4), 63.

[8] Kim, H., Kim, I., & Kim, K. (2021). AIBFT: Artificial intelligence browser forensic toolkit. *Forensic Science International: Digital Investigation*, 36, 301091.

[9] Vatansever, S., Dirik, A. E., & Memon, N. (2019). Analysis of rolling shutter effect on ENF-based video forensics. *IEEE Transactions on Information Forensics and Security*, 14(9), 2262–2275.

[10] Zaharia, M., Konwinski, A., & Stoica, I. (Dec 2008). Improving MapReduce performance in heterogeneous environments. *In 8th USENIX Symposium on Operating Systems Design and Implementation*.

[11] Golec, M., Gill, S. S., Bahsoon, R., & Rana, O. (2020). BioSec: A biometric authentication framework for secure and private communication among edge devices in IoT and industry 4.0. *IEEE Consumer Electronics Magazine*, 11(2), 51–56.

[12] Gill, S. S., Xu, M., Ottaviani, C. et al. (2022). AI for next generation computing: Emerging trends and future directions. *Internet of Things*, 19, 100514.

[13] Yang, H., & Tate, M. (2009). Where are we at Cloud Computing by H Yang and M Tate. Available at: https://aisel.aisnet.org/acis2009/26/ [Accessed 15 July 2022].

[14] Overview of Amazon Web Services. AWS Whitepaper. (2021). Available at: https://d1.awsstatic.com/whitepapers/aws-overview.pdf

[15] Cloud Computing Use Cases White Paper (2023). Available at: http://www.caict.ac.cn/english/research/whitepapers/202208/P020220819513475891365.pdf [Accessed 18 June 2022].

[16] Irving Wladawsky-Berger, Cloud - the Emergence of a New Model of Computing, 2009. Available at: https://blog.irvingwb.com/blog/2009/04/cloud-the-emergence-of-a-new-model-of-computing.html [Online Accessed: 12 April 2023]

[17] Rajkumar Buyya, R. R., & Calheiros, R. N. (June 2009). Modeling and simulation of scalable cloud computing environments and the CloudSim toolkit: Challenges and opportunities. *Proceedings of the 7th High Performance Computing and Simulation Conference.*

[18] NIST. Cloud Deployment models. Available at: http://csrc.nist.gov/groups/SNS/cloud-computing/ [Accessed 10 July 2022].

[19] Incidence Response. Available at: https://www.intrinium.com/managed-it-services/ [Accessed 17 July 2022].

[20] De Chaves, S. A., Uriarte, R. B., & Westphall, C. B. (2011). Toward an architecture for monitoring private clouds. *IEEE Communications Magazine*, 49(12), 130–137.

[21] Craggs, S. (2009). *Cloud Computing Without the Hype; an Executive Guide.* Lustratus Research Limited.

[22] Hurwitz, J., Bloor, R., & Kaufman, M., Halper, Dr. F. (2009). Cloud Computing For Dummies. John Wiley & Sons.

[23] Martini, B., & Choo, K. K. R. (2012). An integrated conceptual digital forensic framework for cloud computing. *Digital Investigation*, 9(2), 71–80.

[24] Velte, A. T., Velte, T. J., & Elsen Peter, R. C. (2010). *Cloud Computing a Practical Approach.* McGraw-Hill. https://books.google.co.uk/books?id=mf0LMXve2gEC&printsec=frontcover&redir_esc=y#v=onepage&q&f=false[Accessed 18 May 2022].

[25] Mather, T., Kumaraswamy, S., & Latif, S. (2009). *Cloud Security and Privacy: An Enterprise Perspective on Risks and Compliance.* O'Reilly Media, Inc.

[26] Ropella, G. E., & Hunt, C. A. (2010). Cloud computing and validation of expandable in silico livers. *BMC systems biology*, 4, 1–13.

[27] Azure proof of concept guide for developers azure whitepapers. Available at: https://azure.microsoft.com/en-gb/resources/minimize-risks-and-costs-with-the-azure-developer-proof-of-concept-guide/ [Accessed 2 July 2022]

[28] Google Cloud Security Overview. Available at: https://cloud.google.com/docs/security/overview/whitepaper [Accessed 2 July 2022].

[29] Kuyoro, S. O., & Ibikunle, F. (2011). Cloud Computing Issues and Challenges. http://eprints.lmu.edu.ng/1390/ [Accessed 3 July 2022].

[30] Vrijders, S., Maffione, V., Staessens, D., Salvestrini, F., Biancani, M., Grasa, E., & Chitkushev, L. (2016). Reducing the complexity of virtual machine networking. *IEEE Communications Magazine*, 54(4), 152–158.

[31] Gonzalez, N., Miers, C., Redigolo, F., Simplicio, M., Carvalho, T., Näslund, M., & Pourzandi, M. (2012). A quantitative analysis of current security concerns and solutions for cloud computing. *Journal of Cloud Computing: Advances, Systems and Applications*, 1, 1–18.

[32] Gill, S. S., & Kaur, R. (2023). ChatGPT: Vision and challenges. *Internet of Things and Cyber-Physical Systems*, 3, 262–271.

CHAPTER 13

Centralised and Decentralised Fraud Detection Approaches in Federated Learning

A Performance Analysis

Shai Lynch, Ahmed M. Abdelmoniem, and Sukhpal Singh Gill

13.1 INTRODUCTION

Fraud detection has emerged as an important necessity across several industries, including healthcare, finance, and e-commerce [1]. As the digital landscape continues to develop, fraudulent individuals as well as companies are constantly advancing their techniques, showing formidable challenges to conventional methods of fraud detection. To effectively fight this increasing threat, advanced approaches that can bolster fraud detection while safeguarding data privacy are mandatory [2]. Industries struggling with fraud, more specifically those with stringent regulations surrounding customer privacy and data, face the ongoing issue of thwarting fraudsters who avail themselves of these guidelines to stay one step ahead of techniques for detection. Therefore, any innovative resolution in this arena should carefully include the intricacies of these industries to improve effective strategies for fraud detection. In today's interconnected world, the value of strong fraud detection cannot be overstated, not only because of significant losses of financial capital for businesses but also because of the undermining of consumer trust and the compromise of integrity for the whole system [3]. As fraudsters continually change their tactics, companies should proactively adopt advanced techniques that prioritise the privacy of data to maintain a competitive edge in fighting fraud [3]. Traditional fraud detection methods typically involve centralised storage of sensitive data, which raises privacy and security concerns. Nevertheless, federated learning presents a decentralised approach in which data are kept locally and only model updates are shared collaboratively. This strategy reduces the risks associated with data breaches and unauthorised access while delivering superior fraud detection capabilities [4]. Federated learning is a distributed machine learning approach that enables model training on local data without the need for data centralisation. By leveraging the power of local data sources while preserving privacy, federated learning holds

DOI: 10.1201/9781003467199-18

promise for overcoming the challenges faced by conventional fraud detection methods, which are isolated and less collaborative [5]. Against this backdrop, this chapter aims to explore and evaluate the potential benefits of federated learning for enhancing fraud detection. The research objectives encompass three primary aspects: firstly, to explore the potential of federated learning as a solution to enhance fraud detection systems, and secondly, to address the limitations associated with traditional centralised fraud detection approaches and investigate how federated learning can offer innovative solutions. Through a comparative study between federated learning and traditional methods, this research moves to shed light on the unique advantages and innovations that federated learning brings while ensuring privacy-preserving techniques [6]. This chapter intends to make a number of significant contributions to the field of fraud detection. First, this research will show the unique benefits and new ideas that federated learning brings to improving fraud detection by comparing it with traditional methods. This study also aims to address the limitations of traditional centralised approaches and investigate how federated learning can provide practical solutions to surmount these obstacles. In addition, an important contribution of this study is the investigation of the practical application of federated learning for fraud detection [7]. The goal of this study is to help policymakers and practitioners adopt and integrate federated learning into real-world fraud detection systems by looking into the techniques for making it work, keeping privacy safe, and whether it is even possible to use [8]. The subsequent sections of this chapter will delve into the theoretical foundations, methodologies, experimental evaluations, and discussions to provide a comprehensive analysis of the potential of federated learning in the field of fraud detection.

13.2 RELATED WORK

On a global scale, fraud has a devastating effect on individuals, organisations, families, and financial institutions. Not only do fraudulent activities result in significant financial losses, but they also erode trust, disrupt operations, and impair the economy as a whole [9]. Therefore, there is an ongoing and urgent need for innovative solutions and techniques to effectively identify, prevent, and mitigate fraud-related risks. Current fraud detection techniques range from conventional rule-based systems to sophisticated machine learning algorithms [10]. However, these methods frequently fall behind the evolving nature of fraud, which is characterised by increasing sophistication and adaptability. As a result, researchers and organisations are constantly investigating novel approaches and strategies to enhance fraud detection capabilities and remain ahead of fraudulent activities.

A review of fraud detection techniques outlines the main techniques to include neural networks, decision trees, logistic regression, and clustering techniques [5]. These key techniques currently employed in the field of fraud detection primarily rely on centralised data and systems that leverage customer information and historical fraud cases to identify patterns and detect fraudulent activities. These techniques encompass a range of approaches, each with their own strengths and limitations. Neural networks, for instance, have gained significant attention in fraud detection due to their ability to capture complex nonlinear relationships and handle large volumes of data. Decision trees, on the other hand, are popular for their interpretability and the ability to capture both numerical and categorical variables. Logistic regression, a widely used statistical technique, offers simplicity and interpretability while effectively modelling the probabilities of fraud occurrence [6]. Clustering techniques provide a valuable means to identify groups or clusters of similar transactions, aiding in the detection of anomalous activities. These techniques form the backbone of current fraud detection systems, and understanding their applications and limitations is crucial for the comparative analysis and evaluation conducted in this study.

The benefits of neural networks in fraud detection lie in their ability to handle complex patterns, process large amounts of data, learn relevant features automatically, and adapt to changing fraud scenarios [1]. These capabilities contribute to improved detection accuracy and the ability to identify both known and emerging fraud patterns. However, neural networks can require powerful hardware and specialised infrastructure. The inner workings of neural networks are difficult to understand, which may raise concerns about their usability and ethics, and neural networks are very sensitive to hyperparameter tuning, which can leave them prone to overfitting. The key aim of decision trees is to break down complex problems into multiple simple problems to overcome complex scenarios [5]. Decision trees can be beneficial in fraud detection by offering easy interpretability, handling mixed data types, and capturing nonlinear relationships and interactions. Decision trees provide valuable advantages in fraud detection as they allow analysts to gain insights into fraud patterns, process diverse types of data, and detect complex relationships that may not be easily identifiable with other algorithms. Decision trees can overfit and potentially become too complex with deep trees and multiple branches; they can be sensitive to small changes and variations in input data; and they also struggle with nonlinear relationships, which can be a big issue with fraud detection. Logistic regression can handle both categorical and continuous input variables, provide probabilities for prediction, and provide an interpretable model [11]. Its simplicity, interpretability, ability to handle different types of data, and capacity to capture nonlinear relationships contribute to its effectiveness in identifying fraudulent activities.

However, logistic regression techniques assume linear relationships exist between input variables and the log-odds of the target variable; simpler models may struggle with more complex nonlinear relationships. This can make more complex techniques harder to prevent and stop [12]. Clustering is the process of dividing a population or set of data points into a number of groups such that data points within the same group are more similar to one another than to those in other groups.

Clustering techniques are able to identify groups with anomalies in the cluster and can be useful for identifying groups of fraudulent behaviour, which may be useful in revealing groups with fraudulent intentions and using fraudulent techniques. However, these techniques may require careful algorithm parameters and have limited ability to handle high-dimensional or noisy data. This technique relies on the notion that fraud patterns exist in clusters [1]. Similarly, in the banking industry, work is being conducted in fields where data privacy and confidentiality are highly regulated and of great importance. The medical field is one of the alternate leading areas of research for federated learning. Hospitals tend to only have access to information local to them, as this is where the majority of their patient base will reside. Potential key information, factors, or progress may be missed or not taken full advantage of as the information is limited to a region or organisation. Where patient information must remain confidential, this slows progress in the development of medicine. Centralised methods face this issue continuously and require decentralised innovations to address it. This is a challenge that federated learning aims to address, but key concerns have to be addressed, including collaboration trust, true data privacy, navigating strict regulation, and legislative compliance [13].

Collaboration trust among participating entities using federated learning initiatives is a big concern, as all participants have to rely on the quality and truthfulness of the results without access to the data. For this to be achieved, a collaborative framework that promotes trust and defines roles and responsibilities while addressing potential conflicts of interest is crucial in developing a mechanism for sustained trust and progress throughout the enterprise. Medical data are highly sensitive and subject to very strict privacy regulations. Implementing federated learning initiatives requires an open and documented assurance of privacy and security of patient data across every participating entity in the network and ensuring data are protected from unauthorised access and data breaches. Adequate controls and techniques will need to be utilised and deployed consistently and to a high standard to ensure consistent compliance. Ongoing work in the medical industry is being conducted with a focus on the true viability of federated learning in overcoming data privacy challenges and how these challenges may be overcome.

Navigating strict regulation and legislative compliance is a challenge, and with centralised data in a decentralised enterprise, the challenge will increase for all participants. Strict guidelines, data agreements, and legal considerations must be implemented, along with obtaining proper consent from patients where the data originated. Federated learning permits companies to collaborate as well as leverage data without compromising individual privacy rights [14]. To solve the problems of data integration, efficiency, and privacy protection, future research in the field needs to focus on improving and refining the federated learning system [15]. This will help artificial intelligence (AI) and data analytics reach their full potential in more areas. Federated learning shows promise in the movement towards successful collaboration where strict data security, privacy, and confidentiality remain core principles. The complete step may fall under a different name, but federated learning is an innovative step that will spearhead collaboration initiatives by answering questions and providing clarity on ways of operating [16]. The most attractive aspect of federated learning is its ability to decompose model training into a centralised server and distributed nodes without collecting private data. This kind of decomposed learning framework has great potential to protect users' privacy and sensitive data.

13.3 METHODOLOGY

The chosen methodology for this chapter is the comparative study approach, which has been selected over other potential methodologies, including agile methodology, experimental research methodology, and case study methodology. Each methodology was carefully considered, but the comparative study approach was deemed the most suitable for achieving the research objectives and addressing the specific challenges in enhancing fraud detection through federated learning. Agile methodology was initially considered due to its iterative and flexible nature, which could have facilitated the adaptation and refinement of the research process. However, it was determined that agile methodology is more commonly associated with software development projects rather than research studies. Given the research focus of this chapter, a methodology specifically tailored for research was preferred. Experimental research methodology was also explored as a potential option, considering the need to collect data, build models, and compare the performance of different approaches. While experimental research methodology provides a structured framework for conducting controlled experiments, it may not fully capture the nuances and contextual factors associated with real-world fraud detection scenarios. As the aim of this research is to evaluate the effectiveness of federated learning in a practical setting, a methodology that incorporates a broader perspective was sought. Case study methodology was another viable choice, as it offers an in-depth examination of a specific phenomenon within a real-world context. However, the focus of this research is to compare the performance of different models, rather than delving deeply into a single case. Therefore, the case study methodology was considered less suitable for the objectives of this chapter.

Ultimately, the comparative study approach was selected as it provides a robust framework for evaluating and comparing the performance, privacy preservation, and other relevant factors of federated learning with traditional models. It allows for a systematic analysis and comparison of multiple models using consistent evaluation metrics and datasets. The comparative study approach also enables the exploration of variations within the models being compared, providing a comprehensive understanding of their strengths, limitations, and trade-offs. Acquiring high-quality datasets is a crucial aspect of this research on fraud detection through federated learning. In this regard, Kaggle has proven to be an invaluable resource that offers numerous advantages.

Kaggle provides access to a diverse range of datasets contributed by a global community of data scientists and researchers. This diverse collection includes datasets specifically related to fraud detection, which are highly relevant to this research. These datasets are often well curated, properly labelled, and documented, ensuring their quality and reliability. Using Kaggle saved a significant amount of time and effort in the data acquisition process. Kaggle offers a centralised platform where we can easily browse and search for relevant datasets. The datasets hosted on Kaggle are already collected and made available for public use, allowing us to focus more on the preprocessing, model development, analysis, and experimentation aspects of this research.

Ethical considerations are paramount in conducting fraud detection research, particularly when handling sensitive and personal data. Kaggle has strict guidelines and policies in place to ensure the ethical use of datasets and protect individual privacy. By utilising datasets from Kaggle, we can be confident that the data has been sourced and shared in accordance with ethical guidelines, providing an additional layer of assurance in this research. For a fuller comparative analysis three different datasets have been chosen, the first is made up of simulated data so that the data are not pre-encrypted or altered [16]. The data were curated using the Sparkov Data Generator, a widely used and well-documented tool for generating data [17]. The second dataset was based on real transactions in Europe, and the data have been altered as a result of a Principal Component Analysis (PCA) transformation to remove information that can put personal data at risk. This dataset had no labels, only the letter v followed by a column number [18]. The third dataset has simulated data from Chitwan Manchanda, and all three datasets had documentation and a Kaggle rating over 8.5. The datasets had public usable licenses and heavily skewed fraudulent transaction data [19]. The initial phase revolved around data collection, where distinct datasets were acquired, representing various fraud detection scenarios. Subsequently, a systematic preprocessing procedure was executed to cleanse and prepare the collected data for analysis. This included data cleaning and transformation to ensure consistency and reliability across the datasets. To preprocess and clean the data incomplete rows were removed, duplicates were removed, and non-numerical rows were encoded ready for model training. This is only a basic level of preprocessing as this was not the focus of the study. Post completion of preprocessing the data, the methodology advances into the model development stage. Three fundamental models, including a neural network, linear regression, and decision tree, are meticulously constructed, and trained. This selection aligns with prevalent practices in fraud detection and establishes a solid foundation for comparison. The models were trained on three variations of the dataset including oversampled, under sampled, and unsampled versions. The results from this provide the basis for comparison against the federated learning environment. To ensure methodological rigor, a congruent data preprocessing pipeline is then applied to create analogous datasets for the federated learning experiment. The federated learning scenario simulates a practical real-world scenario with three distinct clients, representing banks, each employing their individual models. These client models collaboratively contribute updates to a federated system, fostering a collective and privacy-preserving learning process.

Neural network models were developed for the federated learning process where ten rounds of training and updates were conducted for final evaluation. This was conducted on the same preprocessed and sampled data used in the centralised versions split over three clients representing three financial institutions taking part. The analysis culminates in a comparative assessment of both the centralised and federated approaches. A set of performance metrics, including F1 score, precision, recall, Area under the curve (AUC), and specificity, are meticulously computed and utilised to gauge the quality of both methodologies. These metrics are particularly chosen to reflect the intricacies of fraud detection tasks, capturing both the model's predictive accuracy and its ability to distinguish fraudulent cases. Due to the highly skewed data, a focus on F1 score, precision, and recall are important. Although other metrics will be important, in terms of fraud classification the importance of classifying true fraudulent cases will be more important compared with specificity. Identifying how many non-fraud cases were misclassified with time inconvenience will be less important to the financial implications of lower precision and recall, as that will suggest more fraudulent cases are missed.

Precision measures the predictive value, and a high precision is good for situations when classifying positive cases such as fraud is of high importance. Recall focuses on how good a model is in effectively identifying real cases, which is slightly less important to precision in context, but this metric still gets results. F1 score combines precision and recall indicating the balance between both, and all three remaining high is very positive. The pursuit of this research methodology was not without its challenges. One significant hurdle arose during the process of selecting appropriate datasets for analysis. Credit card data, which is sensitive and private, presented a considerable ethical challenge. Ensuring the availability of comprehensive datasets that adhered to ethical guidelines proved to be a meticulous process. Moreover, the establishment of a federated learning environment posed another formidable challenge. Despite its potential, the limited and complex documentation surrounding the creation of such an environment using new data hindered the development of suitable experimental settings.

13.4 RESULTS

In this section, we present a comprehensive comparative analysis of the performance of fraud detection models using both federated learning and centralised approaches. Our analysis focuses on key quality metrics, including F1 score, precision, and recall, which collectively capture the effectiveness and robustness of these models. By systematically evaluating the models across these metrics, we aim to provide insights into their strengths, limitations, and potential applications in real-world fraud detection scenarios. The following side-by-side comparison and narrative explanation delve into the details of our findings, shedding light on how these models perform in varying aspects of fraud detection. For the federated learning environment the focus was on a neural network across three banking clients. The previous neural networks achieved consistent competitive F1 scores, can handle complex patterns, and can operate efficiently in a federated environment where data privacy is a requirement. The comparison of F1 scores across models and datasets is given in Figure 13.1.

The linear regression models showed mixed performance across different datasets and sampling strategies, The decision tree model performance was strong across all datasets and sampling techniques. The neural network's performance varied across the datasets and sampling techniques, but the consistency is not achieved across datasets. The federated environment showed a more consistent scoring across datasets and

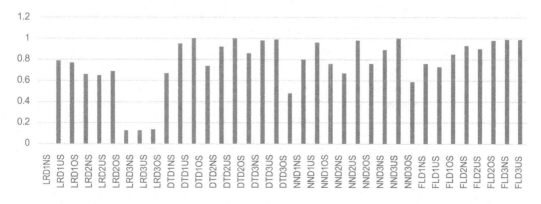

FIGURE 13.1   F1 scores from practical element.

TABLE 13.1   Results of Testing on Dataset 1

Dataset 1 No Sampling			
Model/Metric	LR	DT	NN
F1 score	0	0.667	0.479
Precision	0	0.655	0.691
Recall	0	0.678	0.366
Dataset 1 Under Sampling			
Model/Metric	LR	DT	NN
F1 score	0.788	0.952	0.850
Precision	0.831	0.954	0.902
Recall	0.764	0.950	0.803
Dataset 1 Oversampling			
Model/Metric	LR	DT	NN
F1 score	0.765	0.997	0.962
Precision	0.761	0.997	0.961
Recall	0.769	0.998	0.962

sampling techniques. Table 13.1 shows the results of testing on dataset 1, Table 13.2 shows the results of testing on dataset 2, and Table 13.3 shows the results of testing on dataset 3. Table 13.4 shows the results of the federated learning environments on all datasets.

Some key trade-offs of note presented themselves including the evidence that there is a trade-off between precision and recall for many of the models. As precision increases, recall may decrease and vice versa. This trade-off is particularly noticeable in scenarios where models achieve high precision but lower recall. The performance of models varies significantly based on the dataset distribution and sampling strategy.

TABLE 13.2   Results of Testing on Dataset 2

Dataset 2 No Sampling			
Model/Metric	LR	DT	NN
F1 score	0.657	0.736	0.760
Precision	0.835	0.784	0.772
Recall	0.541	0.695	0.748
Dataset 2 Under Sampling			
Model/Metric	LR	DT	NN
F1 score	0.648	0.920	0.670
Precision	0.959	1	0.504
Recall	0.490	0.846	1
Dataset 2 Oversampling			
Model/Metric	LR	DT	NN
F1 score	0.694	0.996	0.974
Precision	0.999	0.993	0.995
Recall	0.532	0.998	0.955

TABLE 13.3   Results of Testing on Dataset 3

Dataset 3 No Sampling			
Model/Metric	LR	DT	NN
F1 score	0.132	0.863	0.760
Precision	0.987	0.870	0.989
Recall	0.071	0.856	0.617
Dataset 3 Under Sampling			
Model/Metric	LR	DT	NN
F1 score	0.133	0.978	0.887
Precision	0.989	1	0.924
Recall	0.071	0.957	0.947
Dataset 3 Oversampling			
Model/Metric	LR	DT	NN
F1 score	0.135	0.993	0.995
Precision	1	0.996	0.994
Recall	0.072	0.991	0.996

Some models perform exceptionally well with oversampled data, whereas others excel with under sampling. This sensitivity highlights the importance of understanding the characteristics of the dataset and selecting models accordingly to achieve optimal results.

The comparison of recall scores across models and datasets is given in Figure 13.2, and the comparison of precision scores across models and datasets is given in Figure 13.3.

TABLE 13.4   Results of the Federated Learning Environments on All Datasets

Federated Environment No Sampling			
Model/Metric	D1	D2	D3
F1 score	0.586	0.764	0.728
Precision	0.528	0.932	0.473
Recall	0.482	0.723	0.574
Federated Environment Under Sampling			
Model/Metric	D1	D2	D3
F1 score	0.848	0.930	0.902
Precision	0.821	0.835	0.826
Recall	0.797	0.879	0.862
Federated Environment Oversampling			
Model/Metric	D1	D2	D3
F1 score	0.978	0.994	0.992
Precision	0.982	0.987	0.980
Recall	0.987	0.987	0.986

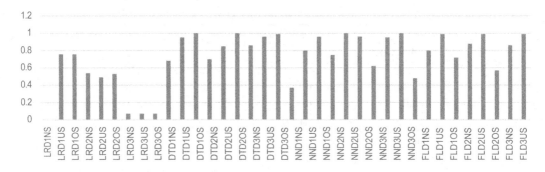

FIGURE 13.2   Recall score chart for all models and datasets.

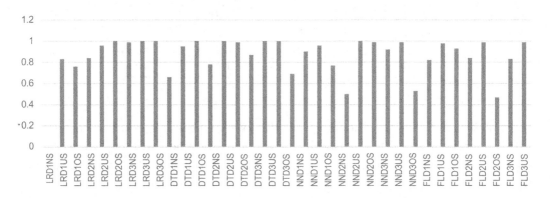

FIGURE 13.3   Graph of precision scores for all models and datasets.

13.5 CONCLUSIONS

This research has undertaken an extensive exploration of fraud detection methodologies, with a specific focus on comparing centralised and federated learning approaches. The analysis of various datasets and models has shed light on both the strengths and limitations of these methods, presenting valuable insights for the field of fraud detection. The results obtained from the centralised models reveal a nuanced picture of their performance across different datasets and scenarios. The decision tree model consistently demonstrated high F1 scores, precision, and recall, positioning it as a reliable choice across various data distributions. Neural network models, particularly in oversampled scenarios, exhibited an ability to capture complex relationships within the data. However, the logistic regression model struggled in situations with limited positive cases, affecting its overall predictive accuracy.

The exploration of federated learning in a collaborative environment has showcased promising results as well. The federated environment, with its emphasis on privacy preservation, displayed competitive F1 scores, precision, and recall. The approach demonstrated its ability to maintain consistent performance across diverse datasets and methodologies.

The research's alignment with theoretical foundations and its translation into practical applications have highlighted the importance of bridging theory and real-world scenarios.

Challenges in applying theoretical knowledge, especially in addressing dataset diversity and practical constraints, underscore the dynamic nature of research and the need for flexibility in approach.

The performance indicated in the results suggests strong competition between the decision tree in a centralised environment and the neural network in a federated environment. While the quality improvement was expected to be better, this does support a hypothesis of a maintained quality in a federated environment. Further research could delve into more data and tuning to better gauge the quality gap and to understand the strengths and limitations of centralised approaches vs. decentralised approaches. However, the consistency of quality in the federated environment does support the place and continued research that this paradigm deserves as a contender for future collaborative efforts.

In conclusion, this research contributes to the ongoing discourse surrounding data-driven research and fraud detection. Whereas centralised models showcase their strengths in certain scenarios, the potential of federated learning for collaborative, privacy-preserving fraud detection is evident. The findings underscore the importance of ongoing research, ethical considerations, and sustainable advancements in the field. As technology evolves and data privacy concerns grow, research efforts such as this play a crucial role in driving innovation and fostering trust in data-driven industries with strict regulation and legislation surrounding sensitive data and its use.

13.6 FUTURE WORK

There are numerous captivating avenues for further study and advancement within the domain of federated learning for the purpose of fraud detection. One intriguing research area pertains to conducting a comprehensive comparative analysis of different federated frameworks to evaluate their relative effectiveness in diverse fraud detection scenarios. This may involve analysing the trade-offs among model complexity, communication efficiency, and predictive performance across various federated systems. Furthermore, exploring the suitability of various privacy-preserving methodologies, such as homomorphic encryption and differential privacy, within the framework of federated learning for the purpose of fraud detection has potential [20]. Several outstanding questions and areas for enhancement in the field of federated learning for fraud detection necessitate careful investigation. One unresolved inquiry revolves around the adaptability of federated models in scenarios when client datasets exhibit substantial variations. Examining the performance of federated learning in scenarios where separate clients have disparate data distributions could yield useful insights into the resilience and generalisation abilities of these models. An alternative approach involves simulating real-world scenarios in which clients utilise diverse datasets, potentially enhancing the understanding of the overall model's performance across varied circumstances [21]. Additionally, investigating methodologies for generating synthetic data to train federated models, which can simulate diverse contexts, presents an opportunity to address the constraints posed by limited data availability.

To optimise the utilisation of federated learning in the context of fraud detection, it is imperative to prioritise both practical implementation and research backing. Enhancing the documentation and exemplification of establishing federated learning environments specifically designed for fraud detection scenarios has the potential to facilitate the adoption process. The expedited advancement of research and the effortless exploration of various configurations can be achieved by developing user-friendly tools and platforms that support rapid setup and experimentation with federated models. Moreover, it would be beneficial to promote the development of benchmark datasets that are specifically tailored for federated fraud detection models [20]. This would establish a standardised foundation for evaluating and comparing models in various research investigations.

The significance of continuous research endeavours in the domain of federated learning for the purpose of fraud detection cannot be overemphasised. In light of the progressively stringent regulations pertaining to data privacy, industries are confronted with the imperative to develop novel methodologies that effectively safeguard both the quality of models and the privacy of individuals. The persistent development of fraudulent individuals' strategies and the wide range of difficulties presented by different data sources necessitate continuous investigation and enhancement of federated learning methodologies [21]. This study makes a significant contribution to the development of fraud detection techniques and also has implications for the wider field of privacy-preserving machine learning. The findings of this research have the potential to be applied in other fields that face similar challenges in sharing sensitive data.

REFERENCES

[1] Gill, S. S., Wu, H., Patros, P. et al. (2024). Modern computing: Vision and challenges. *Telematics and Informatics Reports*, 13, 100116.

[2] Bin Sulaiman, R., Schetinin, V., & Sant, P. (2022). Review of machine learning approach on credit card fraud detection. *Human-Centric Intelligent Systems*, 2(1–2), 55–68.

[3] Gill, S. S. (2024). Quantum and blockchain based serverless edge computing: A vision, model, new trends and future directions. *Internet Technology Letters*, 7(1), e275.

[4] Gao, L., Li, L., Chen, Y., Xu, C., & Xu, M. (2022). FGFL: A blockchain-based fair incentive governor for federated learning. *Journal of Parallel and Distributed Computing*, 163, 283–299.

[5] Chaudhary, K., Yadav, J., & Mallick, B. (2012). A review of fraud detection techniques: Credit card. *International Journal of Computer Applications*, 1645–1653, 41.

[6] Bondok, A. H., Mahmoud, M., Badr, M. M., Fouda, M. M., Abdallah, M., & Alsabaan, M. (2023). Novel evasion attacks against adversarial training defense for smart grid federated learning. *IEEE Access*. 11, 112953–112972.

[7] Li, Y., & Wen, G. (2023). Research and practice of financial credit risk management based on federated learning. *Engineering Letters*, 31(1), 1–8

[8] Li, Q., Wen, Z., Wu, Z., Hu, S., Wang, N., Li, Y., & He, B. (2023). A survey on federated learning systems: Vision, hype and reality for data privacy and protection. *IEEE Transactions on Knowledge and Data Engineering*. 35, 3347–3366.

[9] Gill, S. S., & Kaur, R. (2023). ChatGPT: Vision and challenges. *Internet of Things and Cyber-Physical Systems*, 3, 262–271.

[10] Gill, S. S., Xu, M., Ottaviani, C. et al. (2022). AI for next generation computing: Emerging trends and future directions. *Internet of Things*, 19, 100514.

[11] Domínguez-Almendros, S., Benítez-Parejo, N., & Gonzalez-Ramirez, A. R. (2011). Logistic regression models. *Allergologia et Immunopathologia*, 39(5), 295–305.

[12] Nandhakumar, A. R., Baranwal, A., Choudhary, P. et al. (2024). Edgeaisim: A toolkit for simulation and modelling of ai models in edge computing environments. *Measurement: Sensors*, 31, 100939.

[13] Yang, J., Baker, T., Gill, S. S., Yang, X., Han, W., & Li, Y. (2022). A federated learning attack method based on edge collaboration via cloud. *Software: Practice and Experience.* https://doi.org/10.1002/spe.3180

[14] Rieke, N., Hancox, J., Li, W. et al. (2020). The future of digital health with federated learning. *NPJ Digital Medicine*, 3(1), 6.

[15] Gadekallu, T. R., Pham, Q. V., Huynh-The, T., Bhattacharya, S., Maddikunta, P. K. R., & Liyanage, M., (2021). Federated learning for big data: A survey on opportunities, applications, and future directions. *arXiv preprint arXiv:2110.04160.*

[16] Long, G., Tan, Y., Jiang, J., & Zhang, C. (2020) Federated learning for open banking. *Lecture Notes in Computer Science*, 240–254. https://doi.org/10.1007/978-3-030-63076-8_17

[17] 'Neural Networks (2023). *Cambridge Advanced Learner's Dictionary & Thesaurus.* Cambridge University Press.

[18] Yang, W., Zhang, Y., Ye, K., Li, L., & Xu, C. Z. (2019). FFD: A Federated Learning Based Method for Credit Card Fraud Detection. *Big Data–BigData 2019: 8th International Congress, Held as Part of the Services Conference Federation, SCF 2019, San Diego, CA, USA, June 25–30, 2019, Proceedings 8* (pp. 18–32). Springer International Publishing.

[19] Koko, R. R. Z., Yassine, I. A., Wahed, M. A., Madete, J. K., & Rushdi, M. A. (2023). Dynamic construction of outlier detector ensembles with bisecting k-means clustering. *IEEE Access*, 11, 24431–24447.

[20] Singh, R. & Gill, S. S. (2023). Edge AI: A survey. *Internet of Things and Cyber-Physical Systems*, 3, 71–92.

[21] Walia, G. K., Kumar, M., & Gill, S. S. et al. (2024). AI-empowered fog/edge resource management for IoT applications: A comprehensive review, research challenges and future perspectives. *IEEE Communications Surveys & Tutorials*, 26(1), 619–669

CHAPTER 14

AI-Based Edge Node Protection for Optimizing Security in Edge Computing

Muhammed Golec, Waleed Ul Hassan, and Sukhpal Singh Gill

14.1 INTRODUCTION

In recent years, edge computing has brought revolutionary changes in the way information and data are processed and used. By moving processing power closer to the data source, it offers much better response time and reduces latency in the system, which ultimately increases scalability [1]. Today, millions of sensors produce large amounts of data, and processing this data in traditional cloud computing causes high amounts of latency and bandwidth usage. This may cause unintended service-level agreement (SLA) violations [2]. Edge computing is very useful in such scenarios, as it brings processing power closer to the data source [3]; thus data does not always have to go to the main cloud server for processing, making the overall system very efficient and greatly reducing latency. This model has a wide range of applications in different fields, including the Internet of Things (IoT), smart cities, and industrial automation [4]. Edge nodes have some security concerns because they consist of different devices with variable features and are located in different locations [5]. A great deal of work has been done to solve security concerns in edge computing. One of these is a PIN-based system that allows access to the system with digital encryption. However, if the password is stolen or lost in these systems, security vulnerabilities are revealed. Therefore, higher security methods are needed. Here, biometric authentication methods, one of the artificial intelligence (AI)-based solution methods, come into play [6]. Biometric authentication systems contain unique information such as fingerprints and faces, and unlike pin-based systems, they offer high security. However, reasons such as containing unique information and not being able to reproduce it raise concerns about privacy [7]. For this reason, innovative solutions are needed to ensure biometric data security in authentication applications in edge computing.

14.1.1 Motivation and Our Contributions

In addition to the advantages it offers, edge computing also brings with it some inherent disadvantages, such as security and privacy [8]. It is important to ensure security in edge

DOI: 10.1201/9781003467199-19

applications used in various military and civilian areas. One of the innovative solutions used to ensure security in edge computing is biometric recognition [9]. In biometric recognition applications, face images, which are unique biometric data, are used and cause privacy concerns if stolen [10]. In this chapter, we present the innovative framework AIBioSec, which uses biometric recognition to ensure security at edge nodes while providing cryptographic algorithms to secure biometric data. CompreFace, an open-source application, is used for facial recognition [11]. This application uses a neural network to identify different features of the provided image. It compares the image with existing face records in the database to compare the percentage similarity with each face and shows the best match for the image. The following are the main contributions of this chapter:

- AI-based face recognition is used to ensure security in edge nodes.

- A cryptographic algorithm is used for the security of biometric data.

- DES, 3DES, and AES are compared based on encryption and decryption speeds to find the fastest cryptographic algorithm.

14.2 RELATED WORK

Edge computing has become popular recently because of its ability to bring computation closer to data sources, which reduces latency in different applications. This is especially beneficial where large amounts of sensors or many IoT devices are used to collect data because processing all the data gathered closer to the devices themselves will decrease the latency of the network and ultimately improve the efficiency and scalability of the whole system. But the decentralised system makes the edge nodes less secure, so some innovations are required for the improvement of security in this model and to ensure the system's integrity [12]. This literature review gives an overview of research related to edge computing security, facial recognition, and encryption methods for secure communication channels.

14.2.1 Edge Computing Security Challenges

Because the edge nodes are scattered in different locations they are in danger of unauthorized access, getting stolen, network attacks and privacy violations [12]. The variation of machines for nodes and every machine having limited resources makes securing the system complicated. Researchers have mentioned that these problems must be addressed because this model has been used a great deal in recent years [13].

14.2.2 Facial Recognition for Access

Because of facial recognition's non-intrusive nature and the fact that it supports real-time identification, it has gained a great deal of interest as a biometric authentication [14]. Integrating facial recognition on edge nodes can be a reliable way to create user authentication.

14.2.3 Encryption for Communication Channels

Encryption is very important for maintaining the integrity of sensitive data in transmission channels. Existing encryption algorithms such as Advanced Encryption Standard

TABLE 14.1 Comparison between Other Related Studies

Study	Mechanism	Biometric Authentication	Face Recognition	Encryption
[16]	Remote password authentication	✗	✗	✗
[14]	Face recognition using OpenCV	✓	✓	✗
[15]	AES and DES encryption	✗	✗	✓
[5]	Biometric authentication in edge computing (BioSec)	✓	✗	✓
This study	Facial recognition, Encryption and decryption	✓	✓	✓

(AES) and Data Encryption Standard (DES) provide us with various levels of security and computational costs [15]. To select the appropriate encryption algorithm, we must consider the computational cost and efficiency of the algorithm, as some of our edge nodes may not have good processing power.

14.2.4 Critical Analysis

Table 14.1 shows the comparison of proposed systems with related studies. There are other studies that are focused on facial recognition for authentication, but they are not focused on edge computing, and they are not using encryption for communication channels [10]. Even though there are some studies that are doing biometric authentication and encryption for communications, they are not using the facial recognition system for authentication. We believe that by integrating facial recognition systems and encryption for communication channels, we can improve the security of the edge computing model.

14.3 AIBIOSEC: METHODOLOGY

This system is designed as three layers as shown in Figure 14.1. Raspberry Pi is used as an edge node, one virtual server on Google Cloud Platform (GCP) is used as the closest processing machine, and one machine is used as a server where the face recognition system is hosted. AES-128 encryption is used to secure communication between these layers. Raspberry Pi is hosted on a local virtual machine (VM) on a laptop and given access to the laptop's webcam, which acts as a camera connected to an edge node for authentication and then encrypts the image for privacy [16]. Then it sends an application programming interface (API) call to the GCP server, which is hosting a flask API that receives the encrypted image and uses the key to decrypt the image. Decrypted images are then used for another API call-to-face recognition system for matching with the username.

Face recognition used in this implementation is an open-source application called Exadel CompreFace [17]. CompreFace provides the user with a Graphical User Interface (GUI) for accessing it for face recognition, but in this system, we are using the API they have provided to directly access the functionality of the application for our face recognition system. The GUI consists of many functionalities, including admin access to create subjects, adding images to existing subjects for better face recognition results, deleting existing subjects, or uploading an image for testing to see if it matches with the existing subjects. Only the API is used to do all these actions in our system, not the GUI.

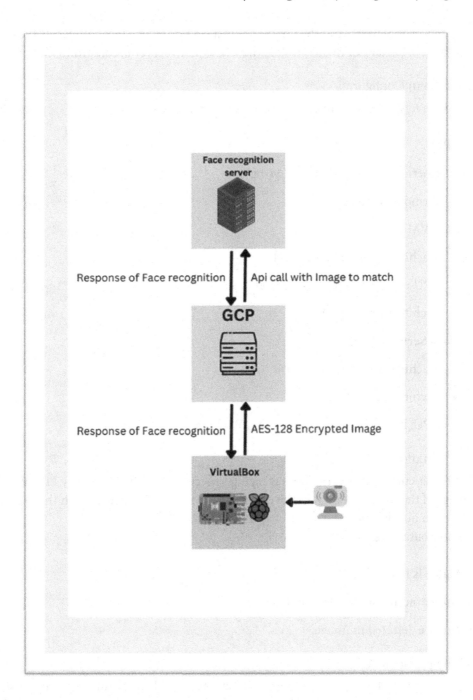

FIGURE 14.1   System design of this implementation.

In the start, the user is asked to enter their username. If the username entered is an admin and the face matches, they are given access to a command for adding a new subject by capturing their image using the webcam and entering their username for the first time in the system. The CompreFace application is hosted using Docker, as explained in their documentation. Settings for saving images to the database are turned off because of the privacy concerns of users, and the images are instead hosted in a local directory; thus there is no chance of leakage of images unless the whole main server is compromised.

14.3.1 System Configuration

We used the following system configurations to run experiments.

1. **RPi:**

   - Operating system: Debain (64-bit)

   - Memory: 4096 MB

2. **GCP VM:**

   - Machine type: n2-standard-4

   - CPU platform: Intel Cascade Lake

   - Architecture: ×86/64

3. **Main Server (GCP):**

   - Machine type: n1-standard-8

   - Architecture: ×86/64

   - GPU: NVIDIA Tesla P100 Virtual Workstation

14.3.2 Workflow

First the user enters the username he is trying to access, then the Raspberry Pi (RPi) takes the image of that user to send it to the closest server to see if it matches with the username registered in our database.

Possible outcomes:

1. Match is found.

2. Username and face did not match.

3. No face detected in image.

14.3.3 Implementation

In the edge node, the OpenCV library for Python is used to capture the image using a webcam connected to the node. The captured image (Figure 14.2) is saved on the local directory in JPEG format. AES is used to encrypt the file we saved using a key and then the encrypted file is sent the GCP VM using Flask API that is hosted in that GCP VM.

In the GCP VM, Flask API receives the encrypted image (Figure 14.3) and saves it temporarily and then decrypts it using the same key after that the decrypted image is sent to the CompreFace application using their API to match the image with the already registered images.

```
1  # Pseudo code for capturing an image from webcam, encrypting it, and performing face recognition
2
3  # Prompt the user for their username
4  username = input("Enter your username and look into the Camera:")
5
6  # Capture an image from the webcam
7  if webcam.detect_face():
8      captured_image = webcam.capture()
9  else:
10     display_message("No face detected. Please try again.")
11
12 # Encrypt the captured image
13 encryption_key = generate_encryption_key()
14 encrypted_image = encrypt(captured_image, encryption_key)
15
16 # Send the encrypted image to the remote server for face recognition
17 response = server.send_image_for_recognition(encrypted_image)
18
19 # Process the server's response
20 if response.error:
21     display_error_message(response.message)
22 else:
23     recognized_username = response.get_recognized_username()
24
25     # Compare recognized username with the input username
26     if recognized_username == username:
```

FIGURE 14.2   Pseudo code for encrypting the image and sending it to the VM.

The CompreFace app has five containers:

1. Balancer + UI

2. Admin server

3. API server

4. Embedded servers

5. PostgreSQL

```
1  # Open encrypted input file and create output file
2  open in_file
3  open out_file
4
5  # Decrypt the input file and save to the output file
6  decrypt(in_file, out_file, password)
7
8  # Close input and output files
9  close in_file
10 close out_file
11
12 # Prepare data for POST request
13 file_data = create dictionary with 'file' as key and binary content of image as value
14 headers = create dictionary with 'x-api-key' as key and API key string as value
15
16 # Make a POST request to the specified URL
17 response = send POST request to CompareFaceApi with headers and file_data
18
19 Remove the temporary image file
20
```

FIGURE 14.3   Pseudo code for decrypting the image and sending it to the CompreFace app.

The balancer and UI container runs the Nginx server, which redirects the user's request to API and admin services and acts as a default gateway when accessing the app [17]. The admin server is connected to the database and handles all the UI requests by the user. The API server handles all the API requests for face recognition or registering new subjects. This server is also connected to the database server for storing data. The embedded server container is responsible for running the neural network used for all the main functionalities like face recognition, age detection, and gender detection. This container is not connected to the database and is stateless. As this container is hosting the neural network, it requires more processing power than the other containers. PostgreSQL container is used to host the database, which holds all the data required for the working of the application [17].

14.4 EXPERIMENTAL RESULTS

Experimental results show that the performance of the system is very good. The system is tested by adding two subjects to the face recognition database and asking other people to try to access the system by capturing them on the camera. Whenever someone unauthorized tried to access the system, the image did not match. Here are some example runs of the application. Figure 14.4 shows the response if no face is captured by the camera. Figure 14.5 shows the response if the face and username match.

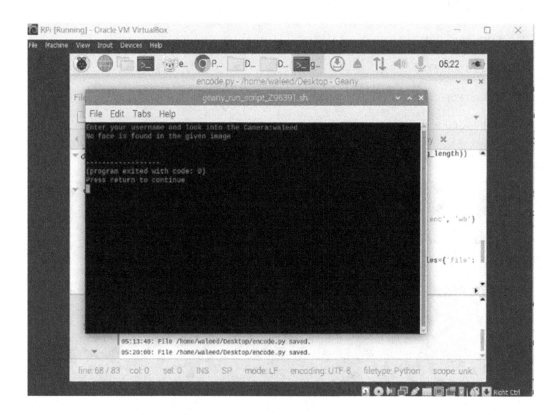

FIGURE 14.4   The response if no face is captured by the camera.

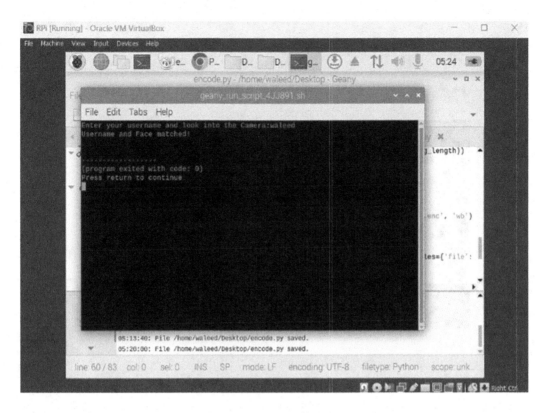

FIGURE 14.5   The response if the face and username match.

Figure 14.6 shows the response if the face and username do not match.

Figure 14.4 is the output the system gave when the camera angle was wrong or the face of the person trying to access the application was captured correctly. Figure 14.5 is when the correct username is entered, and the image captured by the webcam matches with that username in our CompreFace database. Figure 14.6 is when someone tried to access the username that was not their own, so the image did not match with the username they entered and they are denied access to the system. Different encryption algorithms are tested in this study to see what suits this system (Table 14.2). AES, DES, and 3DES are compared in the following Table 14.2 by calculating the time it took each of them to encrypt the image on the RPi side and decrypt the same image on the GCP VM.

With these results it is apparent that AES-128 is more efficient and less time-consuming in our low-end RPi as well as on our cloud VM. So to maintain the efficiency of the edge

TABLE 14.2   Comparison between Various Encryption Algorithms

Algorithm	Bits	Encryption Time (ms)	Decryption Time (ms)
AES	128	1.007	1.137
AES	256	1.161	1.538
DES	64	1960	3491
3DES	192	51756	43521

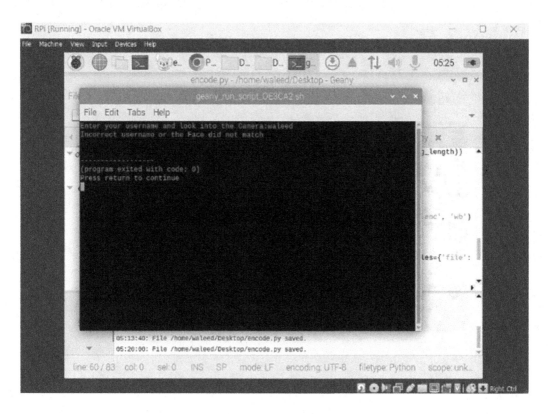

FIGURE 14.6   The response if the face and username do not match.

computing network and not overload the edge nodes with encryption, we can still achieve security by implementing AES encryption for our communication channels.

14.4.1 Effects on End Users

This system is designed with two goals for the user, protecting their privacy and authorizing them to the system. In previous systems, the user was required to enter a pin or text-based passwords, which have a high possibility of being leaked to an unauthorized person. It is also likely that the user can forget the password. These factors make this system more vulnerable. By using this new system with face recognition authentication users will not have to remember their password, only their username, so this makes things easier for the end user and improves the security of the system at the same time. Using the encryption for communication will make sure the user's images are not stolen or leaked putting their mind at ease for any privacy concerns they might have because of the biometric nature of authentication used for this system [18].

14.5 CONCLUSIONS AND FUTURE WORKS

Edge computing is a computing paradigm that offers advantages such as reducing latency and unnecessary bandwidth usage by bringing processing power closer to the data source. In addition to the advantages it offers, the heterogeneous structure of edge nodes raises some concerns such as security. To solve this problem, this chapter introduces AIBioSec, a new framework based on face recognition to ensure security for edge nodes. If the biometric data used in face recognition is stolen, privacy issues as well as the security of edge nodes arise. For this reason, AIBioSec encrypts biometric data in communication channels with the AES-128 bit algorithm. A multi-biometric authentication model, in which more than one biometric feature is used for authentication, can be used in the future to further increase the security of the system. The processing load on edge nodes can be alleviated by using faster cryptographic algorithms to encrypt the transferred data.

REFERENCES

[1] Gill, S. S., Xu, M., Ottaviani, C. et al. (2022). AI for next generation computing: Emerging trends and future directions. *Internet of Things*, 19, 100514.

[2] Gill, S. S., Wu, H., Patros, P. et al. (2024). Modern computing: Vision and challenges. *Telematics and Informatics Reports*, 13, 100116.

[3] Singh, R & Gill, S. S. (2023). Edge AI: A survey. *Internet of Things and Cyber-Physical Systems*, 3, 71–92.

[4] Nandhakumar, A. R., Baranwal, A., Baranwal, A., Choudhary, P. et al. (2024). Edgeaisim: A toolkit for simulation and modelling of ai models in edge computing environments. *Measurement: Sensors*, 31, 100939.

[5] Gill, S. S. (2024). Quantum and blockchain based serverless edge computing: A vision, model, new trends and future directions. *Internet Technology Letters*, 7(1), e275.

[6] Bıçakcı, H. S., Santopietro, M., & Guest, R. (2023). Activity-based electrocardiogram biometric verification using wearable devices. *IET Biometrics*, 12(1), 38–51.

[7] Golec, M., Gill, S. S., Parlikad, A. K., & Uhlig, S. (2023). HealthFaaS: AI based smart healthcare system for heart patients using serverless computing. *IEEE Internet of Things Journal*, 10(21), 18469–18476.

[8] Walia, G. K., Kumar, M., & Gill, S. S. (2024). AI-empowered fog/edge resource management for IoT applications: A comprehensive review, research challenges and future perspectives. *IEEE Communications Surveys & Tutorials*, 26(1), 619–669.

[9] Golec, M., Gill, S. S., Golec, M., Xu, M., Ghosh, S. K., Kanhere, S. S., & Uhlig, S. (2023). BlockFaaS: Blockchain-enabled serverless computing framework for AI-driven IoT healthcare applications. *Journal of Grid Computing*, 21(4), 63.

[10] Golec, M., Gill, S. S., Bahsoon, R., & Rana, O. (2020). BioSec: A biometric authentication framework for secure and private communication among edge devices in IoT and industry 4.0. *IEEE Consumer Electronics Magazine*, 11(2), 51–56.

[11] Adler, A., & Schuckers, M. E. (2007). Comparing human and automatic face recognition performance. *IEEE Transactions on Systems, Man, and Cybernetics, Part B (Cybernetics)*, 37(5), 1248–1255.

[12] Chiang, M., & Zhang, T. (2016). Fog and IoT: An overview of research opportunities. *IEEE Internet of Things Journal*, 3(6), 854–864.

[13] Yu, W., Liang, F., He, X. et al. (2018). A survey on the edge computing for the internet of things. *IEEE Access*, 6, 6900–6919. Available at: https://doi.org/10.1109/access.2017.2778504

[14] Sirivarshitha, A. K., Sravani, K., Priya, K. S., & Bhavani, V. (2023, March). An approach for face detection and face recognition using OpenCV and face recognition libraries in Python. *2023 9th International Conference on Advanced Computing and Communication Systems (ICACCS)* (Vol. 1, pp. 1274–1278). IEEE.

[15] Susanto, C. (2020, October). Using AES and DES cryptography for system development file submission security mobile-based. *2020 8th International Conference on Cyber and IT Service Management (CITSM)* (pp. 1–7). IEEE.

[16] Hao, Z., & Yu, N. (2010, September). A Security Enhanced Remote Password Authentication Scheme Using Smart Card. *2010 Second International Symposium on Data, Privacy, and E-Commerce* (pp. 56–60). IEEE.

[17] Exadel-Inc GitHub - exadel-inc/CompreFace: Leading Free and Open-Source Face Recognition System. Available at: https://github.com/exadel-inc/CompreFace.

[18] Gill, S. S., & Kaur, R. (2023). ChatGPT: Vision and challenges. *Internet of Things and Cyber-Physical Systems*, 3, 262–271.

VI

Telecom Sector and Network

Predictive Analytics for Optical Interconnection Network Performance Optimisation in Telecom Sector

Suganya Senguttuvan and Sukhpal Singh Gill

15.1 INTRODUCTION

Telecom operators can efficiently manage network resources thanks to predictive analytics and machine learning (ML), which improve overall system performance and user experience [1]. Network managers can anticipate network traffic patterns, spot potential congestion points, and effectively manage network resources by using ML algorithms to analyse large amounts of data [2]. This proactive approach not only makes it feasible to arrange preventive maintenance in advance, which reduces downtime and boosts network reliability, but also ensures quick and continuous data transfer. To provide telecom companies with critical insights into the changing demands of their networks, predictive analytics and ML are utilised [3]. This enables them to expand and change their infrastructure as needed. By leveraging historical data and ML models, network operators may estimate future network traffic and enhance resource allocation, resulting in the cost-effective and efficient use of network assets. This improves operational efficiency and decreases expenses while also improving network performance [4]. The identification and mitigation of potential issues before they have an impact on network performance is made feasible by the use of predictive analytics and ML in optical interconnection networks [5, 6]. By proactively spotting anomalies and irregularities, operators may take corrective action, such as re-routing traffic or re-allocating resources, to avoid service outages and ensure continuous connection. Predictive analytics, ML, and optical interconnection networks are all used by the telecom sector to help operators meet growing network demands. By offering their consumers top-notch, trustworthy services, telecom companies may maintain a competitive edge in the

DOI: 10.1201/9781003467199-21

market and ensure customer contentment. To develop the telecom sector as a whole, this study intends to investigate the potential of predictive analytics and ML approaches in enhancing optical interconnection network performance [5, 7].

The complexity and dynamic nature of optical interconnection networks are frequently beyond the scope of traditional techniques of network management and optimisation [8]. Predictive analytics and ML algorithms have emerged as possible solutions as a result of the demand for more sophisticated methods to efficiently allocate network resources, reduce latency, and increase total system throughput. A strategy that combines the strength of ML algorithms with predictive analytics has shown promise in addressing the difficulties related to telecom network performance optimisation. Telecom operators may acquire important insights into network activity, predict future traffic patterns, and make wise decisions about resource allocation and network layout by utilising historical data and powerful ML models [1]. The proliferation of linked devices, multimedia content, and future technologies like the Internet of Things (IoT) and 5G networks is driving a considerable growth in data volumes in the telecom sector [9]. Managing network performance and capacity faces unprecedented problems as a result of this exponential increase. By giving network operators the capacity to predict traffic needs, improve network topology, and ensure effective resource use, predictive analytics and ML algorithms provide a possible answer to these problems [5]. The implications of using ML algorithms for network performance optimisation go beyond the immediate improvement in network efficiency [10]. By reducing network congestion, optimising resource allocation, and reducing latency, telecom operators may enhance the overall quality of service, which will boost customer satisfaction and retention. Additionally, operators may make strategic planning and data-driven choices thanks to ML algorithms' insights on the functionality and behaviour of their networks. The enormous growth of data traffic and the changing nature of consumer expectations in the telecommunications sector provide network operators with ongoing challenges [11]. Predictive analytics and ML algorithms provide a solid basis for resolving these issues by allowing operators to forecast network traffic, improve network design, and ensure efficient resource utilisation [12]. By using historical data and ML models, network operators may estimate future network traffic patterns, make data-driven decisions, and optimise resource allocation for reasonably priced and efficient network operation.

Optimising the performance of optical interconnection networks, which are essential for continuous communication and data transmission, is a difficult task for the telecom industry [13]. Effective connectivity between processors and data centres is made possible by these networks, providing dependable and fast communication in the telecom industry [14]. However, a number of variables, including bottlenecks, ineffective routing protocols, and latency problems, prevent these networks from operating at their best. These difficulties have a direct influence on user experience and system throughput, resulting in inefficient resource allocation and network dependability worries [15]. The telecom industry has always depended on reactive solutions that only address problems after they have already occurred for network management and improvement. The dynamic nature of optical connectivity networks and the constantly rising needs of network traffic cannot be properly addressed with this reactive strategy. As a result, telecom operators struggle to pinpoint potential bottlenecks, mitigate them, improve routing schemes, and reduce latency in real time [16].

Thus, the unsatisfactory performance and inefficiency of optical interconnection networks in the telecom industry are the issues addressed in this research work [17, 18]. Lack of proactive efforts to spot bottlenecks, improving routing protocols, and reducing latency prevents the best use of network resources and jeopardises network dependability [19]. The goal of the research work is to look into the proactive use of predictive analytics and ML algorithms to enhance the performance of optical interconnection networks in the telecom industry [20]. This research aims to give a thorough knowledge of how these cutting-edge solutions may successfully handle the listed challenges by examining the possibilities of predictive analytics and ML algorithms [21]. The objective is to provide a framework that enables telecom operators to forecast network traffic patterns, proactively manage network resources, and improve routing schemes for dependable and efficient network operation [22]. The goal of this study is to advance our understanding of network performance optimisation while offering telecom companies, academics, and other experts in the field useful advice on how to improve the efficiency of optical interconnection networks.

15.1.1 Motivation and Contributions

Embarking on this research journey delves into the future of telecom's optical interconnection networks with a sense of purpose and innovation [23]. The prospect of harnessing ML and predictive analytics to elevate these networks to new heights is nothing short of inspiring. As we explore the intricate dance of point-to-point messaging between central processing units (CPUs)s through message passing, we are reminded of the power that lies within optimisation. Through the lens of historical data and ML models, we glimpse into the future of network traffic estimation and optimal resource allocation. This is not just a research work; it is a gateway to a more cost-effective, efficient, and agile network infrastructure. We stand on the precipice of enabling network managers to foresee, adapt, and lead in the face of growing demands.

15.2 RELATED WORKS

Due to their capacity to evaluate enormous amounts of data, spot patterns, and provide precise predictions, ML algorithms have attracted a great deal of interest in recent years. ML models can accurately forecast future traffic patterns, foresee probable congestion sites, and intelligently distribute network resources by using previous network data [5]. Numerous benefits may be derived from the use of ML and predictive analytics in optical interconnection networks. A more effective use of network resources is ensured through better resource allocation, increasing system throughput, and increasing network dependability [11]. Network operators may reduce latency and provide high-quality services, which will boost customer satisfaction, by proactively resolving bottlenecks and optimising routing techniques.

By linking different network components, such as servers, switches, and routers, they act as the backbone architecture that enables effective communication between them. This section begins by discussing the basic ideas of optical connection networks, such as the advantages of employing optical fibres for data transfer and the fundamentals of optical communication [12]. Following that, a full discussion of the architecture of optical interconnection networks is given, with an emphasis on key components such as optical transceivers, switches, and wavelength division multiplexing (WDM) techniques. The performance factors that impact the efficiency and reliability of optical link networks are also covered in this section [13]. Throughput, latency, and scalability are among the significant qualities that are examined, and it also sheds light on the challenges that network operators face when attempting to improve these performance parameters. By directing data packets to the appropriate destinations, routers manage the flow of traffic inside a communications network [14]. On the other hand, switches enable the connection between devices within a Local Area Network (LAN) or Wide Area Network (WAN). Servers, which house a variety of services and applications, are responsible for handling data processing and storage [15]. These network components are connected via optical interconnection networks, which are essential. They allow for the exchange of routing data between routers, facilitating effective packet forwarding and routing choices. They make it possible for data to be transferred seamlessly across switches within a LAN, guaranteeing a continuous and unhindered connection [16]. Additionally, servers are linked via optical interconnection networks, allowing for data interchange and access to shared resources. Optical interconnection networks guarantee that data may move smoothly and effectively throughout the telecommunications network by acting as the backbone infrastructure [17]. High-quality services may be delivered to end consumers more quickly and reliably because to the high speed and low latency properties of optical fibres. Optimising optical interconnection networks' performance requires an understanding of their function as the backbone infrastructure [24]. Telecom operators may proactively detect and fix bottlenecks, improve routing schemes, and reduce latency inside these networks by utilising predictive analytics and ML algorithms [25]. The end result of this optimisation is an improvement in system throughput, user experience, and support for the rising needs of contemporary telecommunications [26].

The prediction and management of faults is another important use. Operators can identify trends indicating probable equipment breakdowns by evaluating data from network devices and monitoring systems. To minimise downtime and increase network dependability, predictive analytics algorithms can spot early warning indicators and initiate preventive maintenance. Predictive analytics is also crucial for managing the customer experience [27]. Operators can pinpoint areas for improvement and customise service offers by studying client data such as usage trends, preferences, and complaints. Operators can improve customer happiness, lower customer churn, and proactively address possible service quality concerns thanks to predictive analytics. Predictive analytics may enhance performance in the context of optical interconnection networks by locating and removing possible bottlenecks, improving routing schemes, and reducing latency. Predictive analytics algorithms can find trends that are associated with performance degradation by examining previous network performance data [28]. With this insight, operators may take proactive actions to improve performance and guarantee seamless data transfer, such as re-routing traffic or changing network settings.

TABLE 15.1 Comparison of Proposed Work with Existing Studies

Work	Problem Addressed	Techniques
Arévalo et al.[11] Musumeci et al. [5]	Energy-efficient data transfer	Energy-efficient algorithms
Tonini et al. [12]	Network virtualisation	Software-defined networking (SDN)
Masoudi et al. [13]	CRAN optimisation	Integer Linear Programming (ILP)
Chen et al. [14]	Distributed RAN (DRAN)	Algorithmic placement
Klinkowski [15]	5G optimisation	Fibre-based solutions
Ranaweera et al. [16]	5G optical fronthauls	Optimisation techniques
Fayad et al. [17]	5G optical fronthauls	Heuristic techniques
This work	5G optical network	Predictive analysis

Mobile network operators (MNOs) implementing 5G and future networks face a huge difficulty in designing a cost-effective fronthaul for the Cloud Radio Access Network (CRAN). Recently, research has concentrated on creating CRAN-specific optical fronthaul systems that are both affordable and effective [29]. To reduce network costs, deploy equipment effectively, and improve resource allocation, a number of optimisation techniques have been developed. Integer Linear Programming (ILP) formulations have been used in a few studies to handle the placement issue of baseband units (BBUs) in CRAN [30]. By taking into account variables like the number of active BBU sites or the number of fibres utilised for traffic transfer, these formulas seek to reduce the overall network cost [31]. There is a cost-effective architecture called distributed RAN (DRAN) that uses algorithms to find the best places for network equipment while taking into account backhaul connections like the time and wavelength division multiplexing-passive optical network (TWDM-PON). This architecture has been looked at in other works [32].

The telecom industry has made substantial use of ML algorithms to enhance network performance [33]. This section examines the important ML methods that have been used to improve network performance, including classification, regression, and clustering [34]. Identification of network patterns and network behaviour prediction are both greatly aided by the classification method [35]. Operators can categorise network traffic into distinct categories or states, such as normal or anomalous, by building a classification model using past network data [36]. This makes it possible to quickly take action and enhance network performance by detecting network anomalies like security breaches or performance deterioration in real time [37]. Based on previous data, network performance measures are predicted using regression methods. These algorithms examine and forecast the future values of a variety of network metrics, including bandwidth consumption, delay, and packet loss. Operators may proactively deploy resources, improve network configurations, and guarantee optimal performance by properly anticipating network performance data. Table 15.1 compares the proposed work with existing studies.

15.3 METHODOLOGY

In this work, we lay out the systematic process that was employed to achieve the study's objectives. Our approach focuses primarily on three well-known ML algorithms: logistic regression, random forest, and support vector machine (SVM) [38]. These algorithms were chosen because they are efficient and suitable for use in addressing the specific challenges involved in enhancing the performance of optical interconnection networks. To optimise the performance of the optical interconnection network, preprocessing is essential because the data gathered from diverse sources may be noisy or lacking [39]. The calibre of the data used for training and testing determines how accurate the model is. As a result, the preparation stage should be properly carried out to make sure the data are appropriate for analysis. The main component of every ML endeavour is data. The quality of the training data determines how well an ML model performs. We will be utilising the Kaggle-provided synthetic financial dataset for this work, which is a synthetic dataset made up of financial transactions. The dataset includes a number of attributes, including transaction type, sender and receiver information, amount, and more. The data must be processed before being delivered to ML algorithms for training. Preprocessing is a crucial stage when the data are cleaned, converted, and normalised to get it ready for analysis. Figure 15.1 shows the process of data analysis using ML algorithms.

The preprocessing of data for this work [39, 40] will involve the following steps:

1. **Data Collection**: We provide a general overview of the methods utilised to collect the necessary data for the research. Only a few of the network components that are employed as data collection sources for the optical interconnection network include routers, switches, servers, and other relevant hardware. We also include data from performance monitoring tools, network logs, and other real-time data streams to acquire a full picture of network activity and traffic patterns.

2. **Data Preprocessing**: It is crucial to ensure that the data are accurate and suitable for the development of ML models. Beginning with data cleaning to remove any abnormalities, noise, or uninteresting data points that might harm the model's performance, this section explains the various preprocessing techniques employed. The topic of dealing with missing data is also explored; imputation or removal techniques may be used, depending on the degree of missingness and the context of the data.

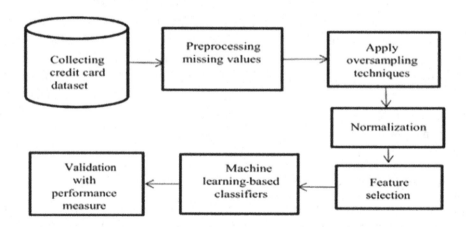

FIGURE 15.1   Process of data analysis using ML algorithms.

3. **Data Transformation**: The resulting data may come in different shapes, sizes, and/or dimensions. To ensure consistency and compatibility with the ML algorithms, data transformation methods are required. All attributes are scaled and normalised to fall within a similar range to remove any bias resulting from the various scales. Categorical data are encoded using methods like one-hot encoding or label encoding to make it simpler for computers to analyse.

4. **Feature Selection**: Finding and selecting the features that have the most bearing on network performance is an essential component of data preparation. We explain how to choose the ideal feature set for ML models in this section. This approach may make use of statistical analysis, correlation analysis, and subject-matter expertise.

5. **Splitting the Dataset**: To appropriately evaluate the ML models, the dataset is split into training, validation, and testing sets. The training set is used to develop the models, the validation set is used to fine-tune the hyperparameters and prevent overfitting, and the testing set is used to gauge how well the models work with untested data.

This part makes sure the data utilised for ML model building and predictive analytics is precise, trustworthy, and reflective of the actual performance of optical interconnection networks in the telecom industry via careful data collection and preparation [39, 40]. This lays the groundwork for the methodology's next phases, producing insightful conclusions and useful recommendations. The preprocessing step helps to improve the accuracy of the model by removing errors and reducing the size of the dataset.

15.3.1 Machine Learning Algorithms

Logistic regression, random forest, and SVM are three effective ML algorithms extensively applied in the Methodology part of the research work [41–43]. In the telecom industry, these algorithms are used to create prediction models that will improve the functionality of optical interconnection networks. Each algorithm contributes distinct advantages and skills to the predictive analytics process, enabling thorough investigation and precise forecasting.

15.3.1.1 Logistic Regression

For binary classification tasks, the supervised learning method of logistic regression is frequently utilised. This technique is used in the research work to forecast outcomes that are binary in nature and have to deal with network performance, such as connection status (up/down), network congestion, or defect detection [44]. The logistic regression model provides an estimate of the likelihood that a specific event will occur, enabling pre-emptive detection of possible problems that might have an impact on network performance. To create a link between input characteristics and a binary output, such as the network condition (e.g., optimum or suboptimal) in our situation, we use the statistical approach of logistic regression [6]. The input characteristics include numerous network metrics that affect the performance of the network, such as connection status, congestion levels, and defect detection indications. Logistic regression helps us to proactively identify possible bottlenecks, optimise resource allocation, and increase the network's overall efficiency by predicting the likelihood of given network situations. We employ logistic regression in a manner similar to that described in the real-time fraud detection use case to optimise optical connectivity networks. To train the logistic regression model, we input historical network performance data, divide it into training and testing sets, and then use the proper learning rate and iterations to train the model [7]. After the model has been trained, we use it to anticipate the state of the network for each incoming data point in real time, enabling us to take prompt action to improve network performance.

15.3.1.2 Random Forest

An ensemble learning method called random forest mixes many decision trees to provide predictions. It excels in both classification and regression tasks, and it handles high-dimensional and complicated datasets very well. Random forest is used in the research work to forecast many network performance measures, including throughput, latency, and packet loss [9]. It is a useful tool for enhancing the performance of optical interconnection networks due to its capacity to manage nonlinear connections and feature interactions. The telecom industry frequently uses random forest, a potent ensemble learning algorithm, to optimise the performance of optical connectivity networks. It works by building several decision trees and combining their predictions to obtain a decision. The method generates a decision tree based on each collection of characteristics and data samples that are randomly chosen from the training data. The final forecast is then created by combining these distinct decision trees using majority voting [10]. Random forest may effectively pinpoint possible bottlenecks, enhance routing schemes, and reduce latency in the context of improving optical connectivity networks. It is appropriate for assessing the enormous volumes of data generated in telecom networks because of its capacity to handle high-dimensional data and spot intricate correlations between variables. Additionally, random forest ensures forecast accuracy and resilience because it is less prone to overfitting. The use of random forest in optical interconnection networks can provide proactive detection of performance problems, enabling network administrators to more effectively distribute resources and boost system throughput [18]. The programme can forecast future traffic patterns and improve resource allocation by examining previous network performance data, resulting in the cost-effective and efficient use of network resources.

15.3.1.3 Support Vector Machine (SVM)

SVM is a potent supervised learning technique that may be utilised for both regression and classification applications. It functions by locating an ideal hyperplane that best divides several classes or forecasts continuous values. In the research work, SVM is used in the optical interconnection network for tasks like traffic forecasting and anomaly detection [21]. SVM helps to improve resource allocation and network dependability by finding trends and spotting abnormalities. Using predictive analytics, SVM, a potent ML method, is used in the telecom industry to enhance optical interconnection network performance. By identifying the ideal hyperplane that optimally separates the data points of several classes, the supervised learning algorithm SVM divides data into distinct groups [27]. SVM is an effective tool for routing strategy optimisation, latency reduction, and possible bottleneck identification in optical interconnection networks.

To make the data points more distinct, the SVM algorithm maps input characteristics, such as previous network performance statistics, to a higher-dimensional space. The hyperplane that maximises the margin between the data points of distinct classes while best separating them is then determined. This hyperplane serves as a barrier for making decisions as to which classes to assign new data points. Telecom operators may more effectively manage resources by utilising the SVM algorithm to proactively identify performance concerns in their optical interconnection networks [28]. The SVM model can forecast future traffic patterns and improve resource allocation by assessing previous network performance data, resulting in the cost-effective and efficient use of network resources. Implementing and analysing these ML techniques can shed light on how well the optical connectivity network is doing [29]. The telecom industry may proactively resolve bottlenecks, enhance routing techniques, and reduce latency by utilising predictive analytics and ML, which will eventually improve system throughput and improve the customer experience.

15.3.2 Implementation and Experimental Setup

The experimental setup describes the dataset, evaluation measures, system settings, and training and testing procedures.

1. **System Configuration**: An Intel Core i5 machine with 8 GB of RAM and a 1 TB hard drive is used in the experimental configuration. Python, Jupyter Notebook, and ML libraries like scikit-learn, Pandas, and NumPy are among the programmes that must be installed.

2. **Dataset**: The dataset consists of 10 columns and 640 rows, representing optical interconnection network performance metrics. Each row contains information about node number, thread number, spatial and temporal distribution, transmitter/receiver (T/R), processor utilisation, channel waiting time, input waiting time, network response time, and channel utilisation.

3. **Evaluation Metrics**: To validate the ML models' performance, evaluation metrics such as accuracy, precision, recall, and F1 score are used. These metrics measure the models' efficiency in optimising optical interconnection network performance.

4. **Training and Testing**: The dataset is split into a test set (30%) and a training set (70%). The training set is used to assess each ML method (logistic regression, random forest, and SVM). For more validation, cross-validation methods are used.

The overall goal of the experimental setting is to evaluate how well ML techniques may improve the performance of optical interconnection networks. The dataset, system design, and assessment metrics are crucial elements in ensuring the accuracy and validity of the findings. On the submitted dataset, ML models are trained and tested as part of the assessment process to ascertain their predictive power and applicability for improving network performance in the telecom industry.

15.4 DATASET STATISTICS

We outline the technical specifics of using ML algorithms on large datasets in the telecom industry to optimise optical interconnection network performance [22, 26, 38]. This section includes the necessary software and hardware setup as well as a step-by-step tutorial for putting the ML models into practice.

1. **Technical Setup**: The establishment of the necessary hardware and software infrastructure is the first step in the implementation process. The essential libraries for the Python-based program are scikit-learn, pandas, NumPy, and matplotlib. The system needs a computer with enough memory and processing capability to handle huge datasets in real time.

2. **Data Preprocessing**: Missing values, outliers, and normalisation are handled in the 10-column, 640-row dataset including optical interconnection network performance measurements. By preparing the data, we make sure that it is suitable for ML algorithms.

3. **Feature Selection**: To determine the most crucial characteristics for network performance improvement, feature selection techniques including correlation analysis, principal component analysis (PCA), and recursive feature elimination (RFE) are used. This aids in lowering data dimensionality and improving the accuracy of ML models.

4. **Evaluation Metrics**: Metrics like accuracy, precision, recall, and F1 score are used to assess the effectiveness of the ML models (logistic regression, random forest, and SVM). These metrics measure how effectively the models improve the performance of optical interconnection networks.

5. **Implementation of ML Algorithms**: Selected characteristics from the training set are used to implement each ML method. Each algorithm's pseudo code is offered, and the hyperparameters are adjusted to enhance the performance of the model. The dataset is used to train and test the algorithms, such as logistic regression, random forest, and SVM.

The methods and strategies used to deploy ML algorithms for improving optical interconnection network performance in the telecom industry are summarised in this section. By ensuring that the models are properly trained and assessed, it enables data-driven decision-making for the improvement of network performance. Important phases in fulfilling the research goals include the technological setup, data preparation, feature selection, dataset splitting, evaluation measures, and implementation of ML algorithms. The dataset utilised for this study on predictive analytics for optical interconnection network performance optimisation in the telecom sector using ML algorithms has 640 rows and 10 columns. The data are collected from an optical interconnection network in the telecom sector and includes various performance metrics related to network nodes, threads, spatial distribution, temporal distribution, T/R, processor utilisation, channel waiting time, input waiting time, network response time, and channel utilisation. The primary data-related activities are as follows:

- **Data Collection**: The optical interconnection network's real-time performance statistics were gathered during the data collection procedure. A thorough dataset could be created since the network was set up to log pertinent performance information on a regular basis.

- **Data Preprocessing**: The dataset underwent a preprocessing procedure to handle any missing values, eliminate outliers, and standardise the data before being used for ML algorithms. The data must go through preprocessing to be in a format that will be useful for analysis and model training.

- **Data Availability**: The dataset is accessible in a structured manner for additional study and analysis. The gathered information provides insightful information about the functionality of the telecom industry's optical interconnection network.

- **ML Model Training**: The division of the dataset into training and testing sets makes it possible to train ML algorithms like logistic regression, random forest, and SVM. After the models had been trained on the training set, they were put to the test using metrics like accuracy.

For researchers and business professionals working to improve the performance of optical interconnection networks, the availability of this information is a wonderful resource [22, 26, 38]. It enables the development and testing of predictive analytics models for improving network performance, strengthening telecom networks' dependability and efficiency.

15.5 RESULTS

The study's findings and the information discovered via data analysis are highlighted in this and next section. The results of the experiment, which tested a number of ML algorithms employed in the real-time fraud detection system, will be discussed here. In this section, the data will also be extensively reviewed, with a comparison of the effectiveness of various strategies and an explanation of the elements influencing them. A description of the results is followed by recommendations for further study to advance predictive analytics for improving optical interconnection network performance in the telecom industry.

15.5.1 Exploratory Data Analysis (EDA)

The used dataset has 640 rows and 10 columns, and it represents various performance parameters in the optical interconnection network utilised in the telecom industry. EDA seeks to learn more about the dataset and the EDA's opening data summary statistics provide a summary of the dataset's main patterns and distributions. Visualisations are used to investigate data patterns and correlations between characteristics, such as histograms, box plots, and scatterplots. Correlation analysis, which identifies the connections between the metrics, directs the selection of features for ML models. In the end, the EDA contributes to informed judgements throughout model construction and analysis by assisting in the discovery of significant patterns, outliers, and possible difficulties. The scatterplot gives a visual depiction of the data points, each of which represents a particular optical connectivity network architecture. The y-axis displays network response time, which evaluates how quickly the network responds to requests, and the x-axis displays processor utilisation, which shows the proportion of the processor's capability that is being utilised. The scatterplot shows how these two variables are distributed and trend over time. It assists in spotting any possible relationships or trends between processor use and network response time. For instance, a grouping of data points with low processor utilisation to the left of the plot may signify periods of low network demand, and vice versa. The scatterplot may be used as a useful exploration tool to learn more about the properties of the dataset and to spot any noteworthy findings or outliers. Researchers can make informed decisions about data preprocessing, feature engineering, and selecting the best ML algorithms for the study's subsequent phases by carefully examining this plot and other visualisations. For the whole EDA process, Figure 15.2 is very important because it helps understand and make sense of the dataset for improving the performance of optical interconnection networks in the telecom industry.

The line plot demonstrates how the channel utilisation statistic varies depending on how many threads are present in the optical connectivity network. The number of parallel threads utilised to carry out processing tasks is represented by the x-axis's thread number, and the percentage of time that each channel is actively transmitting data is represented by the y-axis's channel utilisation. Researchers can identify any trends, patterns, or possible connections between channel utilisation and the quantity of threads used by looking at the line plot. If the number of threads increases along with the channel usage, this might mean that the channels get more crowded as the number of threads increases, which results in a higher utilisation rate.

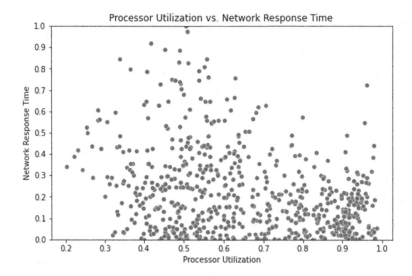

FIGURE 15.2   Scatterplot for processor utilisation vs. network response time.

In EDA, the line plot is essential because it enables researchers to comprehend how the interconnection network functions in various thread configurations. It aids in locating any potential performance hiccups or inefficiencies in the network with regard to channel utilisation and the number of threads employed. This knowledge is important for developing strategies to improve network performance and guarantee effective resource usage in the telecom industry. In general, Figure 15.3 offers insightful information about the connection between channel utilisation and thread number, assisting in the creation of data-driven judgements and further investigation for this work. The box plot graphically illustrates how network response time is distributed among the various spatial distribution categories in the optical connectivity network as shown in Fig 15.4. The y-axis shows network response time, which calculates how quickly a network node responds to incoming requests. The x-axis shows spatial distribution, which shows the sort of network topology used (such as Client-Server). The interquartile range (IQR) of network response time for each category of spatial distribution is shown in the box plot as a series of boxes. The whiskers extending from the boxes reflect the data points within 1.5 times the IQR, whereas the horizontal line within each box is the median reaction time. Outliers are any data points that fall outside of this range and are displayed as separate points. Researchers can identify changes in network response time across various forms of spatial distribution by examining the box plot.

Based on the network structure, possible outliers or differences in reaction time can be identified. Understanding how the network response time changes with spatial distribution can offer insightful information about the network's performance in various configurations, assisting in performance optimisation decision-making (see Figure 15.4).

The box plot, which graphically represents the central tendency, spread, and presence of outliers in the network response time with respect to various spatial distribution categories, is a crucial part of EDA. Researchers may draw conclusions about the optical interconnection network's dependability and effectiveness, which aids in the development of

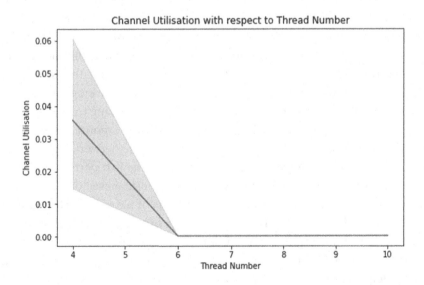

FIGURE 15.3   Line plot for channel utilisation with respect to thread number.

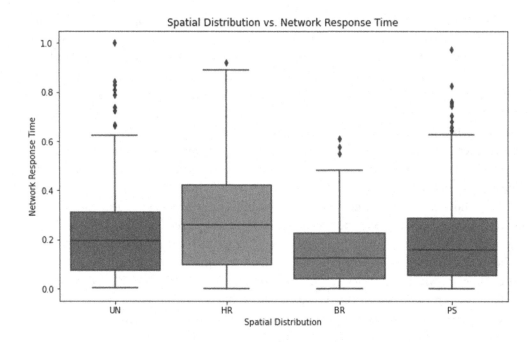

FIGURE 15.4   Box plot for spatial distribution vs. network response time.

ideas and the planning of additional research for network performance improvement in the telecom industry. Overall, Figure 15.5 contributes to the thorough study carried out in the research work by offering important insights into the link between spatial distribution and network response time.

The optical connectivity network's bar plot illustrates the average network response time for each temporal distribution category. The temporal distribution, represented by the x-axis, shows how network traffic is distributed over time periods (such as hourly, daily, etc.). The average network response time, which gauges how quickly network nodes typically reply to incoming requests throughout each temporal distribution, is shown on the y-axis. Each bar in the bar plot represents a distinct temporal distribution category. Each bar's height corresponds to the typical network response time for that specific temporal distribution period. Researchers can notice differences in the average network response time based on the distribution of the network traffic by comparing the heights of the bars.

The bar plot makes it easier to see how the total network response time is impacted by the temporal distribution of network traffic. To optimise the network's performance during peak or off-peak periods, it enables researchers to evaluate if particular time intervals have greater or lower response times. Companies in the telecom sector would benefit from this study as it offers insights on the temporal patterns of network performance that can be utilised to more effectively manage resources and enhance the overall customer experience. Additionally, knowing how temporal distribution affects network response time can be useful in developing measures to prevent possible bottlenecks and guarantee the network's efficient operation during times of high demand. In addition to the thorough study undertaken in the research work, Figure 15.5 adds a clear and succinct picture of the

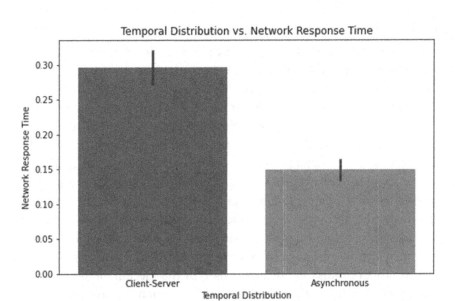

FIGURE 15.5   Bar plot for temporal distribution vs. network response time.

link between temporal distribution and network response time. Making educated choices for network optimisation in the telecom industry is made possible by its contribution to the debate about the performance characteristics of the optical interconnection network.

Accuracy, which is the percentage of properly predicted occurrences out of all the instances in the test dataset, is the main statistic used to assess the effectiveness of the predictive models. Divide the total number of predictions by the number of accurate forecasts to get a percentage representation. After that, multiply the outcome by 100. The accuracy of each model's predictions of the "Spatial Distribution" based on network performance measures is reported in the "Results" section. As shown in Table 15.2, the accuracy values for each algorithm are as follows:

1. **Logistic Regression**: This model has a prediction accuracy of about 45.31% for the "Spatial Distribution".

2. **Random Forest**: This model showed a better accuracy of about 51.56% in predicting the "Spatial Distribution".

3. **SVM**: This model achieved a prediction accuracy of about 44.53% for the "Spatial Distribution".

TABLE 15.2   Spatial Distribution Prediction Using Various ML Algorithms

ML Method	Accuracy (in %)
Logistic regression	45.3125
Random forest	51.5625
SVM	44.53125

15.6 DISCUSSIONS

The discussion section can deeper into these findings and examine the effects of the effectiveness of each algorithm. For instance, it can look at why random forest did better than the other two models, what caused the accuracy gaps, and whether the models' accuracy levels are enough for the particular use case in the telecom industry. The dataset was split into training and testing sets, with the features "T/R", "Processor Utilization", "Channel Waiting Time", "Input Waiting Time", "Network Response Time", and "Channel Utilization" serving as predictors for the "Spatial Distribution". The models were then trained on the training set and their accuracy was calculated on the test set. Overall, the "Results and Discussion" chapter emphasises the three ML algorithms' prognostic potential for enhancing the performance of optical interconnection networks in the telecom industry. By providing insightful information about the advantages and disadvantages of each algorithm, it lays the groundwork for drawing conclusions and making recommendations for the network optimisation strategies used by the telecom industry.

We used three different ML algorithms (logistic regression, random forest, and SVM) to look at a dataset that shows how well optical interconnection networks work in the telecom industry. The "Results and Discussion" section of the research chapter shows and talks about the results.

1. **Interpretation of Accuracy Scores**: To assess each model's performance, accuracy scores must be taken into consideration. The proportion of accurate predictions generated by each model, especially in forecasting the "Spatial Distribution" based on several network performance measures, is represented by the accuracy. The models' accuracy scores — 45.31% for logistic regression, 51.56% for random forest, and 44.53% for SVM — serve as a starting point for more investigation and debate.

2. **Comparing Model Performance**: In this case, the random forest model showed the highest accuracy, indicating that it was the most efficient algorithm among the three for this particular prediction task. Comparing the accuracy scores allows us to identify which model performed the best in predicting the "Spatial Distribution". This discovery might lead to discussions on the root causes of random forest's superior performance to logistic regression and SVM.

3. **Factors Contributing to Model Performance**: This and previous sections ought to go over the variables that affected the differences in model accuracy. For instance, it can look at whether certain network performance measures had a greater effect on one model's accuracy than the others. It may also look at how the algorithms perform differently depending on the size, distribution, and properties of the dataset.

4. **Generalisability and Applicability**: The generalisability and application of the findings should be discussed. It is critical to think about whether the models' accuracy results are enough for the telecom industry's real application of these algorithms. Understanding the possible drawbacks and difficulties of applying these models to real-world situations may be extremely insightful for network performance enhancement techniques.

5. **Recommendations and Future Directions**: Based on the results, the Results and Discussion chapter might make suggestions for improving the performance of the optical interconnection network. This can entail recommendations for the ML algorithm best suited for this particular telecom industry use case or whether combining several models will produce more effective results.

15.7 CONCLUSIONS AND FUTURE WORK

According to the findings of our research, the random forest model had the best accuracy (51.56%), closely followed by logistic regression (45.31%), and SVM (44.53%). Even though these accuracy levels show the promise of ML algorithms for network performance improvement, there are many ways that future research might improve the models' effectiveness and usability. In the future, we advise investigating ensemble strategies that integrate the predictions of many models to take advantage of their unique advantages and achieve higher accuracy. The performance of each model should also be further optimised through hyperparameter adjustments. Additionally, using time-series analysis and data augmentation approaches can help improve model generalisation and capture temporal interdependence in network performance. Other areas of research include using feature importance analysis to find the most important factors affecting network performance, adding anomaly detection methods to find problems before they happen, and making the most of a variety of performance goals, such as lowering latency or cutting down on energy use. Examining the deployment factors and the cost-effectiveness analysis may also make it easier to use the predictive analytics system in actual telecom infrastructure.

The robustness and generalisability of the models to various network contexts may be improved by verifying the models on actual network data and using transfer learning techniques [45]. Last but not least, creating real-time predictive analytics models and permitting human involvement when required would be essential for efficiently managing quickly altering network circumstances. The suggested predictive analytics system can develop into a useful tool for improving optical interconnection network performance in the telecom industry by addressing these areas of future study, which will be advantageous to both service providers and end users.

REFERENCES

[1] Kibria, M. G., Nguyen, K., Villardi, G. P., Zhao, O., Ishizu, K., & Kojima, F. (2018). Big data analytics, machine learning, and artificial intelligence in next-generation wireless networks. *IEEE Access*, 6, 32328–32338.

[2] Gill, S. S. et al. (2024). Modern computing: Vision and challenges. *Telematics and Informatics Reports*, 13, 100116.

[3] Gill, S. S., Xu, M., Ottaviani, C. et al. (2022). AI for next generation computing: Emerging trends and future directions. *Internet of Things*, 19, 100514.

[4] Singh, R. et al. (2023). Edge AI: A survey. *Internet of Things and Cyber-Physical Systems*, 3, 71–92.

[5] Musumeci, F., Rottondi, C., Nag, A., Macaluso, I., Zibar, D., Ruffini, M., & Tornatore, M. (2018). An overview on application of machine learning techniques in optical networks. *IEEE Communications Surveys & Tutorials*, 21(2), 1383–1408.

[6] Ahmed, S. F., Alam, M. S. B., Hoque, M., Lameesa, A., Afrin, S., Farah, T., Kabir, M., Shafiullah, G. M., & Muyeen, S. M. (2023). Industrial internet of things enabled technologies, challenges, and future directions. *Computers and Electrical Engineering*, 110, 108847.

[7] Mohammadi, M., Al-Fuqaha, A., Sorour, S., & Guizani, M. (2018). Deep learning for IoT big data and streaming analytics: A survey. *IEEE Communications Surveys & Tutorials*, 20(4), 2923–2960.

[8] DeCusatis, C. (2013). Optical interconnect networks for data communications. *Journal of Lightwave Technology*, 32(4), 544–552.

[9] Militano, L., Araniti, G., Condoluci, M., Farris, I., & Iera, A. (2015). Device-to-device communications for 5G internet of things. *EAI Endorsed Transactions on Internet of Things*, 1(1), e4.

[10] Ahmad, T., Madonski, R., Zhang, D., Huang, C., & Mujeeb, A. (2022). Data-driven probabilistic machine learning in sustainable smart energy/smart energy systems: Key developments, challenges, and future research opportunities in the context of smart grid paradigm. *Renewable and Sustainable Energy Reviews*, 160, 112128.

[11] Arévalo, G. V., Tipán, M., & Gaudino, R. (2018). Techno-economics for optimal deployment of optical fronthauling for 5G in large urban areas. *2018 20th International Conference on Transparent Optical Networks (ICTON)* (pp. 1–4). IEEE.

[12] Tonini, F., Raffaelli, C., Wosinska, L., & Monti, P. (2019). Cost-optimal deployment of a C-RAN with hybrid fiber/FSO fronthaul. *Journal of Optical Communications and Networking*, 11(7), 397–408.

[13] Masoudi, M., Lisi, S. S., & Cavdar, C. (2020). Cost-effective migration toward virtualized C-RAN with scalable fronthaul design. *IEEE Systems Journal*, 14(4), 5100–5110.

[14] Chen, H., Li, Y., Bose, S. K., Shao, W., Xiang, L., Ma, Y., & Shen, G. (2016). Cost-minimized design for TWDM-PON-based 5G mobile backhaul networks. *Journal of Optical Communications and Networking*, 8(11), B1–B11.

[15] Klinkowski, M. (2018). Planning of 5G C-RAN with optical fronthaul: A scalability analysis of an ILP mode. *2018 20th International Conference on Transparent Optical Networks (ICTON)* (pp. 1–4). IEEE.

[16] Ranaweera, C., Nirmalathas, A., Wong, E., Lim, C., Monti, P., Furdek, M., Wosinska, L., Skubic, B., & Machuca, C. M. (2021). Rethinking of optical transport network design for 5G/6G mobile communication. *IEEE Future Networks Tech Focus*, 12, 1–7.

[17] Fayad, A., Cinkler, T., Rak, J., & Jha, M. (2022). Design of cost-efficient optical fronthaul for 5G/6G networks: An optimization perspective. *Sensors*, 22(23), 9394.

[18] Gill, S. S., & Kaur, R. (2023). ChatGPT: Vision and challenges. *Internet of Things and Cyber-Physical Systems*, 3, 262–271.

[19] Nandhakumar, A. R., Baranwal, A. et al. (2024). Edgeaisim: A toolkit for simulation and modelling of ai models in edge computing environments. *Measurement: Sensors*, 31, 100939.

[20] Walia, G. K. et al. (2024). AI-empowered fog/edge resource management for IoT applications: A comprehensive review, research challenges and future perspectives. *IEEE Communications Surveys & Tutorials*, 26(1), 619–669.

[21] Abbasi, M., Shahraki, A., & Taherkordi, A. (2021). Deep learning for network traffic monitoring and analysis (NTMA): A survey. *Computer Communications*, 170, 19–41.

[22] Hou, T., Feng, G., Qin, S., & Jiang, W. (2018). Proactive content caching by exploiting transfer learning for mobile edge computing. *International Journal of Communication Systems*, 31(11), e3706.

[23] Spagna, S., Liebsch, M., Baldessari, R., Niccolini, S., Schmid, S., Garroppo, R., Ozawa, K., & Awano, J. (2013). Design principles of an operator-owned highly distributed content delivery network. *IEEE Communications Magazine*, 51(4), 132–140.

[24] Zhang, Y., Chowdhury, P., Tornatore, M., & Mukherjee, B. (2010). Energy efficiency in telecom optical networks. *IEEE Communications Surveys & Tutorials*, 12(4), 441–458.

[25] Ramaswami, R., Sivarajan, K., & Sasaki, G. (2009). *Optical Networks: A Practical Perspective*. Morgan Kaufmann.

[26] Benzekki, K., El Fergougui, A., & Elbelrhiti Elalaoui, A. (2016). Software-defined networking (SDN): A survey. *Security and Communication Networks*, 9(18), 5803–5833.

[27] Hadi, M. S., Lawey, A. Q., El-Gorashi, T. E. H., & Elmirghani, J. M. H. (2018). Big data analytics for wireless and wired network design: A survey. *Computer Networks*, 132, 180–199.

[28] Li, F., & Whalley, J. (2002). Deconstruction of the telecommunications industry: From value chains to value networks. *Telecommunications Policy*, 26(9–10), 451–472.

[29] Vassakis, K., Petrakis, E., & Kopanakis, I. (2018). Big data analytics: Applications, prospects and challenges. *Mobile Big Data: A Roadmap from Models to Technologies*, 10, 3–20.

[30] Bega, D., Gramaglia, M., Fiore, M., Banchs, A., & Costa-Perez, X. (2019). DeepCog: Optimizing resource provisioning in network slicing with AI-based capacity forecasting. *IEEE Journal on Selected Areas in Communications*, 38(2), 361–376.

[31] Rony, R. I., Lopez-Aguilera, E., & Garcia-Villegas, E. (2021). Cost analysis of 5G fronthaul networks through functional splits at the PHY layer in a capacity and cost limited scenario. *IEEE Access*, 9, 8733–8750.

[32] Keiser, G. (1989). *Local Area Networks*. Information Gatekeepers Inc.

[33] Kabir, A., Rehman, G., Gilani, S. M., Kitindi, E. J., Ul Abidin Jaffri, Z., & Abbasi, K. M. (2020). The role of caching in next generation cellular networks: A survey and research outlook. *Transactions on Emerging Telecommunications Technologies*, 31(2), e3702.

[34] Musumeci, F., Bellanzon, C., Carapellese, N., Tornatore, M., Pattavina, A., & Gosselin, S. (2016). Optimal BBU placement for 5G C-RAN deployment over WDM aggregation networks. *Journal of Lightwave Technology*, 34(8), 1963–1970.

[35] Yeganeh, H., & Vaezpour, E. (2016). Fronthaul network design for radio access network virtualization from a CAPEX/OPEX perspective. *Annals of Telecommunications*, 71, 665–676.

[36] Marotta, A., & Correia, L. M. (2020). Cost-effective joint optimisation of BBU placement and fronthaul deployment in brown-field scenarios. *EURASIP Journal on Wireless Communications and Networking,,* 2020 (242), 1–26.

[37] Hilt, A. (2019). Microwave hop-length and availability targets for the 5G mobile backhaul. *2019 42nd International Conference on Telecommunications and Signal Processing (TSP)* (pp. 187–190). IEEE.

[38] Xu, Q., Mehrotra, S., Mao, Z., & Li, J. (2013). PROTEUS: Network Performance Forecast for Real-Time, Interactive Mobile Applications. *Proceeding of the 11th Annual International Conference on Mobile Systems, Applications, and Services*, pp. 347–360.

[39] Naseer, S., Saleem, Y., Khalid, S., Bashir, M. K., Han, J., Iqbal, M. M., & Han, K. (2018). Enhanced network anomaly detection based on deep neural networks. *IEEE Access*, 6, 48231–48246.

[40] Priyanka, A., Gauthamarayathirumal, P., & Chandrasekar, C. (2023). Machine learning algorithms in proactive decision making for handover management from 5G & beyond 5G. *Egyptian Informatics Journal*, 24(3), 100389.

[41] Duato, J., Yalamanchili, S., & Ni, L. (2003). *Interconnection Networks*. Morgan Kaufmann.

[42] Fodor, I. K. (2002). A survey of dimension reduction techniques. No. UCRL-ID-148494. Lawrence Livermore National Lab.

[43] Allam, A., Nagy, M., Thoma, G., & Krauthammer, M. (2019). Neural networks versus logistic regression for 30 days all-cause readmission prediction. *Scientific Reports*, 9(1), 9277.

[44] Zheng, K., Yang, Z., Zhang, K., Chatzimisios, P., Yang, K., & Xiang, W. (2016). Big data-driven optimization for mobile networks toward 5G. *IEEE Network*, 30(1), 44–51.

[45] Teoh, Y. K., Gill, S. S., & Parlikad, A. K. (2023). IoT and fog computing based predictive maintenance model for effective asset management in industry 4.0 using machine learning. *IEEE Internet of Things Journal*, 10(3), 2087–2094.

VII

Emotional Intelligence

CHAPTER 16

Machine Learning-Based Emotional State Inference Using Mobile Sensing

Diogo Mota, Usman Naeem, and Sukhpal Singh Gill

16.1 INTRODUCTION

According to the World Health Organization, in 2015 alone, an estimated 322 million people suffered from depression, corresponding to an 18.4% increase compared with 2005 [1]. The latest Global Burden of Disease (GBD) study shows that in 2019, depression was the sixth most common cause of years lived with disability for people aged between 25 and 49 years old and only fourth for 10–24 year olds [2]. Due to the heterogeneity of the disease, diagnosis is often difficult. According to [3], in the United States, the median time to treatment is actually 8 years. This means that the time before a person first shows symptoms of depression and their first treatment session can reach as long as 8 years. During this time the symptoms only worsen, making remission harder to achieve. Even though there are a plethora of effective treatments for depression, ranging from psychotherapy to antidepressants, failure to detect depression is a major cause of a population-level disability. Furthermore, people often do not receive adequate care [4, 5]; in fact, more than two-thirds of diagnosed patients do not actually receive treatment [6].

Smartphones have become an essential, everyday object for humans. These devices allow users to connect with the world. It even has been shown that people create emotional attachments to their mobile phones [7]. It is therefore not surprising that researchers have been investigating important aspects of peoples' interactions with them. Several studies have already investigated the correlation between users' moods and their interactions with their smartphones [8–10]. More interestingly, however, was [11] the investigation of the causal links between users' emotional states and their interaction with mobile phones. It was found that users' emotions have a direct causal impact on different aspects of their mobile phone interactions.

Mobile phones can also be used to help clinicians detect users' emotional states on the fly. As smartphones evolved, we have been able to capture important data shown to link back to depression and its symptom severity. One example is the mobile phone location

DOI: 10.1201/9781003467199-23

sensor data, which [12] has important features that provide reliable predictors of depression symptoms. Smartphones can also be used to infer and alter users' emotional states, as demonstrated by [13]. These researchers developed a mobile app to increase the positive mental health of students in a Swedish university. The mHealth app proved to be more effective than the usual care in increasing students' positive mental health, proving that mHealth solutions are more than an ideology in public mental health promotion.

Wang et al. [14] displayed the monitoring capabilities of mobile phone sensing data when they assessed users' mental health in the StudentLife study. Using a mobile app, they monitored the mental state of a collection of students from Dartmouth University for a period of 10 weeks, using mobile phone and smartphone sensing capabilities. The resulting dataset, comprising a variety of features, such as audio inference, activity inference, call logs, app usage, ecological momentary assessments (EMAs), and survey data was made publicly available online for anyone to use.

Even though a number of studies have shown that smartphones provide continuous monitoring of users' mental states, these are limited to exactly this, monitoring. More often than not, the data extracted from these studies are only used for analysis after the experiment has finished and not during it. This is because the usual goal of these studies is to unobstructedly collect data to infer the participants day-to-day mental state. In contrast, this work, using mobile sensing data collected during the StudentLife study, aims to show that smartphones can be used to monitor a user's mental state as well as to predict user behaviour and provide them feedback to increase user awareness and help them cope with their mental struggles. We show that mobile sensing provides sufficiently reliable features that allow for the construction of machine learning algorithms capable of effectively predicting users' emotional states. This opens the way to the creation of more attentive mobile apps capable of delivering personalised mental health interventions for their users.

16.1.1 Contributions

In light of the difficulty in detecting depression and the challenges current mobile sensing studies present, this work, inspired by the work of [15], uses data produced in the StudentLife dataset to investigate potential, reliable features that allow machine learning models to infer a user's mental state. This work is divided into two main tasks. Firstly, we focus on the prediction of aspects interconnected with depression, such as signs of stress and sleep quality by using and comparing the XGBoost and TabNet models. Secondly, through the implementation of a fully convolutional network (FCN), we attempt to predict signs of depression in students after the completion of the StudentLife study.

16.2 RELATED WORK

This section discusses various related works regarding mobile sensing and machine learning models.

16.2.1 Previous Mobile Sensing Studies

Mobile phones are an everyday item in everyone's lives. Because of their increasingly large complement of sensors, the potential of mobile phones to monitor behavioural patterns that provide insight into a user's mental state has been proven in several studies. A review of the literature was performed to identify key studies that display the capabilities of mobile sensing to both monitor and alter a user's emotional state. The StudentLife study, developed by [14], assessed the mental health of a collection of students during a 10-week term at Dartmouth College. Influenced by a number of previous experiments, such as the friends and family study [16] and the reality mining project [17], researchers developed a mobile app to collect a range of sensing data types and had participants answer several EMAs and fill out a set of surveys with the intent to assess students' mental health. With the purpose of implementing classifiers to infer some users given states, they built upon previous work. For instance, they implemented a sleep classifier developed in [18, 19] to unobtrusively infer sleep duration. Another example was the activity classifier [19, 20], implemented to infer stationary, walking, running, driving, and cycling states. Other types of data were collected using mobile sensing such as app usage, Bluetooth, Wi-Fi, and EMA and survey data. Results from this study showed multiple significant correlations between mobile sensing data and mental health and educational outcomes. Furthermore, they identified a term life cycle in the University of Dartmouth. The StudentLife experiment worked as a basis for several new studies that attempted to show the applicability of mobile sensors to monitor mental health [21]. The data produced were also used to predict the students grade point average (GPA) in another study [22]. As previously stated, smartphones can also be used to alter the users' mental states. This was the case of a study [13] that consisted of a two-arm, single-blind, parallel group randomised controlled trial that aimed to test the feasibility of an mHealth mobile app to increase the positive mental health of a group of students from a Swedish university. The primary outcome of the experiment was positive mental health and the secondary was depression and anxiety symptomatology. Participants were randomly assigned to either an intervention group or a control group. For the duration of the study (10 weeks), the intervention group had access to an mHealth positive psychology app, which aimed to enhance users' positive mental health and was developed based on empirical evidence. The application was comprised of information regarding well-being, self-help exercises, brief tips, self-monitoring, and personalised feedback. Participants allocated to the control group were notified of their position through text message, which also included all essential contact details to their local health centre, primary care centre, and governmental national health website. At the 3-month follow-up, data from both groups were collected and showed that positive mental health, measured by the Mental Health Continuum Short Form (MHC-SF), was substantially higher in the intervention group compared with the control group. On one hand, the study proved the viability of using a fully automated mHealth app to enhance users' mental states. On the other hand, it is important to note that the interventions given were not tailored for different individuals. All participants were given the same interventions and no adjustments were made to attend to users' preferences. If feedback from the participants had been collected, a machine learning algorithm could have been deployed to inform what given intervention was better suited for a given participant. With the goal of discovering the reliability of mobile phone Global Positioning System (GPS) and app usage sensing for the prediction of both signs and levels of depression, work [15] consisted of an experiment comprised of 40 participants, which in a span of 2 weeks provided GPS and phone usage data from a data acquisition app named Purple Robot [23]. Based on the collected data, they defined a given number of features and built classification and regression models to investigate their relationship with depressive symptom severity. To determine whether the obtained features would provide useful insight regarding users' depressed symptoms, correlation analysis between the different features and the Patient Health Questionnaire (PHQ-9)scores was performed. Additionally, participants were divided into those with depressive symptoms (PHQ-9 >5) and those without (PHQ-9 ≤5). With this they tested whether it was possible to distinguish people with depressive symptoms from those without. Two types of models were created for two different tasks. To estimate the PHQ-9 score of the participants, a regression model was built, using the features extracted from the data. Also, a logistic regression classifier was built to identify participants with depressive symptoms. The regression model predicted the scores with an average error of 23.5% and the logistic classifier performed with an accuracy of 86.5%.

16.2.2 The XGBoost and TabNet Models

All the data produced in the previously discussed studies, more importantly the StudentLife dataset are tabular. Up until recently gradient boosting machines (GBMs) were the heavy favourite for classification problems involving tabular data because, when compared to neural networks, they require less coding, perform better in smaller datasets (neural networks often require very large datasets), are faster to train, and easily interpretable (whereas neural networks are often considered black boxes). At the top of GBMs stands the XGBoost. Introduced in [24], the XGBoost is a speed-and performance-oriented implementation of gradient boosted decision trees. At its core, XGBoost is an ensemble tree method in which each tree boosts the attributes that led the previous tree to a misclassification. However, XGBoost improves upon standard GBMs with its novel system optimisations: parallelisation (the process of sequential tree building is parallelised by interchanging the order of the loops used for building base learners); tree pruning (uses the max depth parameter and starts pruning trees backwards improving performance); hardware optimisation (by introducing cache awareness and out-of-core computing); and algorithmic enhancements, such as regularisation (uses both L1 and L2 regularisation methods to prevent overfitting), sparsity awareness (to handle sparsity patterns in the data more efficiently), weighted quantile sketch (to be able to handle weighted data), and cross-validation (incorporated at each iteration). With these novel changes, XGBoost currently outperforms state-of-the-art decision tree-based algorithms. However, after the introduction of TabNet, the paradigm has shifted. TabNet, a deep neural model, tackled all the previous disadvantages of neural networks compared with GBMs. Developed in [25], the TabNet, although complex, is a highly interpretable model. Its design allows it to inherit the explainability of tree-based methods, while still providing the key benefits of deep learning models. It possesses a set of unique features that allowed it to stand out from other architectures: it is able to input raw data, without any need for preprocessing, which currently constitutes a major step for data scientists when developing machine learning models; it is trained using gradient descent; it uses sequential attention to choose features at each decision step (with a built-in

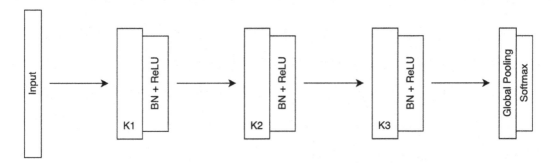

FIGURE 16.1   Example of an FCN architecture, where K1, K2, and K3 represent the filter sizes of each convolution block.

explainability in the form of masks); and it employs single deep learning architectures and enables two types of interpretability, such as global through the quantification of feature contributions and local by visualising the importance of features and how they are combined for a single row.

16.2.3 Fully Convolutional Networks for Multivariate Time-Series Classification

Besides tabular, large amounts of data are stored in the form of time series, such as, stock market data, weather data, electroencephalography results, etc. The tabular data produced in the StudentLife dataset can also be viewed as several time series, one per data type, per student. When it comes to the task of time-series classification, more specifically, multivariate time-series classification, FCNs have shown to be a very effective architecture. Usually, image classification is the common association when talking about convolutional neural networks (CNNs). However, the less famous one-dimensional (1D) convolutions allow for a more generalised use of CNNs. According to [26], a study that explored three different types of networks for time-series classification such as multilayer perceptron (MLP), FCN, and the residual network (ResNet), the FCN achieved premium performance. Its basic block is a convolutional layer (the convolution is performed by three 1D kernels) followed by a batch normalisation (to increase convergence speed and improve generalisation) and a ReLU activation layer. After the convolution blocks, the features are passed to a global average pooling layer, instead of a fully connected layer, to greatly reduce the number of weights. Finally, the prediction is produced by the softmax layer (Figure 16.1).

16.3 METHODOLOGY

This research comprises two main tasks, yielding a total of three classification tasks. The first task was focused on predicting key aspects that influence users' emotional states, such as whether a student, on any given day, will show signs of stress and whether a user, on any given day, will be able to sleep the recommended amount of hours. The second task is aimed at using the data in the form of time series to predict signs of depression in students. We therefore propose the methodology presented in Figure 16.2. The first step consists of preprocessing the data: all missing values are imputed using a K-nearest neighbours

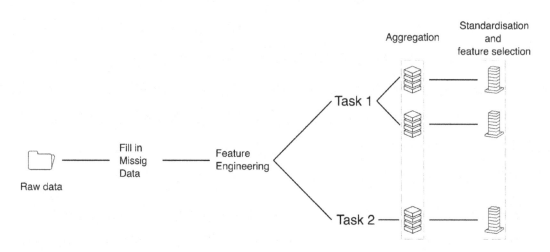

FIGURE 16.2   Schematic representation of the adopted methodology.

(KNN) approach. Secondly, through feature engineering, we extract statistical features from the chosen data types. Thirdly, we aggregate the data depending on the given task. For both tasks, the features are organised by data type and then aggregated by day. Specific to each task is how the data are organised. In the first task, we joined the features from all participants and, given the existence of restrictive data types that shortened the final size of the dataset, we created two datasets: dataset A, which excluded the restrictive data types, and dataset B which included them. For the second task, each data instance is a set of time series that corresponds to a given student. Fourthly, the features are standardised by removing the mean and scaling to unit variance. Moreover, to optimise our models' performances, we removed unnecessary or conflicting features using recursive feature elimination (RFE) for the first task and selected the set of features that allowed the largest dataset possible for the second.

16.3.1 KNNImputer

The sklearn KNNImputer method provides imputation for filling in missing values using the KNN approach. Using the euclidean distance metric, the nearest neighbours of the missing values are found. Each missing value is imputed by averaging (either uniformly or weighted) the available features of the corresponding KNNs.

16.3.2 Feature Engineering

From the plethora of available data types in the StudentLife dataset, we selected the following: Call log, EMA, Sensing, SMS, and Survey. Details regarding the types of data and their collection can be found in [14]. The reasons for this particular subset of data types vary: many data types had a large amount of missing values, details regarding the meaning of the data or how it was collected were not given, or the data was not related to a user's emotional state.

From the Call log data we had access to the duration of all the calls in a day. During the 10-week experiment, students responded to psychological and behavioural EMAs on their smartphones. These EMAs ranged from stress, mood, sleep, social aspects, physical exercise, time spent on different activities, short personality item, and photographic affect meter (PAM), where users identified from a set of images that they found best described how they felt. Due to the vast amount of missing values and being related to specific events, such as the Boston bombing, several EMAs had to be excluded from being used to extract features. Of the 27 EMAs collected during the experiment we used only 4. For the sensing data there are a total of ten different sensor data, eight of which were used to extract features: physical activity, audio inferences, conversation inferences, light sensor, GPS, phone charge, phone lock, and Wi-Fi location. From the SMS data we were only interested in knowing the amount of SMS exchanged per day. Survey data were only used for the purpose of predicting depression signs in the students. These were only collected twice, once before the study began and again when it ended. For the majority of the collected data types, the standard procedure for feature engineering was aggregating the available values by day and extracting statistical features such as the mean, median, standard deviation, minimum and maximum values, the skew, and the variance. Any other processes used include the following:

- **Call log data:** With the duration of the calls received/taken in a given day, the standard procedure was applied to obtain features.

- **Sensing data:**

  - **Activity**: There were four possible values for the activity inference: 0 (stationary), 1 (walking), 2 (running), and 3 (unknown). With these values collected on a daily basis and often collected more than once a day, the standard procedure was applied to obtain the features. As an additional feature, the sum of these values per day was calculated.

  - **Audio**: The same procedure as for the activity inference data was used. There were also four possible values for the audio inference: 0 (silence), 1 (voice), 2 (noise), and 3 (unknown).

  - **Conversation**: The conversation duration was calculated for each day these data were available. Afterwards the standard procedure was applied. The light sensor calculated the amount of time the phone was in a dark environment and executed the standard procedure.

  - **GPS**: Using the latitude, longitude, altitude, bearing, speed, and travel state values the standard procedure was performed. Note that the travel state values were encoded as 0 if the value was "stationary" and 1 if it was "moving".

  - **Phone Charge**: Once again we calculated the amount of time the phone was charging and used the standard procedure to extract features.

  - **Phone Lock**: An analogous procedure was performed on the phone charge data.

  - **Wi-Fi Location**: The amount of different locations a user visited during a day was calculated.

- **EMA data:**

  - **PAM**: With the indexes of the images students chose, we followed the mentioned standard procedure to obtain features.

  - **Sleep**: This EMA was comprised of three questions whose IDs were hour, rate, and social. For each of these questions the standard procedure was applied.

  - **Social**: This was comprised of only one question. We applied the standard procedure for feature extraction. For stress the same process as for the social EMAs was applied.

- **SMS data:** For SMS data we calculated the amount of messages exchanged in a given day and used this as the feature.

Specific to the second task is the preprocessing of the survey data. Students were required to fill in a set of surveys at the beginning of the study and again at the end (10 weeks after). One of the surveys filled was the PHQ-9 [27], a self-administered questionnaire, scoring each of the nine Diagnostic and Statistical Manual of Mental Disorders, 4th ed. (DSM-IV) criteria as "0" (not at all) to "3" (nearly every day). Scores lower than 5 indicate no signs of depression, whereas scores equal or above include mild (5), moderate (10), moderately severe (15), and severe depression (20).

16.3.3 Data Standardisation and Feature Selection

Feature standardisation is an essential step of data preprocessing because it allows for different features to have similar weights between each other. Without it, different features that have larger values carry more weight when compared with smaller features. The final step used to build the datasets for the first task is called feature selection. To optimise the models' performances we removed unnecessary or conflicting features using RFE. This automated feature selection algorithm trains a model on a gradually smaller set of features. In this work, the RFE trained a random forest classifier. Because this method requires a specific number of features, which usually is not known, we added cross-validation. This way, the algorithm selects the best subset of features for the given estimator and then selects the best subset based on the cross-validation score of the model.

16.3.4 Models

Both the XGBoost and the TabNet models have many hyperparameters that need to be tuned so we can get the best possible performance out of them. A schematic representation of the set of hyperparameters tuned, per model, is presented in Figure 16.3. All of the mentioned hyperparameters were tuned and only the best set was used for the classification tasks.

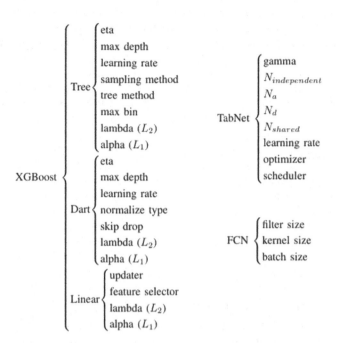

$$
\text{XGBoost}
\begin{cases}
\text{Tree}
\begin{cases}
\text{eta} \\
\text{max depth} \\
\text{learning rate} \\
\text{sampling method} \\
\text{tree method} \\
\text{max bin} \\
\text{lambda } (L_2) \\
\text{alpha } (L_1)
\end{cases} \\
\text{Dart}
\begin{cases}
\text{eta} \\
\text{max depth} \\
\text{learning rate} \\
\text{normalize type} \\
\text{skip drop} \\
\text{lambda } (L_2) \\
\text{alpha } (L_1)
\end{cases} \\
\text{Linear}
\begin{cases}
\text{updater} \\
\text{feature selector} \\
\text{lambda } (L_2) \\
\text{alpha } (L_1)
\end{cases}
\end{cases}
\qquad
\text{TabNet}
\begin{cases}
\text{gamma} \\
N_{independent} \\
N_a \\
N_d \\
N_{shared} \\
\text{learning rate} \\
\text{optimizer} \\
\text{scheduler}
\end{cases}
\qquad
\text{FCN}
\begin{cases}
\text{filter size} \\
\text{kernel size} \\
\text{batch size}
\end{cases}
$$

FIGURE 16.3 Set of hyperparameters tuned per model. For the XGBoost we experimented with the three available boosters and tuned their respective hyperparameters. Both Dart and Tree booster are tree-based methods, and Linear applies linear functions. The most important hyperparameters were the ones focused on tackling overfitting such as eta, alpha, lambda, and max depth. Being a deep learning model, TabNet has some familiar parameters: optimisers (methods to change the attributes of the neural network) and schedulers (to change the learning rate during training). Other parameters unique to TabNet include Nd (width of the decision prediction layer), Na (width of the attention embedding for each mask), N_{steps} (the number of independent [$N_{independent}$]) and shared (N_{shared}). Gated Linear Unites layers at each step, the momentum (for batch normalisation) and an extra sparsity loss coefficient. For the final task, based on the implementation of [28], a custom FCN was created and its standard CNN hyperparameters tuned.

16.4 RESULTS AND DISCUSSION

This section regards the results and discussion from each experiment. The first two sections correspond to predicting signs of stress and whether a given student will sleep the recommended hours in a day. As previously mentioned, the data used for this task were organised by day. We noticed that including both the SMS and Call log features reduces the number of data instances from 397 (dataset A) to 117 (dataset B), therefore one question arose: Are the restricting features important or reliable enough to compensate for the difference in dataset sizes? To answer this question we trained and tested the XGBoost and TabNet models with and without the SMS and Call log data. The final section corresponds to the task of multivariate time-series classification where we used an FCN to predict signs of depression in students after the study was completed. Note that since the analysis in the first two subsections are very similar, only the first subsection presents the produced plots.

Similarly, the TabNet Loss, Accuracy, and Learning rates plots were also placed in the Appendix because their analysis is meant to simply show adequate training.

16.4.1 Stress Prediction

To predict signs of stress we turned to the responses of the stress EMA. Students had to fill in the following sentence: "Right now, I am..." with one of the available answers:

- A little stressed [1]

- Definitely stressed [2]

- Stressed out [3]

- Feeling good [4]

- Feeling great [5]

With these answers we obtained the mean stress level of each student per day. Afterwards, we encoded these results to obtain the labels: based on the meaning of the available responses of the stress EMA, we defined showing signs of stress if the mean level of stress $\in$ [1, 4]. Levels above meant no signs of stress. For the rest of the section we will be presenting and discussing the obtained results: feature correlation, model performance, feature importance, and model explainability. When it comes to feature correlation, both datasets yielded small values of correlations between the features and the mean level of stress a student experiences in a day. Based on the work of [12], we hypothesised that features related to the users' movements, such as the number of distinct locations, activity inferences, and GPS features, which would yield the highest correlation values. When using dataset B, we observed a general increase in feature correlation. Furthermore, features related to Call logs appear in the top 5 correlated features, indicating good predictor reliability. Unexpected was the lack of correlation between stress-related features and sleep and vice versa. This of course can be due to a plethora of reasons: the feature engineering process yielded only statistical features that could have destroyed any correlation or not explored an existing one, or it could additionally be due to the way the data was collected. Interestingly, the features with the highest correlation values were not the ones the models found to be the most important (Figure 16.4). In fact, the importance distribution links the association between sleep and stress we were looking for, which is in accordance with the literature. When trained with dataset A, the TabNet model attributed the most importance to the mean hours of sleep. According to [29], the tendency to experience stressful thoughts is associated with sleep complaints. Furthermore, [30] found that using a mindfulness-based stress reduction program not only significantly reduced stress, but also improved sleep quality in patients. In addition, the second most important feature for both models supports the previously stated link between GPS data and stress because it corresponds to the maximum value of the latitude, for the TabNet, and the median value of the latitude, for the XGBoost.

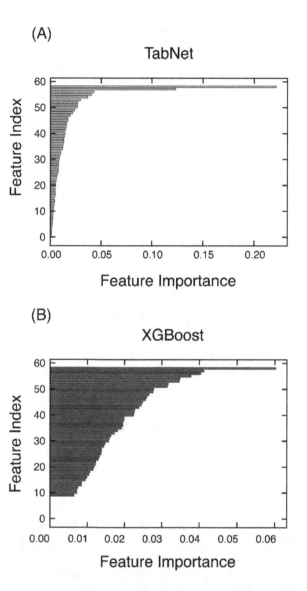

FIGURE 16.4   Feature Importance histogram for dataset A. One advantage of using a tree ensemble and TabNet is their explainability. These models allow for feature exploration so we can better understand how and why a model makes a given prediction. As previously stated, TabNet was designed to learn a "decision tree-like" mapping to benefit from the explainability of tree-based models. (A) Feature importance histogram using the TabNet model. (B) Feature importance histogram using the XGBoost model.

Both models performed exceptionally well and were able to predict signs of stress with an accuracy significantly above chance (Table 16.1). When trained on dataset A, the TabNet, even though very slightly, was able to outperform the XGBoost model. However, this difference is practically negligible. It is also important to note that the performance of both models increased when we included the SMS and Call log data (dataset B), meaning that their reliability allowed for a better model performance (Table 16.1).

TABLE 16.1   Model Performance When Predicting
Whether a User Showed Signs of Stress

Model	Dataset A	Dataset B
XGBoost	0.830	0.890
TabNet	0.833	0.850

The fact that the XGBoost performs better than the TabNet is expected given that the size of the dataset decreased drastically and deep neural networks tend to perform worse with small datasets due to their high number of parameters. This requires a large number of iterations to find all optimal values. Consequently, using a high number of iterations with small datasets often results in overfitting. We are unable to compare feature importance when using dataset B because the best performing model of the XGBoost is obtained using the Linear booster, which implements linear functions and the concept of feature importance is specific to tree-based methods. Even though GBMs have a good level of explainability, TabNet provides a deeper look at feature importance through masks. From Figure 16.5 we can observe three matrices, each corresponding to one decision step of the TabNet when trained on dataset A. Each row of these matrices corresponds to a test sample and a column to a feature. By looking at these matrices we can investigate which features were given more importance per prediction. For instance, if we look at the first decision step (Mask 0) we see that for the majority of predictions, the highest importance was given to the last two features, which are sleep-related features (median of the hours sleep and the minimum of hours of sleep, respectively).

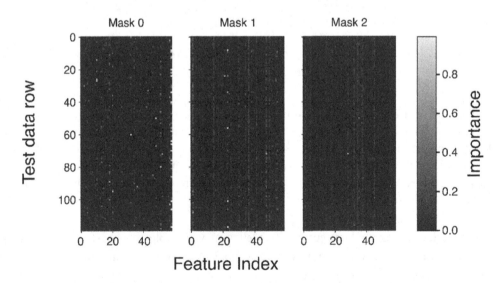

FIGURE 16.5   TabNet feature importance masks for dataset A. Each mask corresponds to a decision step during the testing stage of the TabNet. These masks allow us to understand which features were the most important on an individual prediction level.

16.4.2 Sleep Prediction

From the sleep EMA we used the results of the question "How many hours did you sleep last night?" and calculated the average score of the answer, which corresponds to a given number of hours slept, therefore calculating the mean number of hours a person sleeps in a day. According to a significant body of research [31–33], the recommended sleep duration for adults is between 7 and 8 hours, therefore, we encoded the mean hours of sleep the following way: if the mean hours of sleep were higher than 7, the given student slept the recommended amount of time that day, otherwise they did not. Analogously to what was done in the previous section, we performed the same set of experiments during this task.

Table 16.2 shows that the features with the highest correlation values are all related to phone usage. This finding is expected because several studies have already concluded that phone usage impacts both quality and sleep duration. Such is the case of the work of [34], who found that nighttime usage of mobile phones was significantly associated with difficulty in waking up, waking up tired, and other related effects. Given that we were able to associate sleep with signs of stress, we looked to replicate the finding in this experiment; however, we were unsuccessful. Similarly to what occurred in the previous section, most of the features awarded with the most importance were not the highest correlated ones. This time around, for dataset A, both the TabNet and XGBoost attributed more importance to features related with motion, audio inference, and some phone usage features (not coincident with features with high correlation values). However, the XGBoost gave most importance to the PAM (mood inferences)-related features, which according to [35] are connected with sleep quality. Similar conclusions about model performance can be made as in the previous section: both models predicted if a student slept the recommended number of hours significantly above chance. When trained on dataset B, the XGBoost outperformed the TabNet model. Even though the feature importance distributions behave similarly as in Figure 16.4, the XGBoost achieves a higher performance, leading us to believe that distributing importance more equally, despite being a TabNet characteristic, does not translate to better performance. Table 16.2 also supports this finding because the difference between model performances is practically negligible.

16.4.3 Depression Prediction

Similarly to what was done in [15], the post PHQ-9 scores were encoded as 0 if the score was less than 5, meaning no signs of depression, and 1 otherwise. Because this task is user specific, meaning that each student has a set of time-series (one per feature) that are unique to them, the size of the dataset was particularly small. Furthermore, we are using an FCN as our machine learning model, which presents a previously mentioned problem: neural

TABLE 16.2   Model Performance When Predicting
Whether a User Slept the Recommended Amount of Hours

Model	Dataset A	Dataset B
XGBoost	0.86	0.81
TabNet	0.842	0.723

networks tend to perform poorly on small datasets. An additional constraint was the amount of days' worth of data each participant had. The post PHQ-9 scores were obtained at the end of the study, 10 weeks after the study began. This means that for our predictions and analysis to be credible we needed at least 50 days' worth of data for each student. To tackle the first problem we tuned the hyperparameters as per the Models subsection in the Methodology section. As for the latter constraint, the following approach was taken: to maximise the number of features used as well as the number of days' worth of data (for every user) we determined the lowest amount of data types we could use where, after feature engineering, the majority of the students would have more than 50 days' worth of data. The result was three data types, activity inference, audio inference, and conversation duration, which yielded a total of 23 features per student for a total of 33 students. Moreover, the model was trained using fourfold cross-validation to test the model's ability to generalise and predict new instances of data and to flag issues such as overfitting. The FCN was able to predict depression signs with an accuracy slightly above chance of 53.5%; however, with an average false-negative rate of 54.2% (false-positive rate was 33.3%). This underwhelming performance is mainly due to the size of the dataset. Nonetheless, it shows that mobile sensing features are reliable enough to predict depression signs in students, as per [15]. With a larger dataset, we firmly believe the model would provide a satisfactory performance.

16.5 LIMITATIONS

During the feature engineering process it became clear that, although extremely rich, the StudentLife dataset lacked quality. This is not due to the design of the experiment, but due to the participants. As it is common in "in-the-wild" experiments, as the study progresses participant adherence decreases. This results in several gaps in the daily collection of data that resulted in a heavy size constriction of the datasets built in this study. This was a problem during the prediction of signs of depression because the more features we used fewer students were found to have sufficient days' worth of data. This resulted in a model with an underwhelming performance displaying a high false-negative rate (a common issue as stated in [12]). Furthermore, the feature importance analysis performed is restricted by the feature selection process. Even though we implemented a five-step cross-validation, different uses of the RFE with cross-validation (RFECV) resulted in different selected features, consequently influencing which features the models find the most important.

16.6 CONCLUSIONS AND FUTURE WORK

Regardless of these limitations, the present work displayed the potential and reliability of mobile sensing features to predict both interconnected aspects of depression (stress and sleep), extending the work of [15], and depression signs. We show that it is possible to accurately predict both signs of stress (83.3% and 89.0%) and if a given person will sleep the recommended amount of hours (86.0% and 81.0%). Given the richness of the StudentLife dataset, future work could study further associations between mobile sensing and a user's emotional state, for instance, predicting the amount of people a given user will meet the following day, based on the previous day's set of features. Given the unsatisfactory performance of the FCN, additional architectures should be tested, namely the ResNet and long short-term memory (LSTM) [36]. Furthermore, given the size constriction of the dataset, either a new, refined version of the StudentLife should be performed to increase the dataset quality, or merging similar datasets to increase the final dataset size should be done [37]. All in all this work shows that mobile sensing features can and should be used in either a clinical environment to help track patient progress [38], or in mobile applications to increase user awareness of their mental state and mitigate the time between first showing depression symptoms [39] and the first treatment session and to tailor user interventions to optimise their effectiveness.

REFERENCES

[1] W. H. Organization (2017). Depression and other common mental disorders: Global health estimates. Tech. Rep., World Health Organization.

[2] Vos, T., Lim, S. S., Abbafati, C., Abbas, K. M. et al. (2020). Global burden of 369 diseases and injuries in 204 countries and territories, 1990–2019: A systematic analysis for the global burden of disease study 2019. *The Lancet*, 396(10258), 1204–1222.

[3] Wang, P. S., Berglund, P., Olfson, M., Pincus, H. A., Wells, K. B., & Kessler, R. C. (2005). Failure and delay in initial treatment contact after first onset of mental disorders in the national comorbidity survey replication. *Archives of General Psychiatry*, 62(6), 603–613.

[4] Boenisch, S., Kocalevent, R.-D., Matschinger, H., Mergl, R., Wimmer-Brunauer, C., Tauscher, M., Kramer, D., Hegerl, U., & Bramesfeld, A. (2012). Who receives depression-specific treatment? A secondary data-based analysis of outpatient care received by over 780,000 statutory health-insured individuals diagnosed with depression. *Social Psychiatry and Psychiatric Epidemiology*, 47(3), 475–486.

[5] Wittchen, H.-U., Jacobi, F., Rehm, J., et al. (2011). The size and burden of mental disorders and other disorders of the brain in Europe 2010. *European Neuropsychopharmacology*, 21(9), 655–679.

[6] Kessler, R. C., Chiu, W. T., Demler, O., & Walters, E. E. (2005). Prevalence, severity, and comorbidity of 12-month DSM-IV disorders in the national comorbidity survey replication. *Archives of General Psychiatry*, 62(6), 617–627.

[7] Vincent, J. (2006). Emotional attachment and mobile phones. *Knowledge, Technology & Policy*, 19(1), 39–44.

[8] Alvarez-Lozano, J., Osmani, V., Mayora, O., Frost, M., Bardram, J., Faurholt-Jepsen, M., & Kessing, L. V. (2014). Tell Me Your Apps and I Will Tell You Your Mood: Correlation of Apps Usage with Bipolar Disorder State. *Proceedings of the 7th International Conference on Pervasive Technologies Related to Assistive Environments*, pp. 1–7.

[9] LiKamWa, R., Liu, Y., Lane, N. D., & Zhong, L. (2013). Mood-Scope: Building a Mood Sensor from Smartphone Usage Patterns. *Proceeding of the 11th Annual International Conference on Mobile Systems, Applications, and Services*, pp. 389–402.

[10] Vermeulen, J., Pejovic, V., Mehrotra, A., Hendley, R., & Musolesi, M. (2016) My Phone and Me: Understanding People's Receptivity to Mobile Notifications. *Proceedings of the 2016 CHI Conference on Human Factors in Computing Systems*, pp. 1021–1032.

[11] Mehrotra, A., Tsapeli, F., Hendley, R., & Musolesi, M. (2017). MyTraces: Investigating correlation and causation be- tween users' emotional states and mobile phone inter- action. *Proceedings of the ACM on Interactive, Mobile, Wearable and Ubiquitous Technologies*, 1(3), 1–21.

[12] Saeb, S., Lattie, E. G., Schueller, S. M., Kording, K. P., & Mohr, D. C. (2016). The relationship between mobile phone location sensor data and depressive symptom severity. *PeerJ*, 4, e2537.

[13] Bendtsen, M., Müssener, U., Linderoth, C., & Thomas, K. (2020). A mobile health intervention for mental health promotion among university students: Randomized controlled trial. *JMIR mHealth and uHealth*, 8(3), e17208.

[14] Wang, R., Chen, F., Chen, Z., Li, T., Harari, G., Tignor, S., Zhou, X., Ben-Zeev, D., & Campbell, A. T. (2014). Student life: assessing mental health, academic performance and behavioral trends of college students using smartphones. *Proceedings of the 2014 ACM international joint conference on pervasive and ubiquitous computing*, pp. 3–14.

[15] Saeb, S., Zhang, M., Karr, C. J., Schueller, S. M., Corden, M. E., Kording, K. P., & Mohr, D. C. (2015). Mobile Phone sensor correlates of depressive symptom severity in daily- life behavior: An exploratory study. *Journal of Medical Internet Research*, 17(7), e175.

[16] Aharony, N., Pan, W., Ip, C., Khayal, I., & Pentland, A. (2011). Social fMRI: Investigating and shaping social mechanisms in the real world. *Pervasive and Mobile Computing*, 7(6), 643–659.

[17] Eagle, N., & Pentland, A. S. (2006). Reality mining: Sensing complex social systems. *Personal and Ubiquitous Computing*, 10(4), 255–268.

[18] Chen, Z., Lin, M., Chen, F., Lane, N. D., Cardone, G., Wang, R., Li, T., Chen, Y., Choudhury, T., & Campbell, A. T. (2013). Unobtrusive Sleep Monitoring Using Smart-Phones. *2013 7th International Conference on Pervasive Computing Technologies for Healthcare and Work - shops* (pp. 145–152). IEEE.

[19] Lane, N. D., Mohammod, M., Lin, M., Yang, X., Lu, H., Ali, S., Doryab, A., Berke, E., Choudhury, T., & Campbell, A. (2011). Bewell: A smartphone application to monitor, model and promote wellbeing. *5th international ICST Conference on Pervasive Computing Technologies for Healthcare*, pp. 23–26.

[20] Lu, H., Yang, J., Liu, Z., Lane, N. D., Choudhury, T., & Campbell, A. T. (2010). The Jigsaw Continuous Sensing Engine for Mobile Phone Applications. *Proceedings of the 8th ACM Conference on Embedded Networked Sensor Systems*, pp. 71–84.

[21] Sano, A., Phillips, A. J., Amy, Z. Y., McHill, A. W., Taylor, S., Jaques, N., Czeisler, C. A., Klerman, E. B., & Picard, R. W. (2015). Recognizing academic performance, sleep quality, stress level, and mental health using personality traits, wearable sensors and mobile phones. *2015 IEEE 12th International Conference on Wearable and Implantable Body Sensor Networks (BSN)* (pp. 1–6). IEEE.

[22] Wang, R., Harari, G., Hao, P., Zhou, X., & Campbell, A. T. (2015). SmartGPA: How Smartphones Can Assess and Predict Academic Performance of College Students. *Proceedings of the 2015 ACM International Joint Conference on Pervasive and Ubiquitous Computing*, pp. 295–306.

[23] Schueller, S. M., Begale, M., Penedo, F. J., & Mohr, D. C. (2014). Purple: A modular system for developing and deploying behavioral intervention technologies. *Journal of Medical Internet Research*, 16(7), e3376.

[24] Chen, T., & Guestrin, C. (2016). XGBoost: A Scalable Tree Boosting System. *Proceedings of the 22nd ACM SIGKDD International Conference on Knowledge Discovery and Data Mining*, pp. 785–794.

[25] Arik, S., & Pfister, T. (2021) TabNet: Attentive Interpretable Tabular Learning. *Proceedings of the AAAI Conference on Artificial Intelligence*, Vol. 35, No. 8, pp. 6679–6687.

[26] Wang, Z., Yan, W., & Oates, T. (2017). Time series classification from scratch with deep neural networks: A strong baseline. *2017 International joint conference on neural networks (IJCNN)* (pp. 1578–1585). IEEE.

[27] Kroenke, K., Spitzer, R. L., & Williams, J. B. (2001). The PHQ-9: Validity of a brief depression severity measure. *Journal of General Internal Medicine*, 16(9), 606–613.

[28] Ismail Fawaz, H., Forestier, G., Weber, J., Idoumghar, L., & Muller, P.-A. (2019). Deep learning for time series classification: A review. *Data Mining and Knowledge Discovery*, 33(4), 917–963.

[29] Hall, M., Buysse, D. J., Nowell, P. D., Nofzinger, E. A., Houck, P., Reynolds, C. F., & Kupfer, D. J. (2000). Symptoms of stress and depression as correlates of sleep in primary insomnia. *Psychosomatic Medicine*, 62(2), 227–230.

[30] Carlson, L. E., & Garland, S. N. (2005). Impact of mindfulness - based stress reduction (MBSR) on sleep, mood, stress and fatigue symptoms in cancer outpatients. *International Journal of Behavioral Medicine*, 12(4), 278–285.

[31] Hirshkowitz, M., Whiton, K., Albert, S. M. et al. (2015). National sleep foundation's sleep time duration recommendations: Methodology and results summary. *Sleep Health*, 1(1), 40–43.

[32] Hirshkowitz, M., Whiton, K., Albert, S. M. et al. (2015). National sleep foundation's updated sleep duration recommendations. *Sleep Health*, 1(4), 233–243.

[33] Panel, C. C., Watson, N. F., Badr, M. S. et al. (2015). Recommended amount of sleep for a healthy adult: A joint consensus statement of the American academy of sleep medicine and sleep research society. *Journal of Clinical Sleep Medicine*, 11(6), 591–592.

[34] Gupta, N., Garg, S., & Arora, K. (2016). Pattern of mobile phone usage and its effects on psychological health, sleep, and academic performance in students of a medical university. *National Journal of Physiology, Pharmacy and Pharmacology*, 6(2), 132–139.

[35] Finan, P. H., Quartana, P. J., & Smith, M. T. (2015). The effects of sleep continuity disruption on positive mood and sleep architecture in healthy adults. *Sleep*, 38(11), 1735–1742. 10

[36] Gill, S. S., Xu, M., Ottaviani, C. et al. (2022). AI for next generation computing: Emerging trends and future directions. *Internet of Things*, 19, 100514.

[37] Gill, S. S. Wu, H., Patros, P. et al. (2024). Modern computing: Vision and challenges. *Telematics and Informatics Reports*, 13, 100116.

[38] Singh, R. & Gill, S. S. (2023). Edge AI: A survey. *Internet of Things and Cyber-Physical Systems*, 3, 71–92.

[39] Gill, S. S., & Kaur, R. (2023). ChatGPT: Vision and challenges. *Internet of Things and Cyber-Physical Systems*, 3, 262–271.

VIII

Internet of Things (IoT) and Mobile Applications

CHAPTER 17

Social Event Tracking System with Real-Time Data Using Machine Learning

Muhammad Usman Nazir and Sukhpal Singh Gill

17.1 INTRODUCTION

In any modern city or state where large amounts of people are living there have always been social events. These events can be grouped into multiple prominent categories ranging from corporate events, exhibitions and fairs, sporting events, parties, festivals, concerts, and other seasonal markets. Each of these events has a huge target audience that likes to visit similar events. The event industry in the United Kingdom alone is worth £70 billion with over 85 million annual attendees [1]. Conferences, exhibitions, and festivals rank amongst the most valuable categories of events with a combined worth of £35.3 billion [2]. The UK Events Report 2020 lists the millennials to become the biggest group of event goers and travellers by 2024 due to their increased familiarity with technology and its use [1]. However, with a diverse population in urban cities, there are certain demographics of people that influence their interests in certain types of events apart from their age divides. According to a research by Billeto, most prominent demographics include a person's age, gender, educational level, background ethnicity, and marital status, amongst others [3]. These are some of the most prominent factors that can be used to group together people that may have interest in certain types of events. With an enormous amount of data available and massive potential for generating useful insights, the importance of having a technological platform where these insights can be accessed and visualised vis-à-vis utilised in improving the social event experience is a sheer panacea. According to research by EventMB, 51.5% of planners say the inability to have adequate live event data is the most frustrating thing when it comes to sourcing event tech [5]. In addition to this, around 48% of event organisers are concerned about reaching new attendees that may be interested in their events [5]. With no data-based approach utilised to monitor and capitalise this opportunity, there is an imminent need to take a data-based approach to attract new attendees while improving the current event management experience. Technology can be efficiently utilised in this regard to ensure that tech and data processing is used to find a

DOI: 10.1201/9781003467199-25

better solution for this problem. Having a platform that ensures that both the attendees and the organisers have access to real-time curated data that can provide insights into the events happening live in the area is a substantial requirement. The insights obtained from this platform can be utilised to make better decisions by both the attendees and the organisers. While event attendees can get information about what to expect at an event before attending, the organisers can make data-based administrative and management decisions depending on the audience at their event. According to research by Bizzabo, 91% of event planners say that using a mobile event app has provided a positive return on investment (ROI) with 58% of business-to-business (B2B) companies utilising such software when organising their events [4]. Event planners state the adoption rate of mobile applications to be around 80% [5]. Therefore, this work aims to develop a platform having a cloud-based back end and an iOS-based mobile front end where users and event organisers can come together to view real-time statistics on the demographic data of people interested in nearby events. Additionally, while 57% of current event management applications provide recommendations to the event attendees, no recommendations are presented to the organisers regarding their events [6]. Thus, this platform also aims to have a machine learning-based recommendation system that provides recommendations to the event organisers regarding the locations that would attract the desired audience for their event.

17.2 RELATED WORK

There is previous research regarding event tracking platforms and mobile applications that aim to help event attendees and organisers with recommendations. The most prominent of these were studied and have been summarised below.

17.2.1 GeSoDeck: Geo-Social Event Detection and Tracking System

GeSoDeck is a social event tracking system where a user can detect events in the surrounding area using a density-based K-means clustering technique [7]. The project provides high efficiency and accuracy, providing real-time tracking of tweets by the representatives of the event in real time as well. The events in the system are located and tracked using keywords, related tweets, and location data. These data are processed through a clustering pipeline to locate various events based on the twitter activity related to that event and the location data associated with the tweets. To achieve such event detection, the system performs collective behaviour modelling where tweets posted in a limited amount of time over various geographical districts are clustered using the keywords associated with the given event. This clustering methodology results in narrowing down to a location coordinate where most of the tweets are originating from and the location of the event on the map is calculated. Once the event is detected, event tracking is performed where each detected event is ranked by the term frequency (TF), which is calculated using the same clustering technique on the retweets instead of the actual tweet. This gives an estimate of the liveness of the event and is used to track the event in the system. This chapter highlighted the use of K-means clustering as well as weighted location coordinate calculation, which was utilised in the location recommendation system. Furthermore, this project provides useful insights regarding the usability of a map-based user interface for event discovery.

17.2.2 City Event Management System Based on Multiple Data Sources

This project is aimed to enable efficient event planning and tracking by using multiple data sources where those data sources are comprised of public monitoring facilities, social media, and crowdsourcing [8]. The system divides events into multiple categories that make distinguishing events easy and robust. These events are clustered together and combined based on similarity and can range from custom-defined events by the end users to the ones identified through automated sources. Event processors are independent and have highly decoupled components performing specific tasks in the system. These components reside in the system back end that feeds data to an android front end that can be used by the user. Once the user has created an event, it can be accessed by other users who can see information pertaining to an event's theme, content, and location. This chapter has been a vital source for highlighting the method of implementing crowdsourcing data into the platform. It not only provides information on what essential data to collect when registering a new event but also information about utilising a map-based visual view to discover the events nearby.

17.2.3 Online New Event Detection and Tracking

This section discusses an approach to online event detection using a single pass clustering algorithm [9]. This approach is similar to the native information filtering methodologies where events are detected by looking through a sequential stream of stories online. For each story, a query is built using feature selection and extraction techniques. An initial threshold of the story is determined by evaluating the new story with the query following, which is then matched with other queries in the system. If a match is found through this comparison, a new event is triggered and added to the system; otherwise, the story is simply matched to one of the existing events already present in the system. This chapter identifies new event tracking as a classification task that can be done using single-pass clustering techniques to show substantial results.

This chapter provided vital inspiration behind the clustering technique that is used in the location recommendation algorithm. Although the application of clustering in social event tracking system with real-time data (SETS) is in a different direction, this chapter provided some useful insights into the most useful clustering algorithms to use. In addition to literature review, existing platforms were also researched and studied to develop a critical analysis compared with our platform, SETS.

17.2.3.1 Eventbrite

Eventbrite is an American event management platform that allows users to create and promote local events [10]. It provides two separate mobile applications, one for attending events and ticketing and the other for organising an event. Eventbrite provides a list of events happening around a person based upon the location of the user, the category of event the user is interested in, and the time at which the user wants to attend the event. The platform provides data pertaining to the number of tickets sold and the revenue generated from those tickets. Users on the platform can scroll through a list of events and either add the event to their wish list or make a booking online. Furthermore, users can follow event organisers and are notified of any new event being created by the organiser that may meet their requirements. The attendance of a user at an event is carried out using QR codes. Each event is generated a QR code that can be scanned by the attendee using their app at the event location to mark themselves present at an event.

17.2.3.2 AllEvents.in

AllEvents.in is an event management platform that allows the creation and promotion of events in an area [11]. The platform provides a list view of all the events happening in a chosen city. Within the platform, users and organisers are separate entities and only registered organisers can host events. These events can belong to multiple categories ranging from parties, workshops and arts, etc. The platform also provides a ticketing mechanism where users interested in an event can get tickets online. Users on the platform can scroll through a list of events and either add the event to their wish list or make a booking online. No particular data are provided by the platform to the users or organisers about the event. Furthermore, users can follow event organisers as well as friends on the platform to keep updated about the event activity happening nearby. AllEvents.in does not provide any attendance mechanism related to the event to provide accurate data analytics calculated on the basis of user attendance.

17.2.3.3 Dice

Dice is a platform designed to connect events with their audiences [12]. To achieve this, the platform provides live streams as well as event tracking and planning. Users can view events in a list where events are categorised by type and date of occurrences. Users can also separately search for events using the price whether they are free or priced. Dice provides details about people interested in an event with waiting lists alongside the ability to stream shows, festivals, and workshops from all around the world. Users can also invite friends, follow each other, and get suggestions for shows that they will both like and can attend together. Moreover, users can save events for later and get reminders for when event dates come close. Additionally, users can also transfer tickets to a friend if they have a spare, cannot make it, or as a gift.

17.2.4 Critical Analysis

There are a number of potential shortcomings present in the existing platforms and literature that prevent the systems from reaching the levels of efficiency and usability that they should. Firstly, none of the existing platforms provide a real-time data analysis of the event and its demographics. Eventbrite only provides the total numbers of check-ins and how they are distributed over time [10]. However, the users who are interested in these events have no clue regarding what to expect from the event and the systems do not keep track of the demographics of such events either before the event is occurring or during its live occurrence. Information such as the number of people expected to attend, their genders, ages, disabilities, and educational backgrounds are completely unknown to the organisers as well as to the other people interested in a particular event. Therefore, both the organisers and the attendees lose an opportunity to better plan themselves and have accurate expectations of what to expect from the event and how to adjust according to the changing attendee demographics. SETS, on the other hand, aims to fill in the gap by providing real-time data when an event is occurring using an efficient heartbeat mechanism. Upon each heartbeat the server and client communicate to ensure that the data being presented are accurate and efficiently calculated.

Furthermore, most of the applications and platforms provide a list of events instead of showing the events on a map [10–12]. While a list does convey the basic information regarding an event, it fails to give the user a visual idea of where an event is located in their surroundings and when to reach the event in time. In contrast, as highlighted by GeSoDeck and City Event Management System, having a map showing all the events happening nearby would greatly improve the user experience as the distance and location is very quickly conveyed to the user resulting in a highly improved user experience [7, 8]. In our implementation, the primary view for discovering events is a map instead of a list. Different categories of maps are represented by different colours for the user to easily distinguish between them. Furthermore, events happening live are further separated by using animated rippling icons for ease of use. The user can also quickly have a look at the expected audience demographics of the event by simply tapping on its icon and observing the quick summary in a view appearing from the bottom. Moreover, a majority of platforms fail to provide accurate statistics regarding the attendance of an event to their users. Most platforms only perform the function of event discovery by listing the events happening nearby and distributing tickets for those events online [10–12]. The estimate of people attending the events is calculated using the data of the tickets sold on the platform. However, this is not very accurate as a single event can be listed on multiple different platforms; thus the attendance data generated at either of these platforms is not fully accurate. Our work, in this regard, aims to use a modification of Eventbrite's QR attendance system to mark check-ins at an event [10]. While creating an event, organisers are provided with an instantly generated QR code that can be scanned by the attendees through a quick scan. This approach ensures that the attendance is marked by the people actually present at the event while making sure that the process is quick and user-friendly. Another important feature missing in existing platforms is the ability to provide both the organisers and the attendees with expected demographics. While Eventbrite and AllEvents.in provide basic attendee count details, when marking an event as interesting, no data-based insights are generated for the event organisers regarding the person who has shown interest in the event [10, 11]. This is a problem as there is a possibility that the person showing interest might have some special needs or disabilities and expectations regarding the event that are not fully communicated to the event organisers. Therefore both the organisers and attendees lack vital information about the event before it has started, which may set up false expectations and lead to problems in a swift execution. Contrarily, our work aims to share anonymous demographics data of the user immediately once the user marks their interest in an event along with providing the organiser predictions regarding what attendee demographics to expect at the event. These data are instantly accessible to the event organisers so they can make preparations well in advance accordingly to better manage the event.

TABLE 17.1   Comparison of Similar Platforms with SETS

Work/Study	Real-Time Data	Expected Data	Live Event Map	Location Recommendations	Attendance Management	Demographic Predictions
GeSoDeck [7]	✓		✓			
City Event Management System [8]	✓		✓			
Eventbrite [10]		✓			✓	
Allevents.in [11]		✓			✓	
Dice [12]		✓			✓	
SETS (this work)	✓	✓	✓	✓	✓	✓

Lastly, none of the platforms provide the event organisers with any recommendations regarding their events to better match their expectations. With a multitude of locations available for an event and a need to have a certain amount of free spaces, it is important to have a recommendation system in place that can advise the organisers to choose a better location such that these expectations are well achieved. This requires a data clustering pipeline similar to the one used in the GeSoDeck section, which would take in an organisers expectations and cluster the data present on the platforms pertaining to different events in the past and advise a location coordinate that would most likely fulfil the event expectations set by the organisers [7]. On the other hand, SETS aims to introduce a novel methodology that uses a clustering-based technique to recommend a location to the event organisers to better suit their needs. Upon adding an event, the system takes data regarding an event's category and the organisers targeted audience numbers to utilise the clustering algorithm. The algorithm clusters together events having similar trends in the past and attendees that had attended those events. Once the most suitable attendees are determined, a weighted technique is used to determine a location on the map near the organiser where they are most likely to attend. This location coordinate is presented to the organiser who can then place the event anywhere in the circle for maximum change to achieve their expectations. Table 17.1 summarises the comparison of SETS with existing platforms.

17.3 TECHNOLOGIES

The following are relevant technologies.

17.3.1 Google Maps iOS SDK

The iOS client uses Google Maps iOS-SDK v5.1.0 to render the map view and show the events happening nearby [13]. Google Maps provides a highly customisable SDK where multiple visual features are provided to the engineer. The application uses this SDK in tandem with Apple's Core Location application programming interfaces (APIs) to present a themed map, fetch and translate to the user's current location, and present custom animated markers for events. Furthermore, the SDK also provides APIs to have the recommended location shown on the map.

17.3.2 Swift

Apple's Swift language v5 was used as the primary programming language on the iOS client application [14]. The choice for this language is inspired by the efficiency of the language on iOS devices and provides multiple high-level classes that can be used to fetch, format, and present data efficiently. The views created to present data have been created using Apple's UI Kit.

17.3.3 Python Django

The primary language used to develop the cloud back end is Python 3.8 [15]. The back end framework used is Django as it provides robust Representational State Transfer (REST) APIs and authentication and can very easily be deployed on any major cloud platform. With the flexibility of Python, Django presents itself as the best option available to build an efficient back end with full error handling support and edge case testing abilities.

17.3.4 Heroku

Heroku was used as the cloud platform to deploy the Django back end [16]. The choice for Heroku stems from its ease of usability and maintenance. Once set up using free dynos, Heroku handles all the workload superiorly well and provides good scalability options as the number of users continues to grow.

17.3.5 Scikit-Learn

Python's machine learning scikit-learn was used to perform linear regression and logistic regression [17, 18]. Version 0.24.2 was utilised in conjunction with the Python library NumPy to prepare data for fitting the machine learning models and making predictions for the incoming data.

17.3.6 Apple Authentication

Apple's Sign in with Apple, was used as the primary authentication mechanism for users [19]. This uses Apple's state-of-the-art Touch ID and Face ID to login a user into the platform. All authentication data are transmitted by SHA-2 secure encryption layers for protected implementation of the process. Moreover, this ensures that only authentic users are logged in on the system to ensure quality of the demographics data used in generating the real-time data for each event.

17.4 METHODOLOGY AND IMPLEMENTATION

In this section, we discuss database schema, client architecture, real-time data algorithm, the location recommendation algorithm, and demographic predictions.

17.4.1 Database Schema

The database has multiple tables to hold the core models and their relationships. With the database designed to be relational, there are multiple one-to-one, one-to-many, and many-to-many relationships between the classes. The two major classes are the User and Event class. The User class holds information related to the user including their name, email, disability, marital status, gender, Universally Unique Identifier (UUID), ethnicity, location coordinates, and age. The Event class, on the other hand, holds information related to an event such as its name, location coordinates, category, and description. Additionally, a number of supporting tables are also generated to ensure that the data are normalised and uncluttered. This ensures that the demographics data as well as the interested and attendance data are kept separately for efficient access.

17.4.2 Client Architecture

The client iOS application is built using the model-view-view model (MVVM) architectural pattern [20]. This pattern splits the components into four major entities; View, View Controller, View Model, and Model as shown in Figure 17.1.

The View holds the User Interface (UI) elements on a particular screen. The View Controller handles the displaying of data on the views and the delegates from user interactions. Moreover, the View Model is responsible for network communication with the APIs through the services and finally, the Model residing in the View Model holds the actual data. The networking architecture is designed using generic programming and has two major components, the Services and the Network Engine. Incorporating protocol-oriented MVVM, there are two protocol-oriented services, the user service and the event service [21]. The user service is responsible for creating the API requests pertaining to the user activity such as fetching updated user models or performing user attendance check-ins. This is designed using generic programming, which allows it to handle all requests within the application and use Apple's codable protocols to generically convert JSON responses to their respective classes using custom coding keys.

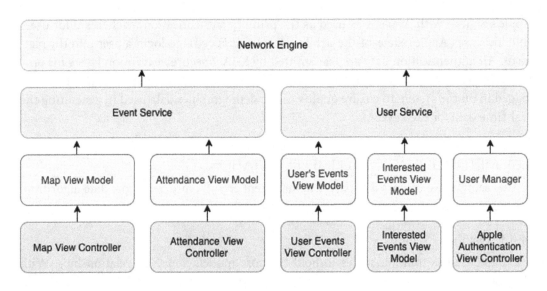

FIGURE 17.1   SETS iOS client MVVM architecture.

17.4.3 Real-Time Data Algorithm

The real-time data updation algorithm is inspired by the Raft consensus algorithm as explained in the chapter "In Search of an Understandable Consensus Algorithm" in [22]. Once an attendance is marked and the user shows interest, the real-time data pertaining to the event is updated to be accurate. These data are stored in their respective demographics tables and a timestamp of the update is stored separately. The iOS client implements a protocol that sends heartbeats to the server to detect any change. These heartbeats are sent every 2 seconds only if the user is actively looking at the data to avoid network overloading. Once the server receives a heartbeat request, it responds with the timestamp of the event. Once the client receives the timestamp, it locally matches it with its most updated timestamp. If the local timestamp is outdated, the client requests the server to provide an updated version of the data. Figure 17.2 presents the heartbeat-based real-time data transfer architecture.

17.4.4 Location Recommendation Algorithm

The location recommendation algorithm is implemented on the server to respond with a suggested location for an event based upon the event's category and desired number of participants. The algorithm follows multiple steps to ensure that an accurate prediction is made based on the X-means clustering technique [23], as shown in Figure 17.3. Firstly, the event data present in the database is passed through a filter to only get the events that are present around the same city as the user. Another filter is applied to only get the ones that belong to the desired category of the event that the user is aiming to create. This data are passed through a layer of feature selection where these events are mapped into a list containing tuples enveloping the event unique IDs and the attendance count, respectively. Secondly, clustering is performed through a distance-based clustering methodology provided by the PyClustering framework [23]. An X-means clustering algorithm is used to identify and cluster similar events based on attendance counts [24].

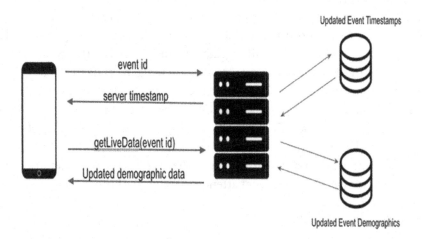

FIGURE 17.2   Heartbeat-based real-time data transfer.

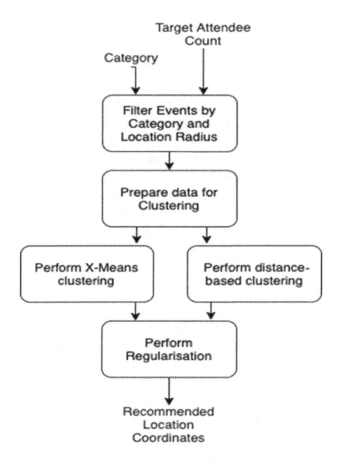

FIGURE 17.3   Location recommendation algorithm.

X-means is seen to provide the most accurate clustering as it automatically calculates the number of clusters accurately. Additionally, a custom regularisation technique using a gradient-based approach is also utilised. This involves creating a gradient-based data space using consistent x-coordinate intervals and calculating gradients between successive attendee counts for the y-coordinates. The algorithm traverses through the sorted space and clusters together events with similar gradient values between the events. If successive values lie between the average of the current cluster's local maxima gradient value with an upper and lower margin of 50%, it is added to the current cluster and the cluster average is recalculated to regenerate the local maxima. Otherwise, the cluster is closed and the value is added to a new cluster. Once all clusters are ready, the final attendee count averages for each cluster is matched with the user's desired attendee count. The closest cluster is picked and location coordinate data of the attendees of the events in that cluster are used to perform a weighted average where frequent attendees are given more value.

17.4.5 Demographic Predictions

SETS utilises a regression-based system to predict demographics for an event. This approach uses both linear regression and logistic regression to make predictions for continuous variables and discontinuous variables. Once an event is created, the data provided including its timing and category are passed to the scikit-learn-based regression models trained on the existing data present in the system [18]. Linear regression is used to predict the continuous demographic variables such as the number of attendees, number of people interested in attending, the predicted median age of attendees, and the predicted number of people with disabilities that may attend the event [25]. Similarly, logistic regression is utilised to predict the most probable demographics pertaining to the marital statuses, educational backgrounds, or ethnicities of the attendees of the event. These predictions are always accessible to view in the iOS application and improve in accuracy as the anonymous demographic dataset increases.

17.5 RESULTS

SETS provides a platform where real-time data can be used to monitor the social events happening in the vicinity. Figure 17.4 shows the multiple screens in the iOS application's

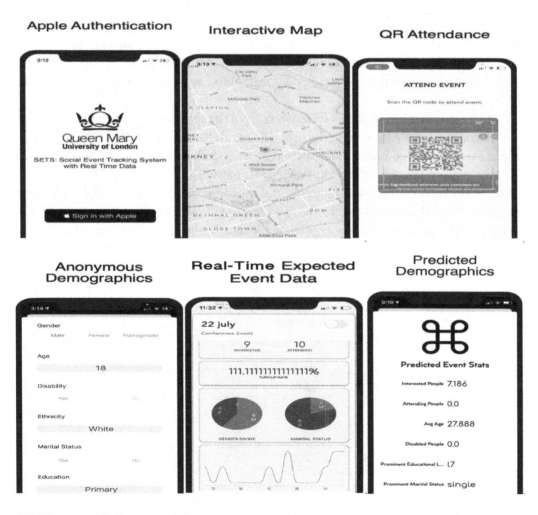

FIGURE 17.4   iOS client application.

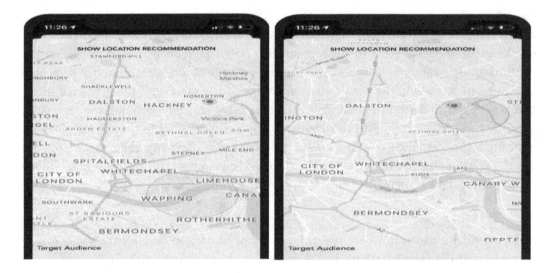

FIGURE 17.5   Location recommendations.

user interface. These screens showcase the ability of the client applications to authenticate users using Apple Sign In, the interactive map to discover events nearby, the QR code-based attendance marking, anonymous demographics, and real-time live and predicted event data.

Furthermore, Figure 17.5 shows screenshots from the application showing how location recommendations are presented to the user. The regularised X-means algorithm is used to generate the location coordinates for these recommendations, which are then highlighted on the map using a circle with a radius of approximately 1 km.

Figure 17.6 represents the accuracy obtained by using multiple different clustering algorithms to cluster the event data effectively. When tested using computationally generated datasets with known clusters, the regularised X-means unsupervised learning algorithm

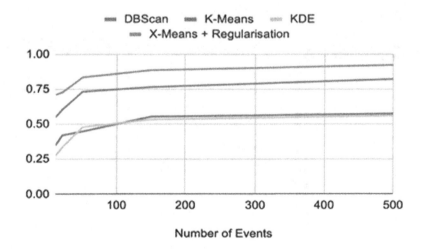

FIGURE 17.6   Performance of clustering algorithms.

performs better than the other algorithms as it can automatically determine the number of clusters effectively. This was followed by DBScan and then K-means and kernel density estimation (KDE) algorithms, which performed poorly on the curated data.

17.6 CONCLUSIONS

In conclusion, we have successfully identified a need in the event planning and management space where it is imperative to know the data related to an event to improve the management and organisation. This need has been answered using this work, which provides a robust and practical approach towards providing real-time data of an event both before and during its lifetime. The system provides useful and real-time insights to both the organisers and attendees of social events. Social events can be discovered on the interactive map and a user can share and observe the expected and live attendee demographics anonymously. These data are not only used to provide real-time insights to the users for better decisions but also utilised to generate location recommendations and demographic predictions regarding an event being hosted. Data privacy and authenticity is ensured using QR-based attendance management and Apple authentication, which makes sure that SHA-2 authentication protocols and private relays are utilised. Furthermore, they ensure data reliability making certain that SETS provides a comprehensive suite of data-based event organising capabilities.

17.7 FUTURE WORK

There are a number of avenues that can be explored to improve further. This includes improving the location recommendation system and the demographic prediction pipeline. Similarly to the category and desired attendee count, further parameters can be used in the clustering process to use values such as the time or gender divide to recommend location coordinates [26]. Moreover, Apple App Clips can be utilised to further improve the iOS application and provide a small, versatile version of the client for check-ins where the users can check in more efficiently and effectively. Additionally, for accurate user data, social media platforms such as Facebook and Google can be integrated for the user to share their online data for linking demographics [27]. Furthermore, an efficient hashing-based consensus algorithm can be implemented that allows the iOS client application and the Python server to communicate using hashes instead of actual data to ensure further data privacy and transferability [28]. Lastly, the Python back end can be deployed to Amazon Web Services or Google Cloud platform to utilise the machine learning libraries that can be used to improve the location recommendation system as well as provide suggestions to the user for events to visit based on their previous activity [29].

REFERENCES

[1] UK Events Report (2020). Online Accessed: 20April 2023. Available at: https://www.excel.london/uploads/uk-events-report-2020---the-full-report.pdf
[2] The Pulse Report: (2019) Event Industry Trends. Online Accessed: 20April 2023Available at: https://www.eventbrite.co.uk/blog/academy/pulse-report-2019-event-industry-trends/

[3] Billeto: 6 Ways to Identify the Target Audience for an Event. (2019) [Online]. Online Accessed: 20April 2023. Available at: https://billetto.co.uk/blog/target-audience-for-event/

[4] Bizzabo. 2020 Event Marketing Report. (2020). Online Accessed: 20April 2023. Available at: https://welcome.bizzabo.com/reports/event-marketing-2020

[5] State of Event Technology. (2020) Online Accessed: 20April 2023. Available at: https://www.eventmanagerblog.com/state-event-tech

[6] State of the Event Industry. (2020) Online Accessed: 20April 2023. Available at: https://www.eventmanagerblog.com/state-of-the-event-industry-report

[7] Gao, X., Cao, J., Jin, Z., Li, X., & Li, J. (2013). GeSoDeck: a geo-social event detection and tracking system. *Proceedings of the 21st ACM International Conference on Multimedia* (MM '13). Association for Computing Machinery, New York, NY, USA, pp. 471–472.

[8] Chunjiao, X., Dianhui, C., & Chunshan, L. (2015 May). City event management system based on multiple data sources. *2015 International Conference on Service Science (ICSS)* (pp. 169–173). IEEE.

[9] Allan, J., Papka, R., & Lavrenko, V. (1998, August). On-Line New Event Detection and Tracking. *Proceedings of the 21st Annual International ACM SIGIR Conference on Research and Development in Information Retrieval*, pp. 37–45.

[10] Eventbrite. (2006) [Online]. Online Accessed: 20April 2023. Available at: https://www.eventbrite.co.uk

[11] AllEvents. (2011) [Online]. Online Accessed: 20April 2023. Available at: https://allevents.in

[12] Dice (2014). [Online]. Online Accessed: 20April 2023. Available at: https://dice.fm

[13] Google Maps iOS SDK (2012). Online Accessed: 20April 2023. Available at: developers.google.com/maps/documentation/ios-sdk/

[14] Swift. (2023) [Online]. Online Accessed: 20April 2023. Available at: https://developer.apple.com/swift/

[15] Python Django. (2023) [Online]. Online Accessed: 20April 2023. Available at: https://www.djangoproject.com

[16] Heroku.(2007) [Online]. Online Accessed: 20April 2023. Available at: https://www.heroku.com

[17] Trappenberg, T. P. (2019). Machine Learning with Sklearn. *In Fundamentals of Machine Learning* (pp. 38–65). Oxford University Press.

[18] Pedregosa, F., Varoquaux, G., Gramfort, A., Michel, V., Thirion, B., Grisel, O., Blondel, M., Prettenhofer, P., Weiss, R., Dubourg, V., & Vanderplas, J. (2011). Scikit-learn: Machine learning in python. *The Journal of Machine Learning Research*, 12, 2825–2830.

[19] Apple Authentication: Sign In with Apple. (2019) [Online]. Online Accessed: 20April 2023. Available at: https://developer.apple.com/sign-in-with-apple/

[20] Luong Nguyen, K. N. (2017). Application of Protocol-Oriented MVVM Architecture in iOS Development. https://www.theseus.fi/bitstream/handle/10024/129037/Nguyen_Luong.pdf;jsessionid=4A12BB5074DFFC8CD62AD0FC0FC8E0C8?sequence=1

[21] Harun, F. B. (2019). Review of iOS architectural pattern for testability, modifiability, and performance quality. *Journal of Theoretical and Applied Information Technology*, 97(15), 4021–4035.

[22] Ongaro, D., & Ousterhout, J. (2014). In search of an understandable consensus algorithm. *2014 {USENIX} Annual Technical Conference ({USENIX}{ATC} 14)*, pp. 305–319.

[23] Novikov, A. V. (2019). PyClustering: Data mining library. *Journal of Open Source Software*, 4(36), 1230.

[24] Pelleg, D., & Moore, A. W. (2000). X-means: Extending k-means with efficient estimation of the number of clusters. *In Icml*, 1, 727–734.

[25] Jolly, K. (2018). *Machine Learning With Scikit-Learn Quick Start Guide: Classification, Regression, and Clustering Techniques in Python*. Packt Publishing Ltd.

[26] Gill, S. S., Xu, M., Ottaviani, C. et al. (2022). AI for next generation computing: Emerging trends and future directions. *Internet of Things*, 19, 100514.

[27] Singh, R. & Gill, S. S. (2023). Edge AI: A survey. *Internet of Things and Cyber-Physical Systems*, 3, 71–92.

[28] Gill, S. S., & Kaur, R. (2023). ChatGPT: Vision and challenges. *Internet of Things and Cyber-Physical Systems*, 3, 262–271.

[29] Gill, S. S., Wu, H., Patros, P. et al. (2024). Modern computing: Vision and challenges. *Telematics and Informatics Reports*, 13, 100116.

Index

Note: Page numbers in *italics* represent figures; page numbers in **bold** represent tables.

Printed in the United States
by Baker & Taylor Publisher Services